Drug Management for Nurses

Drug Management for Nurses

George Downie MSc MPS
Assistant Chief Administrative Pharmaceutical Officer
Grampian Health Board
Aberdeen

Jean Mackenzie RGN SCM DipN(Lond) RCT
Clinical Teacher
Foresterhill College of Nursing and Midwifery
Aberdeen

Arthur Williams MPS
Chief Administrative Pharmaceutical Officer
Grampian Health Board
Aberdeen

Foreword by
Billie Thomson RGN SCM ONC BSc RNT DipNursAdmin
Nursing Officer (Education)
Scottish Home and Health Department
Edinburgh

Churchill Livingstone
EDINBURGH LONDON MELBOURNE AND NEW YORK 1987

CHURCHILL LIVINGSTONE
Medical Division of Longman Group UK Limited

Distributed in the United States of America by
Churchill Livingstone Inc., 1560 Broadway, New York,
N.Y. 10036, and by associated companies, branches
and representatives throughout the world.

First published 1987

ISBN 0 443 03468 0

British Library Cataloguing in Publication Data
Downie, George
    Drug management for nurses. — (Drugs in
    nursing practice)
    1. Chemotherapy
    I. Title   II. Mackenzie, Jean
    III. Williams, Arthur   IV. Series
    615.5'8'024613   RM262

Library of Congress Cataloging in Publication Data
Downie, George, MSc.
    Drug management for nurses.
    (Drugs in nursing practice)
    Includes bibliographies and index.
    1. Chemotherapy. 2. Drugs — Administration. 3. Nursing. I. Mackenzie,
Jean, RGN. II. Williams, Arthur. III. Title. IV. Series. [DNLM: 1. Drug
Therapy — nurses' instruction. 2. Drugs — administration & dosage —
nurses' instruction. QV 55 D751d] RM262.D62 1986   615.5'8   86-9546

Produced by Longman Singapore Publishers (Pte) Ltd
Printed in Singapore

Foreword

One of the most striking features of medicine today is the range and complexity of diagnostic tests, therapeutic agents and technological aids which are used to combat disease. A hundred years ago, only a limited number of remedies, most of dubious effectiveness, were in use. These were often prepared by the prescriber who could not benefit from the expertise of scientists or highly trained health care personnel.

In the past, too, most of the books which nurses used for the study of drug therapy focused on particular aspects such as calculation of dosages, or drug action, side-effects and antidotes, or disease conditions and the drugs appropriate to their treatment. In this book, authors from different health professions have collaborated to produce a text which illustrates the complexity of the subject and they have managed to do it in a simple, easy-to-read style. Information on pharmacology and therapeutics is combined with practical guidance on drug administration and associated procedures. The inter-relatedness and interdependence of several professional groups are also clearly described.

The various professional journals of health workers indicate concern about the need to develop partnership in health care and for professionals to contribute to the education of the public about health maintenance and self-care. The authors share this concern and discuss the arguments for and against issues such as patient information, drug-checking policies and patient compliance with a prescribed drug regime.

The authors do not claim to have written an exhaustive text. Indeed they emphasise that nurses, midwives and health visitors working in specialised fields will need to study books specific to that area. Nevertheless, this book is wide-ranging enough to give an accurate picture of the variety of conditions and settings in which drug therapy is used. At the same time it is sufficiently detailed to provide practical guidance to students and qualified nurses alike.

I congratulate the authors for having managed to tackle a complex subject in such a comprehensive and helpful way.

Edinburgh   Billie Thomson

Acknowledgements

We are indebted to those who have so generously assisted us in writing this book. Among them are senior nurses M. Beattie, S. M. C. Inglis, E. Kerr, H. M. Lemmon, S. Leys, I. MacInnes, P. Miller, K. M. Pedelty and P. R. Runciman. We are grateful to the Grampian Health Board for allowing us to reproduce documents and to Mr G. W. Bell for help with diagrams and photographs. For invaluable assistance with the chapter on nutrition, our thanks go to Miss K. McCall and Dr J. Broom.

Finally it is hard to find words which adequately express gratitude for the amount of secretarial assistance a task such as this entails. To Miss Catherine McEwan especially we say 'thank you' for a job extraordinarily well done.

Aberdeen 1987

G.D.
J.M.
A.W.

Introduction

Every nurse is involved from the earliest days in her career in some aspects of the administration and management of medicines. Although these responsibilities will increase and change with time, the safe and effective management of medicines will remain a high priority for all practising nurses. The importance of establishing a firm basis of learning during the main training period is well recognised, as is the need to progress to wider aspects, once the initial training period is complete. Thus the nurse builds upon the knowledge and skills acquired to prepare herself for the particular responsibilities and duties in her chosen speciality. As with all health professionals the nurse has a responsibility to keep up to date and make her contribution to professional issues of the day. We hope this book will be of value at all stages of the nurse's career, providing information and practical help in addition to being a frame of reference for her own experience. Nurses returning to the profession will, we hope, find a study of the book a useful adjunct to a refresher course. The needs of the community nurse have been considered, as most medicines are prescribed for use in the community. This book will not provide all the detailed knowledge the specialist nurse will require, but will form a sound basis and prepare the way for further study whether learner, experienced, or specialist nurse.

To maintain consistency throughout the text, an approach has been adopted in which nurses are referred to in the female gender and patients in the male gender.

Although it is recognised that the emphasis will vary, depending on the speciality in which the nurse works, the role of the nurse in drug therapy can, we believe, be broadly summarised under the following headings:

- to ensure that the correct dosage is given at the correct time and by the correct route
- to observe/report any side-effects and drug interactions, and to take action to alleviate unavoidable side-effects
- to observe and assess the patient so that medical and nursing decisions can be made
- to participate in education and guidance of patients (and in some cases their relatives) with regard to their drug therapy, in order to promote patient compliance and the achievement of therapeutic objectives

- to take action to help reduce, or remove, the need for drug therapy
- to contribute to the evaluation and development of new treatments, and/or the reassessment of existing treatments
- to follow recognised procedures for the control of medicines and pharmaceutical products at ward or departmental level and to contribute to the development of these procedures and controls in response to changing situations

The nurse's role is much more than a mechanical achievement of objectives. It is a professional role requiring skill, judgment and commitment. In order to assist in the discharge of this role, the nurse should have access to a broadly-based book, which links together aspects of knowledge which are currently only available in separate publications.

Having outlined the current role of the nurse in drug therapy it is important to realise that many changes and developments are taking place both within health care and the health professions. These changes are having, and will continue to have, an increasing impact on the practising nurse whether in hospital or community. Some of the changes are as follows:

- changing patterns in the provision of health care
- increasing complexity of drug therapy in general
- increasing specialisation in the use of drugs, such as cytotoxic therapy and total parenteral nutrition
- the development of new drug delivery systems
- changes in drug presentation, improved packaging, and new drug distribution systems
- increasing concern regarding the side-effects of drug treatment
- a greater interest in alternative medicine
- an increasing emphasis on the need to use resources effectively
- the need to ensure that the person administering drugs is not harmed by them
- a greater awareness of the need to ensure the safe and effective use of medicines by older people
- the increasing use of computers in clinical practice, both in hospitals and the community
- an increasing emphasis on self-care
- the development of ward/clinical pharmacy services
- professional aspirations of health care workers generally.

The practising nurse is becoming more aware of the great benefits and potential dangers of drug therapy. As a result she may become anxious and lose confidence. As the nurse is responsible for her clinical actions, it is essential that she acquires well-founded confidence in what she does. This confidence is achieved through the mastering of practical skills supported by the necessary theoretical knowledge. No matter how careful and expert the prescribing doctor, or dispensing pharmacist, the consequences for the patient may be disastrous if the nurse is ill-equipped to discharge her vital role to the full. We hope that this book will serve both as a ready reference for nurses working in the practical situation and an educational tool for learning and teaching, with the patient being the ultimate beneficiary.

Contents

1 THE ROLE OF THE NURSE IN DRUG THERAPY

Drug therapy in the 1980s can be seen against a very different background of organisation, attitudes, and care from that which existed 20 or even 10 years ago. Care in hospital is now more flexible with a gradual progression towards self-care where possible, including in some wards self-administration of medicines. In psychiatric hospitals and, to a much lesser extent in general hospitals, patients are encouraged to go home for the weekend, and the average length of stay of patients in all hospitals has been markedly reduced. This has led to an increased turnover of hospital patients in hospital wards and consequently there are more acutely ill in-patients than in the past. Society in general is becoming better informed on health matters and as a result of advertising and the influence of educational programmes in schools and through the media, patients' expectations of care and treatment have changed.

The number and range of medicines available is greater than ever and with better anaesthetics, laboratory control and nutritional support treatment in many instances has become much more dynamic. The development of highly sophisticated diagnostic techniques and the growth of specialised units (e.g. renal, neurosurgical, neonatal) have brought with them changes in drug therapy and drug procedures. Psychotropic drug therapy has revolutionised psychiatric care to the extent that many hundreds of hospital beds have been released with the shift of emphasis to community support. The introduction of new drug delivery systems designed to achieve rate controlled drug dosage has made new demands on nurses, calling for alterations in programmes of education. Against these complexities, calculation of drug dosage and the preparation of drugs have, in many instances, been simplified. The ordering of drugs by a pre-printed list compiled by computer is very helpful to nurses, as are improved systems of prescribing and recording of medicines. Probably, however, the greatest impact on ward management of medicines has come with the introduction of ward and clinical pharmacy services. Where these services are not available it may well be that a nurse may spend up to 10 or more hours per week on duties connected directly with the management of medicines.

There is increasing emphasis on care in the community which brings many benefits for patients and, in turn, produces challenges for community nurses and their colleagues. In the first place, the challenge is important since 80% of the national drug bill is incurred by prescribing in the community. In addition, it is one of complexity arising from more flexible provision of care, early discharge from hospital and a wider range of drug treatments being provided at home. Total parenteral nutrition, special inhalational therapy, intravenous antibiotic therapy and other forms of treatment formerly undertaken only in hospitals, are now available to patients in the community. Although the emphasis in this chapter is on the hospital setting, it is intended that the chapter will be helpful to community nurses and their health visitor colleagues.

THE CHANGING PATTERN OF NURSING CARE

With the steady increase in the number of wards where small teams of nurses are assigned the care of patients, the traditional method of administering medicines in a ward needs to be reconsidered. The team approach, coupled with an attempt to care for patients on an individual basis, requires flexibility in the administration of medicines. Systems of medicine distribution need to reflect the aims of patient care in each ward.

Having been allocated a group of patients, the team devises a plan of care for each patient based on an assessment of his needs. The plan, which must be flexible, takes into account not only the patient's condition and management but also any constraints placed upon his care, such as the time available and the number and grade of staff on duty. Medicine rounds carried out in the traditional rigid way are not conducive to this modern approach. The use of task orientated equipment (e.g. the medicine trolley, medicine 'Kardex' and ward drug stocks), may hinder the integration of drug therapy with total patient care. Nurse managers and other health care personnel should work together to ensure that, whenever possible, such barriers to total patient care are removed. Discussion on drug administration as it relates to a 'Nursing Process' approach to patient care appears further on in this chapter.

It is logical to expect the nurse, who knows the minute-by-minute changes in the patient's programme of care, to participate in the administration of medicines and to influence decisions regarding the appropriate use of prescribed medicines for the relief of acute symptoms (e.g. analgesics, anti-emetics). Procedures associated with the administration of certain medicines are also carried out by nurses more effectively. For example, a nurse may give, by mutual agreement with a physiotherapist, a steam inhalation before physiotherapy begins; eye bathing may have to be carried out before instilling eye drops; oral hygiene should precede administration of a medicine for the treatment of oral thrush; assistance to undress may be required to allow application of an ointment. The need for certain medicines (e.g. an analgesic, before performing a surgical dressing or before transporting the patient to another department) can be anticipated by the nurse. Conversely, the nurse may use her discretion in withholding a medicine until a more suitable time, e.g. when she has succeeded in making a dying patient comfortable. Inexperienced nurses require help in making these judgments. They need to learn when it is imperative that the medicine be given but equally when a more flexible approach constitutes good nursing.

It is important to recognise that against the complex and changing background discussed above, the nurse's role in drug therapy will always involve three main interrelated elements — knowledge, skills and attitudes, each of which impinges closely on the other.

KNOWLEDGE

In the course of administering medicines, application of the nurse's knowledge of pharmacology and physiology is required. The nurse must seek certain information about the patient, including any special instructions about his medicines. In order to carry out the tasks involved, a working knowledge of policies, equipment, and procedures is also necessary.

Pharmacology and Physiology
Basic pharmacology includes: drug absorption mechanisms, the metabolic action of the liver, the method by which substances are transported in the bloodstream, cell transport and activity, and the excretory function of the kidneys. The effect of congenital abnormality, metabolic disorders, deficiency states, neoplastic disorders, trauma, infection and degenerative processes on pharmacological activity must be understood. A lack of specialist knowledge of the physiology of the extremes of age may hazard the very young or elderly patient, who is often more at risk from adverse drug reactions than patients in other age groups. Without an appreciation of background physiology, the nurse's comprehension of how drugs act in the body is incomplete and her effectiveness in practice may be open to question.

The Medicines
A working knowledge of the medicines used in each individual ward/department is required. This includes:

- range and presentation of medicines
- ordering/requisitioning procedures
- storage of medicines and disposal of unwanted medicines
- legislation and local hospital policy
- dosage levels
- routes of administration/techniques of medicine administration
- rationale for the particular therapy

- prescribing/recording procedures
- safe handling of drugs known to be hazardous
- methods of promoting effectiveness of and/or reducing the need for drug therapy.

The following additional areas of knowledge are also of importance:

- mode of action of drugs
- recognition of side-effects and methods of minimising unavoidable side-effects and dealing with them
- signs and symptoms of drug toxicity
- methods of dealing with the effects of drug toxicity
- drug/drug interactions
- drug/food interactions
- effects of disease states on drug therapy
- potential dangers of self-medication
- use of clinical reagents
- aspects of research into drugs
- achieving/improving patient compliance.

Legal and Professional Responsibilities
Trained nurses have legal and professional responsibilities as do student and pupil nurses. Legal aspects are discussed in Chapter 5.

All health authorities are required to establish policies and procedures, setting out in detail, instruction and guidance on the administration and storage of medicines. All nurses must adhere to these policies and procedures. Similarly, when prescribing, doctors are required to meet their obligations as defined in the health authorities' policy documents. These policies are derived from statutory sources and circulars of guidance issued by the Department of Health and Social Security (DHSS) and the Scottish Home and Health Department (SHHD).

Nurses must also always work within the professional standards established by the United Kingdom Central Council for Nurses, Midwives and Health Visitors (UKCC), the National Boards for Nursing, Midwifery and Health Visiting, and the Royal College of Nursing (RCN).

The Patient
It is essential that the nurse is aware of the

relevant details about the person who is to receive the medication.

These include the patient's name, age, and hospital unit number as well as the diagnosis, the patient's physical capabilities and his mental capacity. Correct identification of the patient is crucial.

In addition, the nurse must make herself aware of and follow any specific instructions pertaining to the patient. Two examples are cited.

Sensitivity to any drug which is recorded by the doctor on the patient's admission to hospital should be carefully noted by the nurse, since at some future stage this knowledge may prevent an adverse reaction.

Patients (such as those preparing for an anaesthetic or for certain investigations) who are temporarily to be given nothing by mouth, should have oral medicines withheld. An initialled record should be made to this effect by the nurse. If necessary, the doctor should rewrite the prescription completely, stating an alternative route.

Knowledge and information are vital. Acquiring and using knowledge contributes to safety in medicine administration and helps the nurse to develop confidence and to answer patients' questions clearly and correctly. In the interests of the safety and comfort of patients it is also important to recognise that knowledge about medicines and their management keeps changing and that practising nurses have a responsibility to keep pace with new developments. Knowledge alone, however, is not sufficient to guarantee safe practice. Skill is also necessary.

SKILLS

The skills required in relation to complete medicine management are: (1) observational, (2) communicative, (3) teaching (4) motor (5) numerical.

Observational skills
By continuing observation a nurse assesses the patient's condition before and after drug treatment and monitors his response. The nurse is expected to measure, record, and report such values as the blood pressure in a patient receiving an antihypertensive drug, apical and radial pulse rates in a patient receiving anti-arrhythmic drugs or a patient's weight to estimate the effect of diuretic therapy.

Examples of observable changes in a patient following drug therapy are as follows:

- allergic reaction, ranging from skin rash to anaphylaxis
- muscular weakness arising from potassium loss in diuretic therapy
- bruising or overt bleeding arising from too high a dose of an anticoagulant
- euphoria associated with corticosteroid therapy
- depression associated with antihypertensive drug therapy
- anorexia in a patient receiving digoxin therapy.

Communicative skills
From the moment the patient is admitted to hospital his continued wellbeing (and eventual restoration to health) depends on effective communication with the patient and also between health care personnel. Nowhere is this more vital than with all aspects of drug therapy. At a very early stage interviewing skills are essential when eliciting a patient's history. This will involve collecting details of previous drug therapy, whether prescribed or non-prescribed. The patient may reveal some belief in alternative medicine or some form of lay medicine and this should be taken into consideration. Information on a medical condition or drug therapy may sometimes be obtained when a patient is wearing a medical pendant or bracelet.

Throughout the patient's stay in hospital other more general communication skills are used. Instructions to the patient should be clear and concise, offered at a suitable pace, and in a voice that can be heard. A conscious effort should be made to avoid the use of medical or nursing jargon.

Ensuring that the patient is wearing his spectacles and/or hearing aid may mean the difference between success and failure in communicating with him.

An equally important part of the communication process is a willingness to listen. Patients are often happy to talk about their illnesses and treatments and by appropriate questioning and astute follow-up of cues, the nurse can assess how much comprehension a patient has of his disorder and which problems are most real to him. By non-verbal means, such as a gesture, facial expression or mood, the patient can convey respectively the nature or location of pain, his like or dislike of taking a medicine, and the likelihood of his actually taking the medicines.

The nurse also needs to be able to give and receive messages about patients and their medicines to and from doctors, pharmacists and other nurses. In addition the importance of writing out the message in detail serves as an additional check and may also be required in the event of a query arising.

Particular opportunities for communication between nurse and patient arise when medicines are being administered (e.g. when applying a preparation to an area of broken skin, the nurse may help to ease pain by engaging the patient in some topic of conversation so as to divert his attention from the procedure). However, because of the need to ensure that an administered oral dose has actually been swallowed, and that other procedures have been carried out safely, the time of administration may not be the most appropriate to deal with detailed questions. Nevertheless the patient is entitled to know the name of the medicine, why it is being given, the dose he is to have, how often it is to be taken, and, if possible, the length of the course of treatment. Under certain circumstances and following discussions with the doctor, it may be appropriate to advise the patient of any likely side-effects. If possible, the patient's questions should be answered as raised. Those that cannot be dealt with during the medicine round should be noted for attention later, and not forgotten. Any anxiety a patient may feel, especially about a change in his treatment can be reduced by a clear explanation of what the new treatment involves, or why a medicine has been omitted.

The nurse should also be prepared to learn from the patient. Many patients, especially those suffering from chronic conditions, such as asthma, myasthenia gravis or Parkinson's disease will almost certainly have far more practical experience in managing their condition than the nurse. For example, the patient will know by his personal experience what the optimum time of administration of his medicine is.

Teaching skills
Linked with observational and communicative skills are those associated with teaching. Virginia Henderson (1966) states that it is part of the nurse's role to improve the patients' level of understanding and thus promote their health. Rodman & Smith (1974) suggest that nurses should aim to teach about drug therapy so that at the time of discharge from hospital, the patient can display a full understanding of his illness and medicines, and can take his medicines in accordance with the prescription. The assumption is that patient teaching promotes independence by facilitating self-administration of the medication, and thus the achievement of therapeutic benefit. By alerting the patient to potentially harmful situations, (e.g. taking aspirin when receiving warfarin therapy) nurses can contribute significantly to the patient's continued wellbeing. Increased understanding may help the patient in deciding to comply with the prescribed therapy.

If she is to bring about a change in behaviour, the 'teacher', whoever she may be, has a responsibility to guide, stimulate, and occasionally direct the patient to link what he already knows to that which is unfamiliar to him. There must be a willingness to explain, demonstrate, supervise, if necessary draw a diagram and then reinforce as required. Above all, the nurse must both make time and take time for this important part of patient management. Opportunities for teaching need to be recognised and put to use. As so much of what we learn results from copying others, the nurse should display a high level of accuracy and professionalism in relation to all aspects of medicine management and, in effect, teach by the example she sets. Individual factors do, however, influence learning and consequently the approach to teaching. These include the patient's level of intelligence and maturity, knowledge, his past experience, physical ability and degree of motivation. Where a patient is unable to master the necessary skill, the nurse may need to teach a relative or friend.

Some practical points to remember when teaching patients and/or relatives are as follows:

(a) *Make sure the time is right for teaching*
Teaching a patient about his medicines should be carried out at a time mutually convenient to patient and nurse. An explanation of the use of medicines which he is to take when he gets home from hospital should be made well in advance of the time of discharge. In this way, he is less likely to be hurried and there will still be time left to deal with any difficulties which arise (e.g. the occurrence of an unexpected side-effect).

(b) *Avoid giving the impression that you are hurried*
The flustered nurse whose every second glance is at the ward clock can convey anxiety to her patient which in turn may interfere with concentration. By talking to the patient about his medicines from an early stage and continuing to keep him informed of changes until the time of discharge, the task of administering medicines is made more simple and effective. The patient is more likely to assimilate information when the main points are repeated at appropriate intervals. In this way, teaching becomes an integral part of medicine administration.

(c) *Consider whether the patient can hear you*
The noise created by equipment being used in the ward may prevent instructions from being heard. Patients who wear a hearing aid may require assistance in its use.

(d) *Consider whether the patient can see*
Many patients need to wear spectacles for reading and at other times. Good lighting is necessary.

(e) *Maintain eye contact*
This should be achieved as much as possible while talking with the patient.

(f) *Avoid creating a mirror image*
E.g. when demonstrating how to load a syringe, sit or stand alongside the patient rather than facing him so that he can observe the procedure from the stance in which he will perform it.

(g) *Adopt a positive approach*
E.g. 'Hold the syringe this way.'

(h) *Keep speech and demonstration separate*
When learning a skill for the first time, a limited amount of information can be absorbed at one time.

(i) *Break the teaching into stages*
Do this wherever possible and select important points which require special emphasis.

(j) *Do not assume the patient is literate*
Obviously great tact is required to establish the extent of the patient's ability to read and write. People with literacy difficulties often wish to deny them and are skilful at concealing their problems. Conversely do not 'talk down' to patients. Where English is not understood, the help of an interpreter will be required.

In concluding this section, it may be of encouragement to nurses to be reminded that one of the best ways of improving your knowledge of a subject is to teach it to somebody else.

Motor skills
Apart from the specialised situations where hospital inpatients manage their own drug therapy, medicines are administered by nurses using skills acquired through learning and practice. Improvements in drug presentation, (e.g. prefilled syringes and aseptic dispensing services) have simplified and improved the safety of drug administration. On the other hand, further application of modern technology

in clinical areas has placed new demands on nurses' skills and technical abilities. The use of electronically controlled drug delivery systems, pumps, and other devices requires skills quite different from those traditionally associated with nursing. Against this background it is vitally important that the traditional practical skills of the nurse are not neglected.

The degree of skill required in medicine administration will vary considerably, depending on the dosage form used, the route/method of administration, and the extent to which the patient co-operates or is able to co-operate.

The giving of a simple tablet to a relatively well, intelligent, and co-operative patient presents few problems. Administering a small volume of a liquid medicine from a dropper to a mentally handicapped, athetoid child presents a greater challenge. To succeed in administering an intramuscular injection to a very agitated and unco- operative patient demands experience, skill and tenacity. The motor skills required include manual dexterity, co-ordination of hand and eye, coupled with lightness and delicacy of touch. Specialised situations such as those met in dermatology and ophthalmology call for skills which can only be acquired over many years.

Numerical skills

With the increasing potency and specificity of modern drugs it is now more vital than ever before to ensure accuracy when administering medicines. It is essential therefore that the nurse has a sound working knowledge of SI units of mass and volume and can calculate in these units. Recognition by pharmacists that it is important to supply medicines to wards and departments in a suitable range of strengths has reduced the need for calculations prior to the administration of medicines. Nevertheless, a nurse may be called upon to calculate how to obtain a dose of say 50 micrograms from a dosage form that contains 250 micrograms in 2 ml. Attempts to do this have unfortunately resulted in errors of tenfold or even more. Nurses must also have an understanding of proportions and percentages. It is suggested that these alone represent a minimal level of attainment. Nurses working in intensive care units would be expected to have considerably greater numerical skills and knowledge. Guidance on basic calculations is given in Chapter 10.

ATTITUDES

The least tangible part of the nurse's role is her overall attitude to patients and the management of their medicines. Relevant skills and knowledge are vital if the nurse is to discharge her basic responsibilities. However, without an informed respect for drugs generally, the full benefits of drug therapy will not be achieved and drug therapy may fail. This can be discussed under a number of headings.

Firstly, on a professional level, the nurse should have an awareness of the place of all medicines, in the care of the patient. Recognition of the reasons for the need to be systematic in adherence to both national (legal) and local procedural requirements is vital. The recognition should be based on a broad understanding of the principles involved, not merely the mechanical following of a set of rules. An overall sense of the need for security in its widest sense is required, coupled with an appreciation of economic factors. An enquiring attitude of mind associated with a knowledgeable, well-informed approach, will give the nurse confidence to play her full part in ensuring safe and effective drug therapy.

Secondly, it is important to consider those attitudes which are, to a large extent, linked with personal qualities. These qualities include powers of observation and the ability to keep calm and work under pressure. Being selective in dealing with interruptions during procedures involving medicines calls for judgment, patience and, occasionally, a sense of humour. The nurse must exercise judgment, since a degree of flexibility may be called for on occasions; firmness, linked with tact, is a prerequisite. The balanced assessment of one's own knowledge, or lack of it, is important, as is the willingness to ask and seek advice.

Against this background it should not be forgotten that the nurse has a duty to encourage the patient to regard all medicines with respect, without at the same time causing anxiety. In exercising the skills and demonstrating the attitudes discussed above, the nurse sets an example for the patient to follow when he goes home. Special emphasis on certain aspects, such as the need for safe storage of medicines, can be reinforced by the attitude adopted by the nurse and the care and concern she shows. A patient may be reluctant to take the medicines and/or unable to see the need for them. This demands patience and perseverance by the nurse. Often the problem arises with those in greatest need of the treatment. With a responsibility to act as a good role model as health educator, the nurse should respect medicines both in her professional and personal life.

THE EXTENDED ROLE OF THE NURSE

Certain duties and procedures not normally classed as nursing responsibilities are listed in circulars issued by the DHSS and the SHHD. These circulars provide for authorisation (by the medical practitioner involved) of individually named trained nurses to perform defined technical nursing procedures following a period of formal instruction and receipt of a certificate of competence to practise. Of the procedures listed those relating to drug therapy are:

- intravenous and intra-arterial medication
- subcutaneous and intramuscular injections of serum and immunological agents
- tuberculin skin tests (Heaf multiple puncture test and Tine test)
- haemodialysis
  haemoperfusion
  continuous ambulatory peritoneal dialysis.

MEDICINES AND THE NURSING PROCESS

A problem-solving approach to nursing can be used for any or every aspect of care relevant to the individual patient and, therefore, in many instances, involves the question of medicines and their management. Whatever the problem, the components used remain the same (i.e. assessment, planning, implementation and evaluation). Further assessment makes it a cyclical process. Because it is a systematic and logical approach, when properly used, it is efficient. This method applies whether addressing a patient's specific problem, considering the patient and his needs in their entirety, or preparing to teach the patient about his medicines. Illustrations of what is meant follow.

First, a specific problem. The patient complains of a headache. The procedure followed is that the nurse makes an assessment by trying to establish the location, severity and duration of the headache. The nurse then carries out any simple measures to make the patient more comfortable and if this proves unsuccessful she notifies the doctor. The doctor may prescribe an analgesic stating the dose, the method of administration and the frequency with which it is to be given. The nurse administers the medicine accordingly and returns to the patient at intervals to evaluate its effect. Depending on observations made by the nurse (or the doctor) and on opinions expressed by the patient, the prescription may be discontinued or it may continue as before or with an alteration to the choice of analgesic, the dose, the method of administration or the interval between doses. Hence the steps are followed through.

Now to the place of medicines generally in what has come to be known as the Nursing Process. By again using a problem-orientated approach, the nurse is helped in a methodical way to consider aspects of medicine management in relation to the patient as a whole person. As these aspects impinge on every stage of the process, a more detailed study of each stage is necessary.

Assessment
A profile of the patient is compiled during the first 24 hours or so, after admission to hospital. This involves collecting together relevant information some of which will be of assistance during the patient's stay in hospital while the rest will be required when preparing the patient for discharge from hospital. Details can be acquired from a variety of sources such as the general practitioner's letter, previous medical records, relatives and relevant personnel, e.g. the district nurse. Most of the

information, however, is obtained from interviewing the patient.

The profile can be divided into two parts — personal data and an assessment of the activities of living. The patient's personal details including age, address, and family support, are obtained on admission and are useful to know when teaching the patient about his medicines. Of course, medicines do not necessarily feature at this stage. A patient who *is* taking medicines will often spontaneously mention them but the nurse must not rely on him to do so. Patients may not want to talk about their medicines if they fear that this will lead to discussion of their illness e.g. sexually-transmitted disease, malignant disease. The skill of interviewing, not always easy when the patient is unwell, tired or has difficulty with memory recall, involves eliciting accurate details as systematically as possible. Having established that the patient is taking prescribed or non-prescribed medicines, the nurse should enquire whether he is experiencing any difficulty taking them. The examination of medicines brought into hospital by the patient may reveal patient non-compliance.

A list of the activities of living is now a recognised tool which provides a framework for structuring questions about the patient's level of functioning including his ability to cope with medicines. In this way, the patient's physical capabilities are assessed with a view to estimating his degree of dependence on others for assistance including the taking of medicines. Full assessment of the patient's mental capacity is also begun on admission but

Table 1.1

Activity of living	Specific aspect	Nursing implications
Maintaining a safe environment	Support at home	Where compliance is likely to pose a problem, it may be necessary to ask a relative or friend to supervise or assist the patient with his medicines on discharge from hospital.
	Children in the house	Extra emphasis on safety with medicines is essential where there are children.
	Sensitivity	Any drug or medicine sensitivity known to the patient should be clearly entered in nursing and medical records including medicine prescription sheets.
Communicating	Ability to understand	Guidance and instruction in the administration of medicines must be matched to the patient's level of understanding.
	Willingness to co-operate	Nurses must help patients to appreciate the importance of taking medicines correctly. Relatives may be asked to provide further support.
	Ability to see	Many elderly patients have difficulty seeing their medicines. Small white tablets against a white background or clear liquids in a clear medicine glass can be overlooked. Nurses should ensure that good light is provided and that the patient's spectacles are put to use.
	Ability to hear	The successful taking of medicines depends on receiving accurate instruction, most of which is verbal. When patients are weak and depressed, hearing is less acute.
Breathing	Ability to swallow	Where severe breathlessness makes swallowing difficult, an alternative route, such as the rectal route, may have to be used.
Eating and drinking	Ability to swallow	Inability to swallow will necessitate the use of alternative routes of administration (e.g. via nasogastric tube, per rectum or by injection). Patients with dysphagia may require oral medicines in liquid form.
	Ability to retain ingested substances	Nausea and vomiting often prevent successful administration of oral medicines. Patients may indicate ways they have devised to overcome this problem.

Table 1.1 (Con't)

Activity of living	Specific aspect	Nursing implications
	Fluid intake permitted	Care should be taken not to encourage large volumes of fluid where the daily intake is restricted (e.g. in renal failure). Patients taking certain sulphonamides require to take copious amounts of liquid, however.
Eliminating	Degree of continence	Loss of control of the anal sphincter or faecal impaction may make it impossible for the patient to retain rectal medication. Constipation may interfere with the free flow of urine per urinary catheter and may make bladder irrigation difficult.
Personal cleansing and dressing	Interest in personal hygiene/grooming	Lack of interest in personal hygiene or embarrassment may make a patient reluctant to accept treatment for such problems as body odours or head lice.
Controlling body temperature	Ability to recognise changes in temperature	Hyperthermic and hypothermic reactions should be noted in patients taking phenothiazines as these drugs may affect the heat regulating mechanism. Requirements of clothing and room temperature should be adjusted accordingly.
Mobilising	Ability to sit upright	Whenever possible, patients should be in an upright position for taking oral medicines. Great care must be taken to avoid inhalation when giving medicines to patients who have to be nursed in the prone or recumbent position.
	Mobility permitted	Restrictions may be imposed on the patient's mobility so that the nurse must adapt her approach to the administration of medicines accordingly.
	Use of hand(s)	Where there is loss of the use of both hands or where tremor is very severe, considerable assistance will be required with the taking of medicines. Strategies for overcoming the difficulty of mild tremor, stiffness of the hands, or having the use of one hand only, can be taught.
Working and playing	Degree of motivation	Poorly-motivated patients are less likely to take an interest in their medicines. Encouragement should be given to all patients but especially to those who will have to manage their medicines at home. Importance should be attached to drugs which constitute replacement therapy or control of disease.
Expressing sexuality	Degree of embarrassment	Embarrassment may interfere with the satisfactory insertion or application of certain preparations (e.g. pessaries, vaginal creams). The nurse should be tactful in her approach and ensure maximum privacy. Whenever possible, self-administration should be encouraged.
Sleeping	Responsiveness	Very drowsy patients may be unable to co-operate in the taking of medicines, and other routes may have to be used. Special care must be taken to avoid accidental inhalation of medicines.
Dying	Degree of emaciation	In terminal care, injections should be minimised. Where this cannot be avoided, the volume of reconstituting fluid used should be the minimum compatible with the physical and other properties of the drug. A smaller needle may be required for giving an intramuscular injection, e.g. 23G, 1 inch. (for an adult)
	Pain control	Control of pain is achieved through thorough assessment of the pain, careful choice of analgesic, appropriate dosage and administration at regular and suitable intervals. There is no place in terminal illness for 'analgesics as required'.

it may take some time to establish how reliable the patient is in dealing with medicines. Furthermore, the effect that individual drugs are having, or may be suspected of having, on the activities of living should be considered, e.g. the constipating effect of some analgesics may affect elimination; the nauseating effect of an antibiotic may interfere with eating and drinking; a sedative drug may make communication difficult.

The background information gathered then serves as a basis for identifying problems which the patient is experiencing. Table 1.1. shows how the activities of living as categorised by Roper, Logan and Tierney (1985) serve as a checklist. *Note that only topics relating directly or indirectly to medicines are included.*

Planning

In planning a patient's care, the nurse sets individual goals which are aimed at overcoming each of the patient's problems. Decisions are made as to the form care and treatment will take and times or dates are set for reviewing the problems. Medicines are prescribed by the doctor taking into account the patient's age and other factors including body mass, physical and mental condition, and, in some instances, his beliefs. The nurse often assists in suggesting times of administration which will fit in with other activities with which the patient is involved. The presentation of the medicine (e.g. large tablet) may pose a problem and again the nurse can assist by drawing the doctor's attention to the patient's difficulties or preferences. The ward pharmacist can be of great assistance at this stage of the process. The medicines prescribed, if not already in stock on the ward, are requisitioned by the nurse or supplies are arranged by the ward pharmacist.

Implementation

Medicines are administered to the patient most often by nurses in accordance with the prescription. However, medicines seldom are isolated from other aspects of care and it falls to the nurse to integrate them with the rest of the patient's nursing care, investigations, and treatment. Through the system of patient allocation the same nurse (or nurses) looks after the patient for a span of duty. The nurse can plan the patient's programme of care with emphasis on meeting the patient's greatest needs first. For example, the strict time-keeping required to achieve control of pain in terminal illness takes priority over changing the patient's position. Clearly however the exact timing of any medicine comes second to the removal of secretions from the mouth of a patient who is choking. Other aspects of nursing care are carried out in conjunction with the administration of medicines (e.g. a surgical dressing and the application of a topical preparation).

Evaluation

The role of the nurse (and doctor) is to evaluate the effect the medicine has had on the patient. On this basis, the medicine may be discontinued, exchanged for another, continued as before, or continued with some alteration to the prescription.

Hitherto, much of the teaching of patients about their medicines prior to discharge from hospital has been carried out hurriedly in a rather informal and haphazard way. Sometimes it has not happened at all. Using a problem-solving approach once again, the learning needs of individual patients can be met in an organised way. Whether the patient is an elderly person living alone or a child newly diagnosed as having insulin-dependent diabetes, the challenge should be recognised and met, using all the nurse's professional skills to the full.

REFERENCES

Henderson V 1966 The nature of nursing; a definition and its implications for practice, research and education Macmillan, New York

Rodman M J, Smith D W 1974 Clinical pharmacology in nursing Lippincott, Philadelphia

Roper N, Logan W W, Tierney A J 1985 The elements of nursing, 2nd edn. Churchill Livingstone, Edinburgh

2 DRUG FORMULARIES AND THE DEVELOPMENT OF MODERN MEDICINES. ALTERNATIVE AND COMPLEMENTARY MEDICINE

An appreciation of the dramatic increase in the availability of effective medicines during this century can be gained by an examination of pharmacopoeias and formularies of the period. Around the turn of the century (1895) the pharmocopoeia of Aberdeen Royal Infirmary (ARI) contained 76 different preparations, many of which were simple mixtures of inorganic chemicals and extracts of various plant material diluted to a suitable volume with water. The range of presentations was also very limited as illustrated by the following list of contents:

Emulsions	1	Pills	5
Gargles	7	Plasters	1
Inhalations	1	Powders	4
Linctuses	1	Eye drops	6
Liniments	1	Eye washes	4
Lotions	8	Eye ointments	7
Oral mixtures	27	Enemas	1
Ointments	2		

Only Imperial units of mass and volume (e.g. grains and minims) were used. Some alkaloids (active principles extracted from vegetable material) were included, notably atropine, cocaine, morphine, quinine, and strychnine. Mercury compounds were present in some formulations, both oral (for diuretic properties) and topical (for antiseptic properties). Apart from a very limited use of mercury topically, and the occasional use of mersalyl injection, mercury compounds are seldom, if ever, used today. Ginger, peppermint, sulphur, calamine, zinc sulphate, magnesium carbonate and sodium salicylate were commonly used ingre-

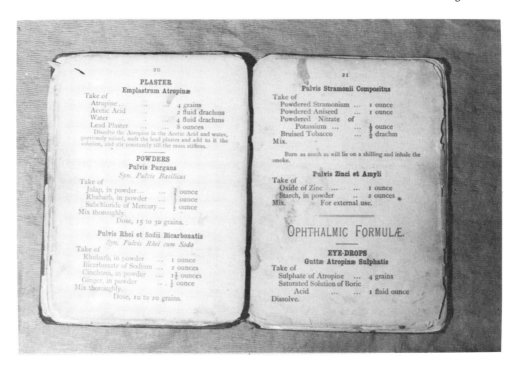

Fig. 2.1 ARI pharmacopoeia in 1895

dients that are still used today as are the alkaloids referred to above. On the other hand, tinctures of squill, senega and lavender, decoction of broom and spirit of juniper, not to mention ipecacuanha wine and tincture of hyoscyamus would hardly be seen outside a museum. The ARI pharmacopoeia, along with others of the day, contained very few medicines which, by current standards, would be considered as having any worthwhile therapeutic activity. Indeed, some of the medicines, especially those containing mercury, would rightly be regarded as dangerous.

Birmingham General Hospital pharmacopoeia of 1908 contained 204 different preparations very similar in composition to those included in the Aberdeen pharmacopoeia but in addition contained solutions for infiltration anaesthesia, the preparation of which included some attempts to produce a sterile preparation. This pharmacopoeia gave metric equivalents to Imperial weights and measures. Information on dosage levels, a guide to the treatment of poisoning, and some information on nursing procedures such as hot air baths, hot and cold packs, and cold sponging were included. Dietary information was also provided, male patients being entitled to receive larger portions than female patients.

Guy's Hospital pharmacopoeia of 1916 was compiled by the Dispensary Committee, no doubt a forerunner of the present day Drug and Therapeutics Committee. This pharmacopoeia is a rather grand publication running to 271 pages which included dietary advice, dosage levels, instructions for feeding an infant, guidance on nursing procedures, urine testing, a bacteriological section and the treatment of poisoning. A wide range of medicines was included, formulated products having both metric and Imperial units. As with earlier pharmacopoeias the medicines consisted mostly of simple chemicals and plant extracts, but were on the whole, slightly more sophisticated. Five vaccines were described in the pharmacopoeia but arsenic and mercury compounds still appeared. An index of proprietary and their non-proprietary equivalents was included.

By 1933 the contents of the pharmacopoeia of Manchester Royal Infirmary demonstrated the advances in therapy that were taking place. The wide range of local anaesthetics, barbiturates, organic arsenical and bismuth injections provided some indication of the therapeutic revolution that was to come. However, Latin terminology was still widely used at this time, and the drugs and pharmaceutical preparations were still fairly crude. A list of proprietary products and their non-proprietary equivalents was included as was dietary advice and procedures for making and applying poultices.

In 1936 (before the NHS was established) London County Council issued an important pharmacopoeia 'for use in the Council's general and special hospitals'. This pharmacopoeia was very much the mixture as before, regarding the drugs and preparations included, since few major advances had taken place. Sections on infectious diseases and clinical pathology were very comprehensive. The administration of drugs by the oral, rectal and parenteral routes was covered in some detail, as was drug administration by inhalation. Procedures for the use of topical applications were fully described and it was recognised that mercury and belladonna were absorbed through the skin 'to enable them to be administered to the patient in this way'.

During the Second World War (in 1941) the then Ministry of Health 'appointed a Committee to prepare a formulary for general use in war time by medical practitioners, pharmacists, hospitals, and others concerned with the prescribing and dispensing of medicines'. The outcome of this work was the publication of the National War Formulary (NWF). Shortages of certain imported and strategic materials were taken into account in drawing up the formulary. Tinctures (and other alcohol-containing preparations) were replaced by aqueous extracts or, in some cases, by concentrated tinctures. The use of liquid paraffin was strictly regulated and the use of liver extracts was controlled by an order that restricted this administration to patients suffering from pernicious anaemia. The shortage of drugs order (SR and 0 1941 No. 273) permitted the pharmacist to dispense the corresponding sodium salts in place of certain

potassium salts, 'unless the prescriber directs otherwise'. The contents of the second edition (1943) of the NWF was essentially an 'economy' version of previous hospital pharmacopoeias, which had been consulted, and reflected the grave difficulties and shortages of that time. In 1947 the National (War) Formulary was issued having been revised in the light of 'the post war position in the supply of drugs'. Existing conditions (even post war), were such that it was still necessary to exercise 'the strictest economy in the prescribing of certain drugs and preparations. Many of importance in medicine, are also required to assist the nation's economic recovery'. This formulary is noteworthy for the inclusion of penicillin ear drops, cream, eye drops, and injections. Guidance was given that penicillin preparations 'should be used under close medical supervision because of the danger of breeding strains of organisms resistant to penicillin'.

The establishment in 1948 of the NHS was a turning point in many ways. Gradually Great Britain began to recover from the devastation of war and by 1955 the National Formulary, although still very much a listing of fairly simple preparations contained some products resulting from the research efforts of major drug companies, although only two antibiotics, penicillin and streptomycin were included.

The next 20 years were times of great advance in the development of effective drugs, although during this time concern regarding the adverse effects of drugs also mounted. An examination of the 1974–76 British National Formulary (BNF) shows that 15 injectable antibiotics were included, a sharp contrast to the 2 included in the 1955 Formulary.

The 1955 Formulary contained no corticosteroids, oral diuretics, oncolytics, or beta-blockers, whereas the 1974–76 edition contains several examples of all these drugs. In order to keep pace with this therapeutic revolution the format of the BNF was totally changed in 1981. There is now much greater emphasis on the clinical use of drugs. The listing of products according to pharmaceutical form is now as archaic as the use of liquid extract of male fern. As a final illustration of the explosion in the availability of powerful and effective medicines, the Aberdeen Royal Infirmary pharmacopoeia of 1895 contained 76 preparations. In 1985 the hospital medicine inventory, held in computer files, includes over 3000 items.

Although the approach adopted in different health authorities will vary district and ward drug formularies are now in widespread use, particularly in light of selected list prescribing introduced into the NHS in 1985.

DEVELOPMENT OF MODERN DRUGS

One of the most dramatic effects of the introduction of modern drugs (and vaccines), has been a significant contribution to the reduction in deaths due to infectious diseases. Effective control of symptoms of many chronic conditions such as asthma and cardiovascular disease is now possible. Nevertheless the search for new and more effective drugs continues. The extent to which further progress is made will depend on many factors, especially the rate at which the fundamental understanding of disease processes develops.

Many stages are involved in the discovery and development of a drug from initial research to large scale manufacture. The whole process now costs many millions of pounds and therefore true innovation is within the capabilities of only a small number of major drug houses worldwide.

A brief outline of the main stages involved in drug discovery and development follows:

1. Medical need, market research, innovative ideas.
2. Initial research programme, e.g. chemical synthesis.
3. Testing for pharmacological activity.
4. Selection of drug(s) with potential, for further basic testing, e.g. toxicity testing.
5. Choice of drug for further development based on outcome of 4.
6. Detailed technical and economic study of drug chosen.
7. Detailed study of the chemical and physical properties of the drug. Detailed

animal pharmacology including toxicity studies.
8. Short term studies in healthy volunteers to establish if effects found in animal studies are also found in man.
9. Studies in patients suffering from the condition for which the drug was developed.
10. Controlled trials, including comparisons with existing treatments.
11. Following further detailed technical and economic appraisal, a large scale manufacturing process is developed and further studies, including international clinical trials are carried out.
12. The whole process takes many years to complete, and is controlled by legislation at all stages. Before the product can be marketed The Committee on Safety of Medicines (CSM) must be satisfied that in the light of all existing knowledge the product is safe for use for its intended purpose.
13. Once a product (medicine) has been licensed the CSM, with the co-operation of the health professions, monitors the incidence of adverse reactions to a product, so that any necessary action can be taken.

The changes in clinical practice resulting from the introduction of modern drugs have been profound, both in terms of benefits for patients and impact on working methods. It is worth reflecting that in the space of 30 years diluted herbal extracts administered by the spoonful have been superseded by highly sophisticated drugs administered in nanogram quantities.

THE FUTURE

Bioengineering techniques have already been successfully used to produce biosynthetic human insulin, and the potential benefit of the interferons will no doubt be exploited. Techniques are being developed to manipulate biological materials in space so as to achieve greater yields of active drug and enhance purity levels. Chemical synthesis will no doubt also continue to yield new drug entities in the future.

Much drug therapy today, although highly sophisticated in many respects, often lacks specificity. The need to target drugs to the affected organ(s) or site(s) of disease has, in some instances, already been met. Drugs can be delivered to the lungs by aerosols and rectal preparations can be used to deliver drugs to the site of lesions in the lower part of the gastrointestinal tract. By delivering drugs directly to the site of the disease, dosage levels can often be reduced, and thus side-effects minimised or even eliminated. New drug delivery systems will no doubt be developed in the future to meet the need that still exists to target drugs to the affected site(s) (e.g. in the treatment of some forms of cancer), the aim being to increase therapeutic benefit while at the same time minimising adverse effects. A liposome drug delivery system has been evaluated and appears to have promise. Techniques have been developed to enable red blood cells to be used as carriers for certain drugs.

A system with a magnetic core and a device based on a miniaturised osmotic pump are examples of drug delivery systems being developed which are designed to achieve and maintain therapeutic levels of a drug in plasma. Mechanical devices, such as specially designed pumps, are already available for drug delivery. It seems likely that, as technology advances, further sophistication will become possible. A combination of new drugs and improved drug delivery systems will no doubt enable therapeutic benefit to be achieved for many more patients in the years ahead.

ALTERNATIVE AND COMPLEMENTARY MEDICINE

Interest in alternative medicine is considerable as evidenced by extensive media coverage and the fact that, at the suggestion of H.R.H. Prince Charles, the British Medical Association has undertaken a detailed study of the value of alternative therapies. Aspects of alternative medicine have even been described as a new growth industry. Whether any or all unorthodox treatments should be regarded as complementary to, or as an alternative to orthodox medicine remains to be seen. Nevertheless a patient who is dissatisfied with modern drug therapy, perhaps because of side-effects, may well see meditation, relaxation therapy, homeopathy, or other form of unorthodox therapy as very real alternatives.

The reasons why people seek treatment by alternative medicine have been examined by Moore et al (1985). A high percentage (97%) of patients interviewed stated that 'failure of conventional medicine' was the reason, and not dissatisfaction with their general practitioner, although some patients felt 'that their general practitioner did not understand their problems'.

Many patients receiving care in conventional hospitals or in the community will, at some time, have sought relief from the symptoms or perhaps even cure outside conventional medicine. This trend towards the use of alternative therapies is being increasingly recognised by health professionals in orthodox medicine. Indeed some doctors are themselves using alternative therapies. Whenever possible, alternative treatment should be given sympathetic consideration. In the community this will generally present few problems, but in hospital, special arrangements may have to be made, in agreement with the doctor, nurse or pharmacist to enable a patient to continue to take say, a herbal remedy the patient finds helpful. The guiding principle at all times will be to ensure that the alternative treatment is complementary to, and not in conflict with, other therapy the patient may need. In a similar way it may be necessary to recognise the possible impact of ethnic medicine on what may be perceived as more conventional treatment. Quite apart from alternative therapies and ethnic medicines, it may be advisable to allow a patient to continue to use a 'lay remedy' again with the proviso that the remedy must not conflict in any way with the conventional therapy.

More than 60 alternative therapies and techniques have been listed by Brian Inglis and Ruth West in their book *The Alternative Health Guide.* Many of these therapies do not of course involve the consumption of any form of medicine, but in some situations a combination of therapies may be used. The best known alternative therapies are osteopathy, acupuncture, chiropractic, naturopathy, homeopathy, (available on the NHS), hypnotherapy and medical herbalism. It may be that alternative therapies will be increasingly used in the years ahead, despite the lack of scientific evidence as to their value.

REFERENCES

Inglis B, West R, 1983 The alternative health guide. Michael Joseph, London
Inglis B, West R 1985 Taking the alternative road to health. The Times 14th March
Moore J, Phipps K, Marcer D, Lewith G 1985 Why do people seek treatment by alternative medicine? British Medical Journal 290: 28–29

3 PHARMACEUTICAL SERVICES

Safe and effective management of modern drug therapy depends on many factors, not least of which is the availability of effective pharmaceutical services. Fortunately for patients pharmaceutical services have been developed in line with the increasing complexity of drug therapy.

The pharmacist's traditional role as skilled intermediary between prescriber and patient remains central wherever he practises, as do his dispensing and supply functions. This role has been enhanced by the provision of information services to patients, prescribers and nurses. Other specialised hospital-based services designed to contribute to the achievement of optimal drug therapy include the compounding of sterile preparations for total parenteral nutrition and cytotoxic drug therapy. Pharmaceutical skills are now widely available in clinical areas. The pharmacist's place within the health care team is firmly established and is likely to develop in the years ahead.

SUPPLY OF PRESCRIBED MEDICINES TO WARDS

Several different methods are used to supply prescribed medicines to wards. The choice of method used will depend on a number of factors including the extent of medicine use, layout of the hospital, geographical considerations and resources available to the pharmaceutical service.

The overall aim of any drug distribution and supply system is to ensure that the necessary medicines of the required quality are available when required in quantities that reflect both current, and to some extent, future usage in the particular ward. No one method of supply is likely to be suitable for use in all situations.

Each method has advantages and disadvantages. An outline of different methods used follows, together with a discussion of how the method used influences the role of nurse and pharmacist.

Total stock system

This is the most basic method of supplying medicines in which the nurse interprets the prescription, checks ward stocks and orders the medicines that, in her judgment, reflect the needs of the ward at that particular time. Medicine orders are then made out by the nurse and met by the pharmaceutical department, usually by pharmacy technicians and assistants, working under the direction of a pharmacist. On receipt of the completed order at the ward, the nurse is responsible for checking the items supplied and ensuring correct storage on the ward prior to administration to the patient.

This total stock system (Fig. 3.1) has superficial advantages in that it is simple to operate and can be used on a temporary basis when staff shortages in pharmacy preclude the use of better methods. It may be the only applicable method where communications are difficult, e.g. when the pharmacy is situated at a considerable distance from the ward. However, the disadvantages of this approach are very significant and far outweigh any marginal advantages. The use of this system does not permit the pharmacist to discharge his full professional role as intermediary between prescriber and patient. There is no opportunity to interpret the prescriptions, check dosage levels or monitor prescriptions for possible drug interactions which may hazard the patient. There is also no opportunity for the pharmacist to advise on aspects of drug therapy prior to decisions being made by the prescriber. In effect, the nurse takes on a role for which she is not fully trained. This is in no way a denigration of the role of the nurse, rather, it is a question of using the specialist skills of health professionals in the most effective way for the benefit of the patient. When using this supply method, the nurse is involved in much clinically unproductive work and at the same time contact on a professional level

between nurse and pharmacist is minimal. As a result there is considerable potential for misunderstanding as to the range and quantities of medicines actually required at a particular time. Although the nurse will be alert to such problems as expiry dates of medicines, the presence of a large relatively uncontrolled ward stock increases the risk of hazard to the patient and may result in wastage of drugs. This method of drug supply is increasingly being replaced by one of the following systems which are designed to overcome the many disadvantages inherent in a system which relegates the role of the pharmacist to that of specialist storekeeper and that of the nurse to a mail order customer.

'Aberdeen System' — ward and clinical pharmacy

With the advent of highly structured documentation for recording the prescribing and administration of medicines, it has become possible for the pharmacist to discharge his professional role at ward level. By visiting the ward on a regular basis the pharmacist is able to obtain readily at first hand, detailed information on the current range of prescribed medicines. He is thus able to contribute his professional skills not only on supply aspects but also on many important facets of the *use* of medicines. The concept of the pharmacist working at ward level has had, and is still having, a profound effect on the management of medicines in hospitals. By becoming a member of the ward team, the pharmacist is able to supervise more effectively the supply of the necessary medicines. In addition he is well placed to advise professional colleagues on a wide range of topics related to drug therapy. Interpretation of the prescriptions, checking of dosage levels and monitoring prescriptions for possible drug interactions have always been an accepted part of the pharmacist's duties but, working at ward level, his contribution becomes much more relevant. By visiting the ward the pharmacist has more information on the patient's condition, special problems, etc. than would be the case when working solely within his department.

It should be noted that with the Aberdeen

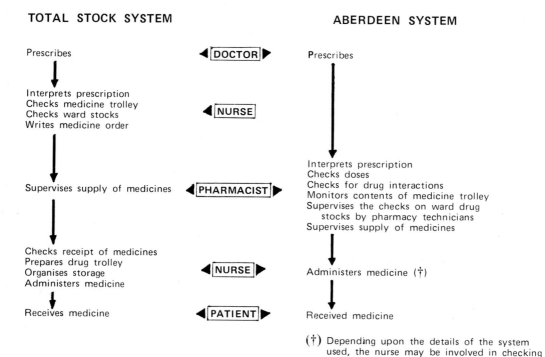

Fig. 3.1 Comparison of total stock system and Aberdeen system

system (Fig. 3.1) the prescription remains on the ward at all times thus eliminating errors that might arise due to its absence. Ward pharmacy services have been described in several official publications, notably in the paper 'Measures for Controlling Drugs on the Wards' HM(70)36 and in 'Control of Medicines in Hospital Wards and Departments' (1972) HMSO. The report 'The Organisation of the In-Patients Day' issued with HC(76)31 also stated that 'ward visits by pharmacists to see prescriptions and offer advice on appropriate medication are now accepted as a valuable contribution to patients' welfare'.

Many refinements and variations are possible within a ward pharmacy service. The pharmacist with the assistance of pharmacy technicians can take complete responsibility for ensuring that the necessary medicines are available both in stock and in the medicine trolley. As with other drug distribution methods, it is possible to use computerised drug management systems to assist in the supply of medicines. In place of time-consuming

traditional handwritten orders, it is possible to use computer-printed medicine order forms (see Fig. 3.2) which reflect the range of medicines used in a particular ward.

Portable microcomputers can also be used to assist in supply procedures, either to produce an order for the required medicines at ward level or to input the order directly into the pharmacy computer (see Fig. 3.3).

The computer can also produce information on use of drugs, range, quantities, costs etc., which can be used as a basis on which to establish ward prescribing policies, ward formularies, or drug stock lists (see Fig. 3.4).

Using the Aberdeen system, the nurse is released from clinically unproductive work and is able to concentrate her skills on the nursing care of her patients. The contribution of the pharmacist at ward level is complementary to, and not in conflict with, the role of the nurse and other clinical staff. A well-organised ward pharmacy service is seen as relevant and worthwhile if not essential, by both medical and nursing colleagues. The development of

ITEM DESCRIPTION	CODE	QTY	ITEM DESCRIPTION	CODE	QTY
ADRENALINE 1-10,000 AMP 10ml x 10	030635_		MAGNESIUM TRISILICATE MIXT 200ml	033995_	
ANUSOL CR 23G	005746_		MEFENAMIC ACID 250mg CAP 50	022888_	
ASPIRIN SOLUBLE 300mg TAB 50	007390_		METRONIDAZOLE 400mg TAB 25	013234_	
BCG VACC BP BNF 1/D 5 x 10 DOSE	037788_		MICROGYNON-30 TAB 21	019240_	
BENYLIN EXPECTORANT 200ml	027081_		MILPAR SUSP 200ml	018899_	
BM-TEST GLYCEMIE 20-800R x50	037796_		MULTISTIX-SG 100	019844_	
CEPHRADINE 500mg CAP 20	048267_		NALOXONE HCL 0.02mg AMP 10	022152_	
CHLORHEXIDINE 0.5% in 70% IMS 30ml	034002_		NON-INJECTABLE WATER [AR1] 1L	024783_	
CHLORHEXIDINE GLUCONATE 0.2% SOLN 250ML	008958_		NORGESTON TAB 35 (Sleeved/Leaflet)	049085_	
CHLORHEXIDINE OBSTETRIC CR 250ml	014885_		NORGESTREL 75mcg TAB 35	036587_	
CHLORHEXIDINE SOLN (Hibiscrub) 500ml	014818_		OXYTOCIN 5iu AMP 10	003999_	
CLINITEST TAB 100	008419_		PARACETAMOL 500mg TAB 50	021032_	
DIMOTAPP ELIXIR 500ml	011207_		PARAFFIN YELLOW SOFT (NON-STERILE) 15G	051268_	
ERGOMETRINE 500mcg/ml AMP 10	027235_		PHYTOMENADIONE 1mg AMP 10	016314_	
ESBACH'S SOLN 100ml	041157_		PROCTOSEDYL OINT 30G	023868_	
EUGYNON-30 TAB 21	012556_		RUBELLA VACCINE 1 DOSE	004170_	
FERROUS SULPHATE 200mg TAB 50	027995_		SAVLODIL SACHET 100ml x 10	040355_	
FLETCHERS PHOSPH ENEMA 130ml	013285_		SAVLON 3.5% SOLN IN 73% IMS 250ml	042528_	
GLYCERIN SUPP 4G x 12	026662_		SENOKOT TAB 50	036633_	
HAND CR 50G	026883_		SODIUM BICARBONATE SOLN 1-160 200ml	028681_	

Fig. 3.2 Computer-printed medicine order form

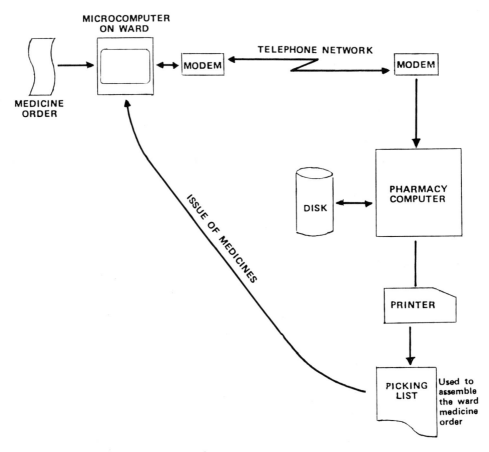

Fig. 3.3 Medicine order system using a microcomputer at ward level linked directly to pharmacy computer

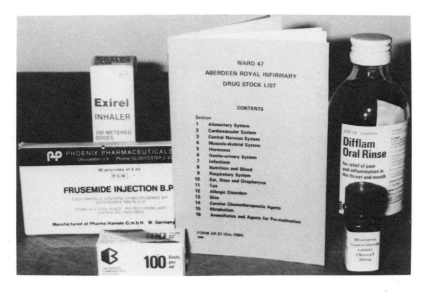

Fig. 3.4 Ward drug stock list

ward pharmacy as described above has provided a basis on which a more clinically orientated pharmaceutical service can be developed.

Clinical pharmacy services can be seen as an extension of ward pharmacy services. The clinical pharmacist's duties are more directly related to the care of the individual patient. The range of these duties is now very wide and includes advising the doctor on aspects of drug therapy, drug history taking, patient counselling, aspects of patient compliance, therapeutic drug monitoring, etc.

Some pharmacists have developed particular expertise in response to the needs of oncology patients, older people, children and other patients in whom optimal drug use is vitally important.

Ward and clinical pharmacy services are compatible with all drug distribution systems. The emphasis placed on a particular aspect will vary according to local needs.

Pharmacists working at ward level may, in the past, have encountered some suspicion or even resentment from nurses, who understandably felt that yet another aspect of their role was being eroded. As ward pharmacy services have evolved each profession has gained a better insight into the role of the other. This has resulted in the establishment of smooth working relationships which have contributed significantly to the safe, effective and economical management of medicines in hospitals. Pressures on nurses are greater than ever before due to many factors including quicker 'turnover' of patients, a shorter working week and highly-stretched staffing resources. Against this background, nurses have to deal with a wide range of problems arising from the ever increasing complexity of drug therapy and drug delivery systems. Nurses now recognise the ward pharmacist as a valuable source of practical help, advice, and support in this important aspect of their work.

Partial stock/individual dispensing system
Under this arrangement prescribed medicines are supplied either as traditional ward stocks, if used regularly, or are dispensed for an individual patient, if seldom used. Confusion can

arise at ward level owing to the presence of these two different categories of medicine in the trolley. The decision as to when a medicine becomes an agreed ward stock item may cause friction especially when an individually dispensed item is retained by the nurse for ward stock. Effective ward pharmacy services will obviate this type of difficulty. Trends in the use of medicines can be closely monitored and agreement reached jointly with ward staff on the range of stock items required.

Individual patient dispensing
With the increasing emphasis on nursing care by allocation and a shift of emphasis away from rounds of tasks to be carried out by nurses there is a need for systems of medication distribution which are compatible with an individual approach to patient care. Dispensing for individual patients meets this need since medicines are supplied, not as communal stock bottles, but for administration only to the patient named on the label of the dispensed medicine. A very limited range of medicines is supplied as ward stock as cover for periods

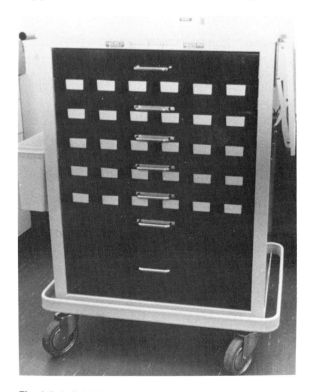

Fig. 3.5 Individual medicine trolley

when the pharmaceutical service is not available.

The dispensed medicines are stored in separate compartments, one for each patient, within a specially designed medicine trolley (see Fig. 3.5). A disadvantage of this method of supply is that it is more labour intensive for pharmacy than (some) other stock systems. However, with good organisation the workload generated can be contained within reasonable limits. Where circumstances permit the trolley can be sent to pharmacy and the prescribed medicines placed in each compartment as appropriate. Some medicine trolleys are fitted with removable cassettes (see Fig. 3.6) which can be sent to pharmacy instead of the complete trolley.

Using this system the nurse makes the selection of medicine(s) to be administered from the patient's own medicines. This is in sharp contrast to the stock system where the selection has to be made from the entire contents of a medicine trolley which may contain 40 or more different preparations (Fig. 3.7). Compared with a stock system the time taken to administer medicines is reduced by up to 50%, where a medicine round is still

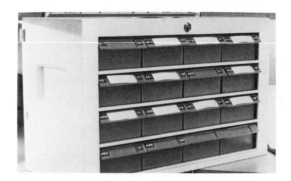

Fig. 3.6 Removable cassette

required. The same care and attention in selecting the medicine against the prescription prior to administration are required as with any other system, but in this case the selection is greatly facilitated. It also gives the opportunity to focus on individual patient's medicines as an entity, which is helpful in teaching sessions that may be undertaken at ward level outwith the medicine round. A further advantage of this system is that it can guide patients in the use of their medicines prior to discharge from hospital. Other aspects of the self-administration of medicines in hospitals are discussed in Chapter 10.

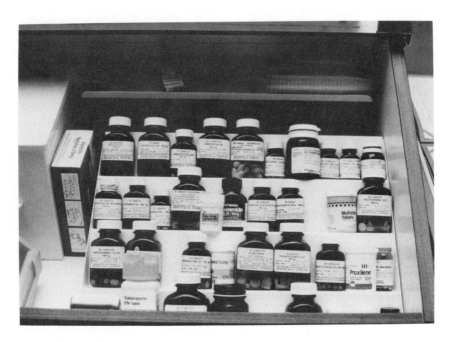

Fig. 3.7 Contents of medicine trolley

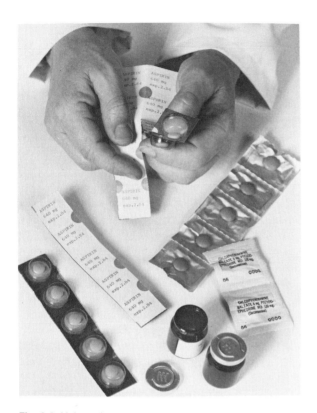

Fig. 3.8 Unit packs

Individual patient dispensing using unit dose presentation

Although widely adopted in American hospitals and some continental hospitals, unit dose systems have not been used on a large scale in the UK. In this system, medicines, both solid and liquid dose forms, are dispensed in unit packs designed to be opened just before administration (Fig. 3.8). As a result, the process of selection of a dose by the nurse prior to administration is greatly simplified. Detailed patient medication records are maintained in the pharmacy and are updated in line with changes in therapy. Using this information the pharmacist is responsible for ensuring that a sufficient number of doses of the correct medicines are available for the individual patient. The pharmacist is therefore playing a very central role in the selection of the particular medicine although the nurse must still undertake the final selection prior to administration. Many advantages are claimed

to derive from the introduction of this drug distribution system.

These include reduction of drug errors, reduction in time spent by nurses on non-clinical work, less wastage of medicines and better control generally, since ward stocks are eliminated. Peak demands on pharmacy can be smoothed out as the supply system is very much under the control of the pharmacist. The disadvantages are, however, quite significant. Unit dose packaging must be undertaken in the hospital pharmacy where the technical problems such as product stability in the packaging system chosen must first have been solved. Heavy demands are placed on staff time both in ward visits by pharmacists and in packaging work. Special medicine trolleys are required which are expensive. Further evaluation of this approach to the supply of medicines is called for.

Controlled dose system

This is a more sophisticated form of individual patient dispensing in which medicines (solid dose forms only) are supplied as courses in multi-blister packs. The advantages and disadvantages are similar to those described with the unit dose system.

Shotley Bridge system

This is a highly structured stock system within which the range and quantities of medicines held in stock are maintained at agreed levels using a system of colour coded cards to record stock levels and issues made by pharmacy. There is also an information card at ward level on each product stocked by the ward.

SUPPLY OF OTHER MEDICINES AND PHARMACEUTICALS TO WARDS

Significant quantities of medicines and related products which are not routinely prescribed are supplied for use in wards. These can be considered broadly under three headings: medicines for emergency resuscitation procedures; products used in nursing care; and disinfectants/antiseptics.

Resuscitation packs

These will normally be supplied by the phar-macy in accordance with the local policy drawn up by a multidisciplinary committee. The pack-aging and presentation of the drugs will normally be a matter for the pharmaceutical service. It is of course vital to ensure that the contents are suitably labelled and that adequate checks are made to ensure the contents are not allowed to pass the expiry date (see p. 31).

Nursing care products

In order to avoid multiplicity of products in use for nursing care procedures such as catheter care, skin care and eye bathing, it is desirable to establish a formulary of nursing care prod-ucts. (see p. 94) Such a formulary contains monographs on the products which are avail-able for use by nurses without medical prescription. The items contained in the formu-lary will normally be supplied on a routine 'top-up' basis.

Diagnostic agents

Clinical reagents are normally supplied on a routine stock basis. Other more specialised agents are supplied on request. A more detailed discussion of diagnostic agents is given in Chapter 4.

Disinfectants, antiseptics, lotions, etc.

It is now standard practice for wards (and departments) to use a range of products as agreed by the control of infection committee. The disinfection policy will normally contain information on the use of products together with supporting technical information. The necessary products are normally supplied on a routine indenting or topping-up basis. A discussion of the properties and uses of disin-fectants appears in Chapter 4.

SUPPLY OF MEDICINES AND PHARMACEUTICALS TO HOSPITAL DEPARTMENTS

The supply of medicines and related products to departments (e.g. to operating theatres) presents a different challenge to the hospital

pharmacist than that posed by ward supply systems. Often considerable bulk is involved, (e.g. antiseptics and disinfectants to operating theatres) and packaging and presentation often require special attention (irrigating solutions). It is important to achieve standardisation since duplication of products is costly and may be confusing to staff. With the advent of compu-terised drug management systems, it is now possible to use pre-printed drug indents for departments which can facilitate the introduc-tion and maintenance of a standard range of products. There is obviously not the same scope for clinical activities as with ward services but the pharmacist must ensure that medicines, etc., are properly stored in depart-ments. This is of particular relevance in the-atres. Visits to check on storage arrangements can also be used to advise on any current tech-nical problems that may present.

Special arrangements are often required in Accident and Emergency departments, such as the provision of 'patient-ready' packs of anal-gesics and antibiotics that can be issued to patients without the necessity of nurses having to undertake 'dispensing'. It is essential to maintain a written record of such issues, which must only be made against a prescription.

TECHNICAL SUPPORT SERVICES

The drug distribution arrangements previously described are usually supplemented by certain specialist technical support services. In essence these are dispensing services which require pharmaceutical expertise and special environ-mental conditions such as those provided in an aseptic dispensing suite. These central, pharmacy-based services, have been developed over the past few years in response to the growing complexity of drug therapy and the need to provide the highest possible standards of patient care.

Intravenous additive services (see also p. 64)

The addition of drugs to intravenous fluids is best performed in an aseptic dispensing suite rather than a ward utility room where adequate aseptic standards are difficult, if not impossible, to achieve. By providing these services centrally, the nurse is relieved of time-consuming manipulative tasks and is able to concentrate her efforts on the direct clinical care of her patients. On occasions it will be necessary to make an addition to an intravenous fluid at ward or departmental level but this should only be undertaken where there is no alternative.

Total parenteral nutrition services (see also p. 142)

The administration of nutrients, vitamins and minerals in combination in a single container presented ready for use represents a far safer method of administration than that obtained by using a series of separate bottles or by attempting to improvise the administration in some other way. By use of the 3 litre (or smaller volume) container prepared under strict aseptic conditions within the pharmacy, infection risks are reduced and accuracy of contents is assured. This is especially important when total parenteral nutrition is required to be administered to neonates.

Cytotoxic reconstitution services (see also p. 167)

The risks inherent in reconstituting cytotoxic drugs without due attention to the safety of the nurse undertaking this task are now fully appreciated. Full protection of operator and product can only be achieved within a specialised unit having all the necessary facilities such as vertical laminar air flow cabinets, air conditioning and facilities for staff to change into protective clothing. As with the other specialist services described above the donor of the medicine is provided with an accurately compounded, fully labelled, ready-to-use sterile product. In cytotoxic reconstitution services the potential hazards to ward staff of the compounding procedures are eliminated. Care will still be required with administering the dose to prevent further hazard.

Radiopharmaceuticals

Major hospital pharmaceutical departments provide a service supplying sterile radioisotope injections for use in specialised diagnostic procedures. The injections are formulated in order to accumulate in a particular organ or part of the body, e.g. phosphate injection becomes concentrated in bone, thiosulphate in the liver, albumin microspheres are temporarily trapped in the lung capillaries. These chemicals are labelled with a short acting radionuclide such as Technetium-99m (half-life 8 hours) which rapidly decays. A camera which is sensitive to the radioactive particles, which are emitted by the technetium, scans the organ or part of the body. This illustrates different concentrations within a particular organ and in this way abnormalities can be located.

Drug information services

The provision of information on many aspects of the use of medicines and properties of drugs is an integral part of pharmaceutical services in hospitals and in the community. The organisation of this service and method of provision will vary considerably, depending on circumstances. In larger acute hospitals, a department under the control of a fulltime specialist pharmacist, will provide the service on a district, area or regional basis. Outwith such centres, in the community and smaller hospitals the pharmacist providing general services will also be the source of drug information. All pharmacists, hospital or community, have access to the specialist hospital-based services to supplement their own local resources. Drug information pharmacists work closely with their clinical colleagues when the nature of the query requires particular clinical expertise. Pharmaceutical manufacturers are also an important source of product information, and professional bodies such as the Pharmaceutical Society of Great Britain provide invaluable support to practising pharmacists in all branches of the profession.

All specialist drug information services are available to health professionals but are not normally available directly to members of the public. With the rapid development of information technology it seems certain that detailed drug information will become much more widely accessible to health professionals in hospital and community practice. Queries received by drug information pharmacists cover a wide range of topics, including dose, route of administration, adverse effects, inter-actions, contraindications and increasingly, costs. Information on drugs is provided on request and also in regular bulletins on specific aspects of therapy, e.g. a review of a particular group of drugs.

The drug information provided by pharma-cists is of course of benefit to patients since it helps to ensure optimal drug therapy. An important part of the practising pharmacist's work is to provide patients with the necessary information to enable the patient to use the medicine(s) in the most effective way. This aspect is discussed in more detail in Chapter 10.

SUPPLY OF MEDICINES IN THE COMMUNITY

The community pharmacist and, in some rural areas, the dispensing doctor are responsible for the supply of medicines to patients in the community. In addition, the community phar-macist is responsible for the provision of a wide range of health care products, surgical appliances, dressings, etc.

Medicines are supplied on prescription and increasingly where legislation permits, are also sold over the counter. In many instances, an individual will seek the pharmacist's advice and guidance on a particular health problem. This may result in a medicine being recommended and sold to the client, or the pharmacist may suggest self-referral to the general practitioner. Surveys have shown that there is considerable use of proprietary medicines by the public and this should always be borne in mind by health care staff in both community and hospital prac-tice. Members of the public often regard purchased medicines as being little more than normal household commodities. As a result, important information on the patient's drug history may be unknown. The community phar-macist, like his hospital colleague, will also provide information on the use of medicines to community health care staff and give invalu-able support and guidance to his clients, especially older people.

For many years the community pharmacist has played a vital part in health care provision. It appears that there is still great potential to extend further the contribution the community pharmacist can make not only in the treatment of illness but in prevention of ill health. With the growing emphasis on self-care and the limitation of prescribing certain products within the NHS it seems likely that many more people will seek the professional advice of the phar-macist for the treatment of minor ailments. This trend has the support of many bodies, indeed government policy is such that it advo-cates the full ultilisation of the pharmacist's professional skills.

More use of computer technology will enable the pharmacist to exercise a monitoring role, maintaining patient drug records, including information on allergies to specific drugs. The provision of information on the use of medi-cines is of growing concern and importance. Again the pharmacist is well placed to provide the necessary information in the most suitable form for patients and their carers. Participation in health education campaigns is clearly a widely accepted part of the community phar-macist's role. There is great potential for an ex-pansion of this increasingly important aspect as the significance of prevention becomes more widely recognised.

4 MANAGEMENT OF DRUGS FOR USE IN AN EMERGENCY; DIAGNOSTIC AGENTS; DISINFECTANTS; VACCINES

MANAGEMENT OF DRUGS FOR USE IN AN EMERGENCY

It is current practice for wards, clinics and operating theatres to have immediately to hand, equipment and drugs needed in the event of cardiac arrest or other medical emergency. Health authorities normally have a policy, which is regularly reviewed, stating the range of equipment and drugs, and where these are sited. Clearly labelled drugs for emergency use are supplied in restricted quantities, since they must be kept unlocked on a tray or trolley for ease of access. While drugs should be retained in their original package complete with batch number and expiry date, there is a real need to be able to identify the drugs easily, perhaps with an additional label, and gain rapid access to them when the emergency arises. An alternative presentation is the IMS Min-i-jet System (Fig. 4.1).

The best possible compromise has to be worked out by staff with regard to what is ultimately in the best interests of the patient.

It is the overall responsibility of charge nurses to ensure that the items required are always readily available and suitable. Checks on equipment and drugs are made according to local policy. In locations where emergencies arise frequently and the range of equipment and drugs is more complex, this may be made once a day, but in others, a weekly check is sufficient. The responsibilities of the nurse with respect to emergency drugs are as follows:

- to carry out checks at regular intervals to ensure that no drug is missing and that

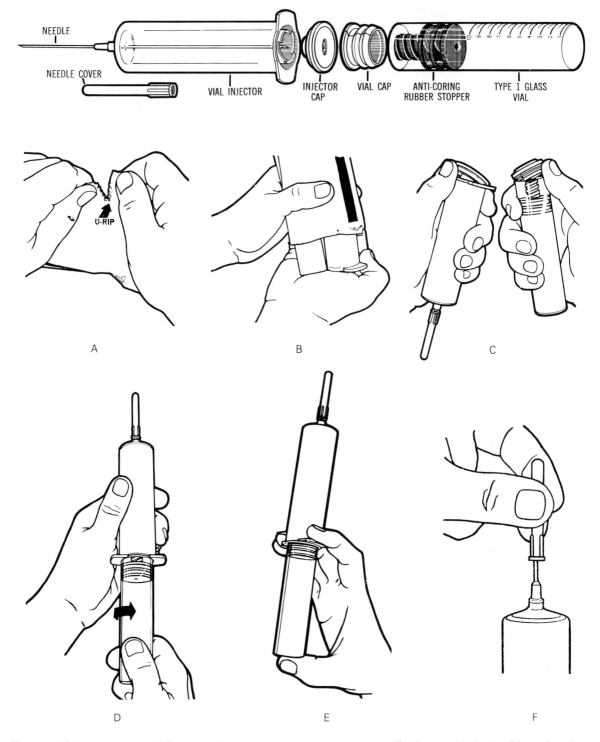

Fig. 4.1 IMS Min-i-jet system (A) Package is torn open at notch indicated by arrow (B) Vial and vial injector slide out into the hand (C) Protective injector and vial caps flip off (D) Vial is screwed into injector — the needle has now penetrated the vial stopper and is in contact with the medication (E) Air is expelled; needle guard is kept in place until ready for injection (F) Needle guard is twisted off to expose sterile needle. After injection, entire unit is discarded.

each drug is in date. It is helpful if the pharmacy department label the drug pack indicating the date of expiry.

- to replenish emergency drug stocks before the expiry date is reached and after each emergency. (Drugs which are no longer suitable should only be returned to pharmacy on receipt of new supplies.)
- to be able to identify each drug and to have some understanding of its use.
- to assist in checking the name, strength and dose of drugs to be given and drawing them up in an emergency.
- to prepare an intravenous infusion ready for use.
- to ensure that clear lines of communication are maintained during an emergency so that there is no misunderstanding of which drug is being given.
- to keep a record of the name and dose of each drug given during an emergency and its time of administration.

Synchronised cardiopulmonary resuscitation on its own is not sufficient. Drugs are required to correct acid–base and electrolyte balance, to improve the function of the heart and to deal with complications such as arrhythmias, hypotension and pulmonary and cerebral oedema. A variety of drugs should be available and these may be classified into those which may be required immediately and those which will be required subsequently. The same drugs are used for children as for adults, although obviously smaller doses will be required. The drugs for immediate use are described here.

Sodium bicarbonate
Administered by intravenous infusion to correct metabolic acidosis which develops as a result of impaired tissue perfusion and inefficient ventilation. Calculated according to body weight and the duration of the cardiac arrest.

Adrenaline
Adrenaline is a cardiac stimulant with a transient action. It produces an increase in myocardial contractility and an elevated perfusion pressure. Defibrillation thresholds are also reduced.

Calcium gluconate
Given to initiate cardiac rhythm in asystole if there is no response to other measures. Calcium ions have a directly stimulating effect on the heart muscle. Converts asystole to ventricular fibrillation to aid defibrillation.

Atropine sulphate
Speeds up the rate of the heart by blocking the vagal stimulus and also stimulates respiration.

Aminophylline
Acts as a myocardial stimulant and reduces venous pressure in congestive heart failure leading to a marked increase in cardiac output. Aminophylline is useful in those patients who are also suffering from asthma and bronchitis because it has a dual action in relieving airways obstruction as well as increasing myocardial contractility. Given too rapidly it can induce convulsions and arrhythmias.

Lignocaine
Suppresses ventricular extrasystoles and ventricular tachycardia following an acute myocardial infarction.

Frusemide
A very powerful loop diuretic with a rapid effect used to relieve pulmonary oedema due to left ventricular failure.

Hydrocortisone sodium phosphate
A glucocorticoid given in large doses to restore the blood pressure in states of profound shock.

Antidotes to certain poisons
In addition to the drugs for immediate use described above, it will be necessary for accident and emergency departments to maintain stocks of specific antidotes. The principles of management of these agents are the same as those applicable to other emergency drugs. It is of course vital to ensure that adequate stock levels are maintained.

Table 4.1 Antidotes to certain poisons

Poison	Antidote(s)	Route of administration
Arsenic, gold, mercury and certain other metals	Dimercaprol	Intramuscular injection
Copper and lead	Penicillamine	Oral
Cyanides	Dicobalt edetate or sodium nitrite followed by sodium thiosulphate	Intravenous injection
Heavy metals (especially lead)	Sodium calcium edetate	Intravenous infusion

DIAGNOSTIC AGENTS

The diagnostic agents used in clinical practice can be broadly classified into three main groups (excluding radiopaque contrast media and radiopharmaceuticals):

1. chemical tests carried out at ward level using clinical reagents
2. chemical substances administered orally or parenterally as part of a biochemical investigation
3. locally applied diagnostic agents.

Clinical reagents

Over the past few years the use of clinical reagents at ward level has become much more efficient and reliable. The availability of ready-to-use test strips has greatly simplified procedures, to a large extent making the use of droppers, spirit lamps and the like unnecessary.

Storage and use

Safe storage of all clinical reagents in a separate locked cupboard is required. It is important to use reagents in accordance with the manufacturer's explicit instructions. Several general points must be remembered. Before using a reagent the expiry date should be checked. To keep the reagents dry and thus effective, the desiccant pack provided should remain in the container and the cap replaced securely immediately after use. If the container

is damp or the contents have altered in appearance they should not be used.

Colour charts used for comparing the colour of chemical reactions should be renewed regularly otherwise they can quickly become faded and dirty. Because of its marked sensitivity, the impregnated end of a reagent strip should not be touched. When reading a multiple reagent strip, care should be taken to hold it horizontally so that urine does not run down the test portions and mix together the chemicals and colours which may affect the result. Care should also be taken to avoid letting the strip rest on the colour blocks on the container leading to alteration of the colours. Reagent tablets should be directly transferred into the cap of the bottle immediately before use and not handled so as to avoid interference with results. Droppers and test tubes should always be rinsed immediately after being used and stored clean and dry ready for re-use.

Specimens should be tested as soon as possible after being voided and certainly before they are 4 hours old. Prolonged exposure to room temperature and light can affect pH and the presence of glucose, bilirubin and urobilinogen and it can also cause false positive results of protein estimation and of blood.

Reagent strips, namely Dextrostix, are now specially designed for use with a glucometer in monitoring blood glucose. This electronic device measures the precise blood glucose concentration and displays the result in large digits in a matter of minutes. Since conventional capillary blood glucose testing involves the reading of reagent strips against a colour chart and colour vision is not infrequently impaired in diabetics, the glucometer is a considerable advantage for self-monitoring where it can be used.

Careful records of results should be kept by nurses and patients as appropriate on completion of any test. Patients who are expected to carry out such tests at home should have the technique and precautions explained to them with the added warning to keep reagents out of the reach of children.

Table 4.2 indicates some of the tests in widespread use.

Table 4.2 Chemical tests in frequent use

Reagent	Test
Multistix	pH, protein, glucose, ketones, bilirubin, blood, urobilinogen
Ketostix	ketones in urine
Acetest	ketones in urine
Clinistix	glucose in urine
Clinitest	reducing substances, e.g. glucose in urine
Diabur 5000 MCP	glucose in urine
*BM-Test Glycemie 1–44	glucose in blood
Dextrostix	glucose in blood
Visidex	glucose in blood
Hema-Chek	occult blood in faeces
*Esbach's solution	albumin in urine

*Procedural details of these tests are given below.

Drugs which interfere in the diagnostic tests
Certain drugs are known to interfere with some diagnostic test results. The effect may be to render the test result falsely negative or positive which could have serious implications for patients.

Ascorbic acid for example, interferes with the tests for glucose in urine and blood. The nature of the interference depends on the type of glucose test being carried out. If a diabetic patient is receiving therapy with ascorbic acid and a blood glucose test is carried out, the result will indicate a blood glucose level *less* than the true value. Conversely, if a urine test is being carried out, the outcome will be a result indicating a *higher* level of glucose than the true value.

Various factors will influence the nature of any interference by a drug or drugs with diagnostic tests, notably the dose of drug the patient is receiving and the type of test being carried out. In general, the doctor initiating the test should be aware of the possibility of the patient's drug therapy interfering with a diagnostic test. Nevertheless the nurse who is alert to the possibilities of problems arising in this way can make a worthwhile contribution in minimising any possible hazard to the patient. It is also important to ensure that the chemical pathology department undertaking the diagnostic tests are made aware of any drug therapy the patient may be taking. Some other drugs that may cause problems are given below:

Cephalosporins increase the test result for glucose in urine
Methyl dopa interferes with the analytical (laboratory) method used to determine glucose in urine.

It should also be noted that drug side-effects can influence the outcome of laboratory tests. *Thiazide diuretics* for example cause blood glucose levels to increase which would be reflected in the test results.

Blood glucose testing
Whenever possible, self-monitoring of blood glucose in diabetics is to be encouraged. The number of tests to be carried out will depend on the clinical condition of the patient.

Requirements
BM-Test 1–44 strips in container with colour scale
Lancets
Autolet if available
Cotton wool
Watch with second hand.

Procedure
1. Wash hands.
2. Explain procedure to patient.
3. Check BM stix fit for use.
4. Wash patient's hand with soap and water, and dry thoroughly.
5. Place test strip on clean surface.
6. Prick side of patient's finger tip with lancet.

7. Gently squeeze patient's finger tip to obtain large suspended drop of blood.
8. Apply drop of blood to cover test area of strip.
9. Start timing using second hand of watch.
10. After exactly 1 minute, wipe off blood carefully and firmly with a clean piece of cotton wool.
11. Gently wipe twice more using clean part of cotton wool.
12. Time for 1 more minute, then compare colours of the 2 test zones with colour scale on container.
13. If after 2 minutes the blood glucose value exceeds 13 mmol wait a further 1 minute then compare again.
14. Safely dispose of lancet, test strip and wool.
15. Wash hands.
16. Record results.

(The comparison colours on the container label are specific to each pack of strips and so it is important to compare the reaction colour with the colour scale on the container of test strips used.)

Esbach's test

For this test an Esbach's albuminometer is used which is a graduated glass tube marked with the letters 'U' and 'R'.

Procedure
1. Pour urine into tube to level marked 'U'. Urine should be acid in reaction (acidify with acetic acid if necessary) and filtered if cloudy. If specific gravity is greater than 1010, the urine should be diluted with an equal volume of water and the final result doubled.
2. Add Esbach's reagent to level marked 'R'.
3. Seal albuminometer with rubber stopper, invert several times to mix well and then place in its stand.
4. Label albuminometer with name of patient, ward, date and time of setting up test.
5. Leave undisturbed for 24 hours.
6. At the end of 24 hours, read level of white precipitate showing amount of albumin in grams per litre of urine.

7. Divide result by 10 to give percentage amount. (If more than 0.4% albumin is present, to obtain a more accurate estimate mix the urine thoroughly and dilute a fresh sample of urine with an equal volume of water then repeat test. Double result.)
8. Wash tube in warm soapy water, rinse and dry.

SYSTEMICALLY ADMINISTERED DIAGNOSTIC AGENTS

The same procedures that are applicable to the administration of medicines apply to the administration of a diagnostic agent. It is normal to prescribe the agent on the in-patient prescription form in the 'once only' section and record the administration accordingly. In many instances very precise instructions regarding the administration must be followed (e.g. timing may be especially important). Some of the following diagnostic agents are also used in the treatment of various diseases.

Orally administered diagnostic agents

Glucose
The oral glucose tolerance test (GTT) is used in the diagnosis of diabetes mellitus. Glucose levels are measured in venous plasma when the patient is fasting and then 2 hours after the oral administration of 75 g of glucose completely dissolved in 250–350 ml of water. A third measurement is made on plasma obtained at an intermediate time. Some physicians request urine samples to be tested for sugar and ketones at 1 hour and 2 hours following administration of glucose. Figure 4.2 shows how the diagnosis of diabetes mellitus is made or excluded.

Metyrapone
This compound is given orally as a diagnostic test of anterior pituitary function. Metyrapone has an inhibiting effect on cortisol production. This results in a fall in plasma concentration of glucocorticoids which stimulates the anterior pituitary to produce more corticotrophin.

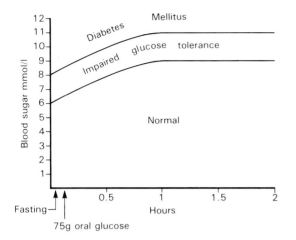

Fig. 4.2 Blood glucose curves following 75 g glucose orally

Precursors of corticotrophin are excreted in the urine where they can be measured. A low level of precursors in the urine would indicate anterior pituitary malfunction if it has been established that adrenal function is adequate.

D-xylose

The xylose absorption test is used in the evaluation of intestinal malabsorption. About 8 hours following an overnight fast, the patient empties his bladder and the urine is discarded. Then 25 g of D-xylose completely dissolved in 250 ml water is given orally followed by a further 250 ml of water. For the next 5 hours the patient continues to fast and *all* urine passed is collected. Since very little xylose is metabolised in the body, a healthy person would excrete 5–8 g in the urine over a 5 hour period under these conditions.

Parenterally administered diagnostic agents

Desmopressin

This long-acting analogue (i.e. a substance with the same actions as the naturally occurring compound with a similar but not identical chemical structure) of vasopressin (antidiuretic hormone) is used in the diagnosis of diabetes insipidus. It is administered by injection for diagnostic purposes and intranasally once treatment is begun. Very careful measuring and recording of urine output are essential.

Edrophonium chloride

This compound antagonises cholinesterase (see p. 79) with the result that naturally occurring acetylcholine is potentiated and muscle power is increased. Intravenous (or intramuscular) injection of this drug is used as a test for myasthenia gravis.

Fluorescein sodium

Administration of fluorescein sodium by intravenous injection is used in the determination of circulation time and the differentiation of healthy and malignant tissue.

Pentagastrin

This analogue of the hormone gastrin has all the physiological effects of the natural hormone. It is used for testing gastric acid secretion. Following overnight fast, a nasogastric tube is passed and its position in the stomach confirmed by X-ray. The gastric contents are aspirated, measured and then discarded. The tube is then connected to a suction pump at 3–5 mm pressure and the secretions aspirated continuously for one hour. This 'basal acid output' is collected and labelled. A subcutaneous injection of 6 μg pentagastrin per kg body weight is administered. Suction is restarted via the pump and the aspirate over the next hour, the 'maximum acid output' is collected and labelled. The specimens are sent for chemical determination of hydrochloric acid levels.

Phentolamine

This is occasionally used as a diagnostic test for phaeochromocytoma (adrenaline-producing tumour). An intravenous injection of phentolamine is followed by a fall in blood pressure, if raised due to excess circulating adrenaline.

Protirelin

Protirelin, thyrotrophic-releasing hormone (TRH) is used as a diagnostic test for hyperthyroidism. An intravenous injection of 200 μg results in a prompt rise in serum levels of thyroid-stimulating hormone (TSH) in normal subjects. Blood samples are taken at suitable intervals and TSH levels measured. Oral administration of protirelin (40 mg), after overnight fasting, is given so that a qualitative assessment of thyroid function can be made.

Skin testing solutions
A wide variety of skin testing solutions (over 200) are available for the diagnosis of allergy. The allergens are often injected intradermally or used with a prick testing method.

Tetracosactrin
This synthetic polypeptide has an adrenocorticotrophin (ACTH)-like action of short duration. It is used as a diagnostic test in the investigation of adrenocortical insufficiency. A blood sample is obtained 30 minutes after an intramuscular injection of 250 micrograms tetracosactrin and plasma hydroxycorticoids measured. This level is compared with the level prior to the administration of tetracosactrin. In normal subjects an increase in the plasma level of hydroxycorticoids is found following the administration of tetracosactrin.

Tuberculin PPD
This is used intradermally for the detection of tuberculin sensitivity in screening for tuberculosis.

Methylene blue
A sterile solution of methylene blue, a dye, is used in a variety of diagnostic procedures including the identification of the parathyroid glands during surgery.

Locally applied diagnostic agents

Fluorescein sodium
A brief description of the use of fluorescein in ophthalmology is given on page 125.

DISINFECTANTS

No group of pharmaceutical products is more widely used than disinfectants. Not only are they used by nursing staff in many aspects of nursing care, be it hospital or community, but also as an integral part of domestic assistants' armoury in wards, theatres and corridors of hospitals. There is a great diversity of products available and this, allied to the marketing pressures brought to bear by the makers of these products, may lead to inappropriate use and wastage of resource. In order to use the correct products in appropriate circumstances, at the correct strength and in the correct manner, it is essential that every hospital has a written sterilisation and disinfection policy. The contents of such a policy consist of clear, concise statements regarding:

1. equipment and areas for which sterilisation is appropriate
2. the purposes for which disinfectants are to be used, and details of the correct disinfectants for particular circumstances
3. where it is appropriate to use disposable equipment.

Sterilisation can be defined as the death of all forms of microbial life on the article to be sterilised. *Disinfection* is the preferential killing of disease-producing microbes in the nonsporing or vegetative state.

Sterilisation

Whenever possible, all equipment or material liable to contamination from patients' exudates, of whatever nature, should be sterilised, not disinfected. The methods of sterilisation utilise dry or moist heat (either in a hot air oven or autoclave respectively), radiation or gassing. Wrapped instruments and operation packs are sterilised by steam sterilisation in a high vacuum autoclave, maintaining the contents for 3 minutes at 134 °C. Oil impregnated gauzes, for which steam sterilisation cannot be used, must be sterilised in a hot air oven at 170 °C for at least 1 hour.

If articles to be sterilised are affected in some way by high temperatures and radiation sterilisation is unavailable or inappropriate, the alternative method is low-temperature steam (70°–75 °C) mixed with formaldehyde gas. If this is not suitable because of the gaseous environment, then the next most suitable treatment may have to be pasteurisation (immersion of dismantled instruments in a thermostatically controlled bath of distilled water for 10 minutes at 75 °C). This is a type of disinfection, not sterilisation, and is permissable only in clearly defined circumstances.

Certain types of cystoscopes can be treated in this way.

Only when none of the above mentioned processes is possible is it legitimate practice to attempt cold disinfection by liquid chemicals.

Disinfection

Disinfection should never be regarded as a substitute for good domestic cleaning which should always precede any attempt to disinfect. Disinfection demands a rational choice of treatment. The correct disinfectant must be chosen for the particular microbial problem and for the type of surface to be treated, whether animate or inanimate.

Properties desirable in disinfectants
1. effective against a wide spectrum of micro-organisms
2. readily soluble in, or miscible with, water at the effective concentration
3. effective in the presence of organic matter such as blood, pus, sputum and faecal material
4. chemically stable and non- corrosive
5. economical in use
6. non-irritant.

No single disinfectant is suitable for all situations. However, in formulating a disinfection policy, it is desirable to carefully select a core of cost-effective preparations. These will be available from the pharmacy, some ready to use and others in a concentrated form which require to be diluted with water. In hospital it is desirable that all disinfectant solutions are supplied by the pharmacy in a form ready for use. Dilution of concentrated disinfectants at ward level may result in solutions that are too weak and therefore ineffective, or solutions may be stronger than required with resulting waste of resources.

Examples of disinfectants

Phenolics. These disinfectants in low concentration disrupt the cytoplasmic membrane causing leakage of bacterial cellular constituents and also affect membrane permeability. Not only are phenolics good bactericides, but they also have the desirable property of stability, remaining active after mild heating and prolonged drying. As a result, subsequent application of moisture to a dry surface previously treated with a phenolic can redissolve the chemical so that it again becomes effective. In addition, concentrations of the order of 2–3% maintain a high bactericidal potency in the presence of soiled fabrics, blood, faeces, urine and other organic matter. A commercial preparation of dimethyl phenols is available formulated in an alcoholic/anionic detergent base and this detergent system effectively helps the bactericide to reach embedded organisms. Under normal conditions of use phenolic preparations are non-injurious to wool, cotton, nylon, terylene, rubber and many common plastics. Wiping metal surfaces is unlikely to cause damage, but the addition to the solution of a corrosion inhibitor, such as sodium nitrite, is recommended where there is prolonged contact with metals.

Unpleasant odour and tissue irritation preclude their useful application on the skin and on objects which come in intimate contact with mucous membranes e.g. anaesthesia equipment. However, the phenolics, in a dilution of 2–3%, are very effective for a wide range of inanimate objects and surfaces, e.g.

1. bedpan shells between patients
2. incubators (which must then be thoroughly dried)
3. theatre floors between cases
4. theatres or wards where areas are splashed with patients' exudates
5. wet string mops (as an alternative when daily laundering cannot be carried out).

Alcohols have the ability to denature bacterial proteins. This is more marked in the presence of water and concentrations of 70% alcohol in water are effective. Both ethyl alcohol and isopropyl alcohol are used as skin disinfectants and also for the disinfection of ampoule necks, vials and rubber closures on infusion fluid bottles. They are also commonly used in combination with other disinfectants such as iodine or chlorhexidine. In this way a synergistic or additive effect is produced.

Iodine has a marked oxidising effect on the amino acid components of respiratory enzymes found in the membranes of micro-organisms. It is a good bactericide and fungicide but stains fabric and tissue. Iodine (2.5%) in 70% ethyl alcohol is the first choice for rapid skin disinfection as ordinarily required in preparation for incision or needle puncture. This is the only liquid skin disinfectant which will both dry off completely and disinfect the skin surface within 15–20 seconds. Oral or rectal thermometers common to all ward patients should be cleaned, then immersed for 10 minutes in 2.5% iodine in 70% alcohol.

To disinfect the mucous membrane in the mouth, the surface is firstly dried then 2.5% iodine in 70% alcohol is immediately applied. A 10% aqueous solution of povidone-iodine followed by sterile water is used to douche and clean fresh wounds where there is much tissue damage, ingrained soil and dirt. This product is also effective in reducing heavy contamination on abnormal skin (e.g. pre-operative preparation prior to amputation involving diabetic gangrene of the foot). This is a special problem requiring prophylaxis against post-operative gas gangrene or tetanus. A compress soaked in alcoholic solution of povidone iodine 10% is applied for at least 30 minutes prior to operation. This will greatly reduce the number of spores commonly present in such tissue.

Chlorine compounds. Hypochlorites are the most useful chlorine-containing components for practical disinfection in hospital. Their bactericidal power is dependent upon the release of free hypochlorous acid. All hypochlorite solutions deteriorate with time, consequently each container will be labelled with an expiry date. Their bactericidal efficiency is reduced in the presence of organic matter. Non-abrasive hypochlorite powder can be used for cleaning bath and wash basin fixtures. Floors and walls of theatres or wards, which have become contaminated with blood or exudate from identified carriers of hepatitis virus, should be cleaned with specific antiviral disinfectant such as a detergent solution of sodium hypochlorite 7%. Care must be exercised when using this solution since at this concentration it is corrosive and has a bleaching action.

Glutaraldehyde. Aldehydes act by combining with the amino groups of proteins in the bacterial cell. Glutaraldehyde is an effective disinfectant frequently used to disinfect lensed instruments, many of which cannot be autoclaved. 10 minutes in glutaraldehyde 2% is required to kill vegetative pathogens, excluding *M. tuberculosis*, which requires 1 hour; 3 hours is required to kill all resistant spores.

Acridine dyes. Basic dyes inactivate bacteria by reacting with acid groups in the cell. Acridines impair the function of cellular deoxyribonucleic acid (DNA) thus interfering with the reproduction of bacteria. Since the acridine dyes remain active for many hours in the presence of pus and blood they are used to disinfect abscess cavities, infected sinuses, etc. The abscess cavity or sinus is packed with gauze soaked in Emulsion of Proflavine BPC.

Surface active agents These are strongly absorbed onto the negatively charged bacterial surface. This is followed by damage to the cell membrane and cytoplasmic leakage. The cationic surface active agent cetrimide is still widely used, mainly in combination with chlorhexidine.

Chlorhexidine has a wide spectrum of antibacterial activity. Activity is reduced in the presence of serum, blood, pus and other organic matter. Chlorhexidine 4% in detergent is used as a surgical scrub and 0.5% chlorhexidine in 70% ethyl alcohol disinfects lensed instruments in 3 minutes. Care must be taken as longer exposure may damage some lenses. A preparation containing chlorhexidine gluconate 1.5% and cetrimide 15% is available as a liquid concentrate (Savlon Hospital Concentrate). A 3.5% dilution of this in 70% ethyl alcohol is used for rapid skin disinfection, or to disinfect trolley tops between dressings. Aqueous dilutions (1%) can be used as a vaginal douche or to clean fresh wounds with minimal contamination. A sterile, single-use plastic sachet of this dilution is now widely used when volumes up to 100 ml are required. Storage of such packs in a warming cabinet should not exceed one week since loss of water can occur through the plastic.

The concentrate containing chlorhexidine gluconate 1.5% and cetrimide 15% is also available in 25 ml bath sachets. In bathing, disinfectants are not required routinely. Furthermore it is an expensive and paticularly pointless gesture to add a sachet or two of this concentrate to a bathful of water — the dilution factor is so great that the disinfectant action is nil. It is literally money down the drain.

Some factors affecting disinfectant action

Time of contact. In order to be effective, disinfectants must be in contact with the organisms for a certain minimum time called the time of contact. Iodine 2.5% in 70% ethyl alcohol has a contact time of 15–20 seconds for skin disinfection. Glutaraldehyde 2% has a contact time of 10 minutes to 3 hours.

The number of surviving organisms decreases with time as illustrated in Figure 4.3. Curve A is the ideal relationship. Curve B is the most usual. There are three stages:

1. Initial slow stage during which sensitive micro-organisms within a population die
2. Response due to the death of micro-organisms of average sensitivity within the population.
3. Slow death stage due to resistant micro-organisms.

Concentration of disinfectants. For a given disinfectant at a particular temperature there is an exponential relationship between concentration and the time taken to kill the micro-

organisms, i.e. doubling the concentration more than doubles the efficiency.

Temperature. There is a direct relationship between efficiency of a disinfectant and temperature — if temperature is increased then efficiency is increased.

VACCINES

Immunity is defined as resistance to attack by micro-organisms and depends on the presence of modified globulins, known as antibodies, in the serum of the immune individual. The immunity provided by these antibodies may be acquired naturally as a consequence of infection, or artificially as the result of vaccination. The invasion of microbes into host tissue stimulates the production of antibodies that counteract the infection. This subsequently provides immunity to further infection by the same species of micro-organism and is known as *active immunity*. These antibodies are transferred across the placenta during pregnancy ensuring that the newborn infant is immune to those infections to which the mother is immune. Since there is no production of antibody by the infant, this form of immunity is termed *passive immunity* and gives protection for a number of months, as long as the antibodies are present.

Immunity can be conferred on an individual by the use of vaccines. The vaccine stimulates the production of antibody in a similar manner as a natural infection. Vaccines are designed to produce specific protection against a particular disease. They may consist of:

1. An attenuated form of an infective agent. For example the vaccines used against virus diseases such as poliomyelitis and measles. Attenuated vaccines contain living micro-organisms which have been manipulated in such a way as to greatly reduce the virulence.
2. Inactivated preparations of the virus or bacteria, e.g. influenza, pertussis or typhoid vaccines. Influenza virus for vaccine manufacture is prepared in embryonated hens' eggs. The resultant

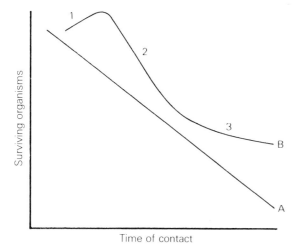

Fig. 4.3 Relationship between time of contact of a disinfectant and the rate of kill of micro-organisms

material is purified, killed with formaldehyde and concentrated.

3. Extracts of, or exotoxins produced by, a
micro-organism e.g. tetanus vaccine. This
is prepared by growing the bacteria in a
suitable liquid medium. After incubating
for 7–10 days the organisms are filtered
off. The filtrate containing the toxin is
purified and treated chemically to produce
the vaccine.

Vaccines are given by injection with the
exception of live attenuated poliomyelitis
vaccines given orally. Immunisation, using
vaccines consisting of living agents, is generally achieved with a single dose, but 3 doses
are required with oral poliomyelitis vaccine.
Live virus multiplies in the body and produces
immunity which may not last quite so long as
that of the natural infection. Inactivated
vaccines may require 'booster' doses at an
appropriate interval after the primary, in order to
raise the antibody titre to an adequate level.

Side-effects
Some vaccines such as poliomyelitis vaccine
produce virtually no reactions, while others
such as typhoid vaccine may produce swelling,
pain and tenderness about 2–3 hours after
subcutaneous or intramuscular injection.
Systemic reactions such as fever, malaise and
headache may also occur and usually last for
about 48 hours after injection. Anaphylactic
shock is discussed on page 88.

Contra-indications
In general vaccines should not be given to
individuals if they have a febrile illness or if any
active infection is present or suspected. Live
virus vaccines, especially rubella vaccine,
should not normally be offered to pregnant
women because of possible harm to the fetus.

They should not be given to patients whose
immune system is compromised either naturally,
or as a result of radiotherapy or treatment with
immunosuppressive drugs.

Storage
All vaccines must be stored in a refrigerator
according to the directions given on the packaging or the package insert, otherwise the
preparations may become denatured and
totally ineffective. Ampoules and vials of
vaccine should be shaken before use to ensure
uniformity of the contents. Where large
numbers of people are to be vaccinated, it will
be more cost effective to use a multi-dose vial.
Where a portion remains in the vial after a
vaccination session has ended it should be
discarded. Once opened, the contents of
multidose vials with no preservative should be
used within an hour, or within 3 hours where
a preservative is present, otherwise the
remainder should be discarded. Single dose
polio vaccine is now routinely available and this
should be utilised where individuals or small
numbers (up to 7 or 8) have to be vaccinated.

Immunoglobulins
The injection of immunoglobulins produces
immediate protection. There are essentially
two types of human immunoglobulin preparation. Human normal immunoglobulin is
prepared from plasma of at least 1000 donors.
Specific immunoglobulins e.g. for tetanus or
rabies are prepared by pooling the blood of
convalescent patients or of immunised donors
who have been recently boosted. Normal
immunoglobulin injection is used for protection
of susceptible contacts against hepatitis A
virus, measles and, to a lesser extent, rubella
and poliomyelitis.

5 GUIDE TO CONTROL OF MEDICINES IN HOSPITALS AND THE COMMUNITY

The supply, storage and use of medicinal products are controlled by the following Acts:

Medicines Act 1968 (Part III)
Misuse of Drugs Act 1971

Previous legislation having been repealed, the position today reflects the sophistication of modern therapy, e.g. the term 'scheduled poison' no longer has any relevance in hospital practice.

Classes of Medicinal Products
There are three classes of products under the Medicines Act 1968:

1. General Sale List Medicines (GSL) — Medicines which can be bought in a general store
2. Pharmacy Medicines (P) — Medicines which may be sold only under the supervision of a pharmacist.
3. Prescription only medicines (POMs) — Medicines that can be sold or supplied on prescription only.

Controlled Drugs are discussed on pages 42–49.

Certain legal requirements apply to the sale, supply, dispensing and labelling of each class of medicinal products. These requirements are primarily applicable in the community, e.g. sale/supply of medicines by community pharmacists and others. The above terms do .not have great practical relevance in hospitals but are useful reference points when discussing the control of medicines.

Detailed Aspects of Controls

Administration of POMs

The Medicines Act provides that* 'no one may administer a POM otherwise than to himself, unless he is a practitioner or is acting in accordance with the directions of a practitioner.'

This aspect is normally covered by a health authority policy statement which permits medicine administration *only* in accordance with the written prescription of a medical or dental practitioner. In hospital practice all drugs are treated in the same way, no distinction being made between the different classes of drugs listed above.

Prescribing of POMs

In hospital practice the in-patient prescription also includes directions to the nurse for administration of the medicine. If a prescription is written for an outpatient more details of the patient are required than would be the case for an inpatient.

Emergency supply of POMs

A community pharmacist, can, under certain carefully laid down conditions, supply POMs in an emergency without a prescription, on the request of a doctor or an individual patient.

Labelling of medicines and medicinal products

Standard labelling particulars are described in the Act. This is largely a matter for the pharmacist, but is very important to the nurse also. The main particulars are listed below:

- The name of the product — this may be an approved name or a proprietary name
- The pharmaceutical form, e.g. tablets, capsules, etc.
- The strength of the product, distinguishing between active and non-active ingredients
- The quantity in the container expressed in appropriate terms e.g. in the case of tablets the number of dosage units and in the case of an ointment the weight contained in the pack

*Certain exemptions to this rule are made in the case of life-saving drugs, e.g. adrenaline, certain antihistamines, antidotes etc. Normally this exemption would not apply in hospitals.

- Any special storage and handling instructions
- A date after which the product should not be used (expiry date)
- Name and address of supplier and product licence number.

Special labelling requirements apply to *dispensed* medicines. It is common in hospital practice for the pharmacist to add other information to labels in response to local need.

Storage of medicinal products (see also Controlled Drugs below)

Although different classes of drugs are recognised under the Medicines Act, in hospital practice *all* medicinal products are treated in the same basic way, i.e. secure storage in locked cupboards. In many instances, the controls applied to the different types of medicines in hospitals exceed the basic legal requirements. This is of course necessary to ensure the protection and safety of both patients and staff. Health authorities have a duty to ensure that regulations are drawn up and applied to all aspects of the use of medicines (Circular ref. no. NHS 1979 (GEN) 11).

Outline of storage arrangements. Separate locked cupboards are provided for the following:

> internal medicines
> external medicines
> disinfectants/antiseptics
> clinical reagents.

A lockable refrigerator is also required. Separate sections will be required within a cupboard, e.g. to segregate oral preparations from injectables. The legal classifications referred to on page 41 are not relevant to these storage arrangements. Other storage facilities are provided for larger volume sterile solutions.

CONTROLLED DRUGS

The Misuse of Drugs Act 1971 regulates the importation, export, sale and use of narcotics such as morphine, diamorphine and other drugs of addiction. Other aspects covered by the Act include the establishment of an

Advisory Council on Misuse of Drugs. The Medicines Act is primarily concerned with regulating the legitimate use of medicines; the Misuse of Drugs Act is primarily concerned with the prevention of the abuse of Controlled Drugs. The use of Controlled Drugs in medicine is permitted by the Misuse of Drugs Regulations 1973. Different levels of control are applied within the regulations. The main controls are as follows:

1. Licence is needed to import or export.
2. Compounding/manufacturing is permitted by a practitioner or pharmacist.
3. A pharmacist may supply to a patient on the prescription of an appropriate practitioner.
4. These drugs may be administered to a patient by a person acting in accordance with the instructions of a doctor or dentist.
5. Safe custody and record keeping are required.
6. The following persons are also authorised to be in possession of and to supply Controlled Drugs:
   Medical or dental practitioner
   Matron or acting matron of a hospital or nursing home (see also below)
   The sister, or acting sister, for the time being in charge of a ward, theatre or other department. The authority is limited to obtaining ward stocks from no other source but the pharmacist engaged in dispensing medicines in the particular hospital. In some situations, where there is no on-site pharmacy, the hospital pharmacy normally providing the pharmaceutical service is regarded as being within this provision.

Limitations are applied to the authorisations, in that they apply only so far as is necessary for the practice or exercise of their profession. (It should be noted that apart from health care personnel, other groups of workers are permitted to possess/supply Controlled Drugs, e.g. Masters of a ship, person in charge of a recognised laboratory, manager of an offshore installation.)

Supply of Controlled Drugs to addicts
Special regulations are applicable to the supply of Controlled Drugs to persons who are addicted to these drugs, e.g. a doctor may only prescribe Controlled Drugs for an addicted person if he holds a licence issued by the Secretary of State. (Any doctor may prescribe Controlled Drugs to an addicted person who is suffering from injury or organic disease.) A special prescription is used to enable addicts to receive daily supplies of Controlled Drugs.

Barbiturates and appetite suppressants
As from January 1985 certain orders and amendments to the list of drugs controlled under the Misuse of Drugs Act 1971 came into effect. This resulted in certain barbiturates and appetite suppressants (e.g. diethylproprion) becoming Controlled Drugs. All the requirements for prescription writing, ordering, recording and storing Controlled Drugs apply to the following drugs (amongst others):

amylobarbitone
butobarbitone
cyclobarbitone
methylphenobarbitone
pentobarbitone
quinalbarbitone

The regulations covering phenobarbitone are not so comprehensive, in that the handwriting requirements (see p. 44) do not apply nor do the storage and recording requirements for Controlled Drugs. This is because of the use of phenobarbitone in the treatment of epilepsy.

Controlled drugs in hospitals
1. A sister, or acting sister in charge of a ward, theatre or department may not supply any Controlled Drug other than for administration to a patient in accordance with the prescription of a doctor (or dentist).
2. Strictly according to the Regulations the sister or acting sister is not required to keep a drug register. However, in practice the keeping of a drug register at ward or departmental level is always required by the health authority.

Storage
Controlled Drugs are required to be stored in a separate locked cupboard constructed to prevent unauthorised access to the drugs. It is customary for this cupboard to be within another locked cupboard.

Prescriptions for Controlled Drugs
As stated above, a prescription is normally written on the drug Kardex for an inpatient. *For out-patients, (or patients on discharge from hospital), the following information is required.*

It is not lawful for a practitioner to issue a prescription for a Controlled Drug, or for a pharmacist to dispense it, unless it complies with the following requirements. The prescription must:

1. be in writing and signed by the person issuing it with his usual signature and be dated by him
2. be in ink or otherwise so as to be indelible
3. except in the case of an NHS or local health authority prescription, specify the address of the person issuing it
4. have written on it, if issued by a dentist, the words 'for dental treatment only'
5. specify (in the handwriting of the person issuing the prescription) the name and address of the person for whose treatment it is issued
6. specify (again in the prescriber's own handwriting) the dose to be taken and (a) in the case of preparations, the form and, where appropriate, the strength of the preparation, and either the total quantity (in both words and figures) of the preparation, or the number (in both words and figures) of dosage units to be supplied; (b) in any other case, the total quantity (in both words and figures) of the Controlled Drug to be supplied.
7. in the case of a prescription for a total quantity intended to be dispensed by instalments, contain a direction specifying the amount of the instalments which may be dispensed and the intervals to be observed when dispensing.

Records
Normally records relating to Controlled Drugs must be kept for 2 years.

Destruction of Controlled Drugs
Certain persons are authorised by the Secretary of State to witness the destruction of Controlled Drugs. In hospital practice the pharmacist normally undertakes this role at ward level, when small quantities are involved. A record of the destruction is normally made in the ward register and witnessed by the ward sister. Larger quantities of Controlled Drugs must be destroyed in the presence of an inspector of the Pharmaceutical Society, drug squad oficer, Home Office inspector or (in Scotland and in Wales) the Chief Administrative Pharmaceutical Officer.

Some problems can arise at ward level with Controlled Drugs brought in by patients on admission. These will have been obtained by the patient on prescription. Technically it is illegal for the ward sister to receive these drugs from the patient. However in such situations the pharmacist may lawfully accept such drugs for destruction. On rare occasions a patient may be in possession of illicit Controlled Drugs. This is obviously a very delicate matter and is dealt with having regard to all clinical and legal considerations. At the present time it is illegal for the pharmacist to receive such drugs and it may be necessary to call in the police to deal with the matter.

General points
Certain of the legal requirements concerning drug control do not apply in hospitals. However, health authorities are required to institute safe procedures in accordance with official circulars, reports etc. Failure to institute or comply with these procedures would leave the health authorities or individual liable to legal action. In practice, a positive attitude to all aspects of the safe use of medicines will benefit patients and safeguard health care workers.

Procedural Aspects
Legislation and responsibility of staff
Procedures involved in the handling of

Controlled Drugs are drawn up by health authorities against the background of the legal and professional responsibilities defined in the documents listed below and may be supplemented where necessary in accordance with local requirements:

The Misuse of Drugs Act 1971
Misuse of Drugs Regulations 1973
The Aitken Report — Control of Dangerous Drugs and Poisons in Hospitals 1958
The Roxburgh Report — Control of Medicines in Hospital wards and departments 1972.

Ordering of Controlled Drugs
Controlled Drug supplies for hospital wards and departments may only be ordered by a sister or acting sister using the order book (ref. no. 90–500) provided for the purpose. For each product, the name of the preparation (in block letters), the formulation, the strength (in figures and words) and the total quantity (in figures and words) should be entered using a separate page for each product (Fig. 5.1A). The nurse placing the order enters her signature and designation, and dates the order.

The whole order book is sent to the pharmacy department where the pharmacist prepares the order and signs the requisition. The person acting as messenger for the return

of the drugs to the ward or department also signs the requisition. The original requisition is then retained in the pharmaceutical department. Replacement order books are obtained from pharmacy departments.

Delivery and receipt of Controlled Drugs
Delivery of Controlled Drugs may be made in a locked box or by a designated messenger. If Controlled Drugs are collected from the pharmacy, the appropriate section should be completed by the messenger. Careful consideration should be given as to persons suitable to act as messengers of Controlled Drugs. It is prudent to restrict nurses, who at times may have to act as messengers, to those who have received theoretical instructions in the handling of Controlled Drugs.

On receipt of supplies of a Controlled Drug and the order book by a ward or department, a registered or enrolled nurse should check the drugs against the copy requisition. If all is found to be correct, the copy requisition is signed (Fig. 5.1B) and the order book retained in the ward or department. If there is any discrepancy, the pharmacy should be notified at once.

An entry is then made in the ward Controlled Drugs record book (ref. no. 90–501) with details of the new supply, keeping records of the different forms and strengths of each prep-

Name of Preparation	Strength	Quantity
DEXTROMORAMIDE TABLETS	10 mg (TEN)	25 TABS (TWENTY FIVE)

(Each preparation to be ordered on a separate page)

Ordered by...... *K. Stewart* S/N   Date...... 15/9/85
(Signature of Sister or Acting Sister)

Supplied by...... *J. Hutchison*   Date...... 15/9/85
(Pharmacist's Signature)

Accepted for delivery...... *M. Duncan*   Date...... 15/9/85
(Signature of Messenger)

TO BE RETAINED IN THE PHARMACEUTICAL DEPARTMENT

Fig. 5.1 A Order form for Controlled Drugs

Name of Preparation	Strength	Quantity
DEXTROMORAMIDE TABLETS	10 mg (TEN)	25 TABS (TWENTY FIVE)

(Each preparation to be ordered on a separate page)

Ordered by...... *K Stewart* S/N ...... Date...... 15/9/85
(Signature of Sister or Acting Sister)

Supplied by...... *J Hutchison* ...... Date...... 15/9/85
(Pharmacist's Signature)

Accepted for delivery...... *M Duncan* ...... Date...... 15/9/85
(Signature of Messenger)

Received by...... *Angela Rhind* ...... Date...... 15/9/85
(To be signed in the ward in the presence of the Messenger)

TO BE RETAINED BY THE SISTER

Fig. 5.1 **B** Copy order for Controlled Drugs

aration in separate sections or pages (Fig. 5.2A). The page is headed with the name of the preparation (in block letters), its form and strength. The columns are filled appropriately to include the number of tablets or vials, or the volume of liquid received, the date and the serial number of the requisition. Where there is continuity of use of a page or section, the existing stock balance is added to the new supply. When it is necessary to start a new section or page the index is amended accordingly.

When an enrolled nurse receives a Controlled Drug in the absence of a registered nurse, the drug should be checked and witnessed in the presence of the senior registered nurse on duty in the unit. The drugs are locked in the Controlled Drugs cupboard.

Storage of Controlled Drugs
All Controlled Drugs must be stored within a locked Controlled Drugs cupboard set aside for the purpose. Preferably, the cupboard should be sited where it is visible to nursing staff on duty. With this recommendation however there is the disadvantage that 'visible' cupboards are also often in the busiest parts of a ward, for example, at the nurses' station or within the patient area of a Nightingale-type ward.

These locations are not conducive to a clear, uninterrupted environment in which to concentrate on checking drugs and so extra care is essential. A warning light indicating when the cupboard is open is normally provided. The key(s) to this cupboard must be held in the possession of the trained nurse in charge of the ward.

Spare keys for Controlled Drugs cupboards are generally kept in the hospital pharmacy. If there is no pharmacy on site, local arrangements are usually made for spare keys to be held in the safe keeping of the senior nurse manager concerned. In departments where Controlled Drugs are stored but which do not have 24 hour supervisory cover such as outpatient clinics, arrangements for the safe keeping of the key(s) to the Controlled Drugs cupboard out of working hours must be made.

Loss or suspected loss of keys should be reported in the first instance to the senior nurse manager on duty whose duty it is to inform a senior member of the pharmacy staff and, if necessary, the security officer for the hospital.

As with other drugs, Controlled Drugs should not be transferred to other containers but must be retained in the original container which should not be defaced in any way.

5

NAME, FORM OF PREPARATION AND STRENGTH...... *DIAMORPHINE INJECTION 10mg*

AMOUNT(S) OBTAINED			AMOUNTS ADMINISTERED						
Amount	Date Received	Serial No. of Re-quisition	Date	Time	Patient's Name	Amount Given	Given by (Signature)	Witnessed by (Signature)	STOCK BALANCE
20 AMPS	7/8/85	07							20 AMPS
			9/8/85	7.20 AM	A. Patient	10mg	J Milne	E Walker	19 AMPS
			9/8/85	11.45 AM	A. Patient	20 mg.	J Milne	E Jones	17 AMPS
			10/8/85	—	STOCK CHECKED and found correct S. Smith, Sister				17 AMPS
10 AMPS	16/8/85	08							27 AMPS

Fig. 5.2 A Extract from ward Controlled Drugs record book

Prescribing of Controlled Drugs

Hospital in-patients. Controlled Drugs are prescribed for in-patients in the normal manner (see p. 150).

Theatre and day units. The required dose is prescribed and recorded in the patients' notes.

Patients on pass and discharge. Preparations which are subject to the prescription requirements of the Misuse of Drugs Regulations 1973 are distinguished throughout the British National Formulary by the symbol CD (Controlled Drugs). The principal legal requirements relating to these prescriptions are listed on page 44).

Procedure for administration in hospitals

The basic procedure for giving any medication applies also to giving a Controlled Drug.

Instructions relating specifically to Controlled Drugs are as follows:

1. Two persons must be involved in the administration of a Controlled Drug, one of whom must be a trained nurse or a registered doctor. Some local policies state that the nurse must be registered and not enrolled.
2. The keys to the Controlled Drug cupboard are obtained from the nurse-in-charge.
3. The stock amount of the drug to be used is checked against the last entry in the Controlled Drug record book.
4. After the dose is selected, the remaining stock is returned to the cupboard which is then locked.
5. The date, the name of the patient, the

amount of the drug to be given and the stock balance are entered in the record book (Fig. 5.2A).

6. Both persons involved take the prepared drug to the patient, one to administer the drug, the other to act as witness.
7. The time of administration and the signatures of the two persons are entered in the record book.
8. The keys of the Controlled Drug cupboard are returned to the nurse-in-charge.

Keeping the ward or department Controlled Drug record book

The record book must be kept in accordance with the guidance given on page 45. Replacement record books are available from the pharmacy department.

When Controlled Drugs are dispensed by the pharmacy for a named individual in-patient, each supply should be recorded in a separate section of the ward Controlled Drugs record book.

When arriving at a stock balance of liquid oral medicines it may not always be possible to obtain exactly the theoretical number of doses from each container. Accordingly records may be made as illustrated in Figure 5.2B.

Checking stock balances

By nurses. This is undertaken in accordance with locally agreed procedures. Regular checks are part of ward drug management. The intervals vary from on a shift basis or daily to weekly.

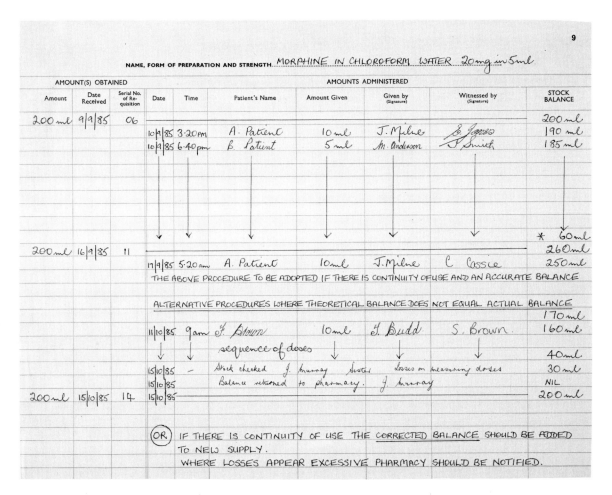

Fig. 5.2 B Extract from ward Controlled Drugs record book

Suitably written records are made of the checks carried out (Fig. 5.2A).

By pharmacists. These checks are made at least at 3 monthly intervals but may be required more frequently. A written record of the check is made in the ward Controlled Drug record book by the pharmacist carrying out the check.

Procedure to be adopted if
(a) The Controlled Drug order book and/or ward Controlled Drugs record book and/or (b) Controlled Drugs are missing. In the event of loss or suspected loss of these, the nurse-in-charge of the ward or department should contact the senior nurse manager on duty who will inform the senior pharmacy manager if this becomes necessary.

Disposal of Controlled Drugs
An individual dose of a Controlled Drug which is prepared and is unsuitable for taking back into stock should be destroyed in the ward or department and its destruction recorded in the ward Controlled Drugs record book. The destruction must be witnessed by a registered nurse. The same procedure should be adopted where only part of the contents of an ampoule is required for administration. Any accidental breakage should be dealt with in the same way.

Unwanted or time expired drugs. These should be returned to pharmacy, having made suitable records in the ward Controlled Drugs record book.

Retention of records
All Controlled Drugs order books and record books must be retained for 2 years after the date of the last entry. After this time, such documents should be destroyed by burning or shredding.

REFERENCES

Dale J R, Appelbe G E 1983 Pharmacy law and ethics. Pharmaceutical Press, London
Department of Health and Social Security 1958 Report on control of dangerous drugs and poisons in hospitals by a joint sub-committee of the standing medical, nursing and pharmaceutical advisory committees, Central Health Services Council (Aitken report) HMSO London
Department of Health and Social Security 1977 Health circular (77) 16. DHSS, London
Scottish Home and Health Department NHS Circular No. 1979 (GEN) 11
Royal College of Nursing 1983 Drug administration — a nurse's responsibility. RCN, London
Scottish Home and Health Department 1972 Report on control of medicines in hospital wards and departments by a joint group appointed by the standing pharmaceutical, medical, nursing and midwifery advisory committees of the Scottish Health Services Council (Roxburgh report) HMSO, Edinburgh

6 SYSTEMIC DRUG THERAPY

DRUG OR MEDICINE?

A drug is a pure chemical substance prepared synthetically or extracted from animal, vegetable or fungal tissue, which produces a pharmacological response. A medicine, is a compounded form of the drug with other substances, suitable for administration to patients. The nature and range of substances included in a medicine will depend on the presentation. Tablets require disintegrating agents to ensure the tablet breaks down in the gut; liquid oral medicines will require a vehicle such as water or a mixture of water and alcohol, flavouring agents, preservatives and perhaps colour. Steps have to be taken to ensure that the product is stable and suitable for the purpose. The distinction between a drug and a medicine is not always made in practice. For the purposes of this chapter the word drug will be used to describe both the active ingredient and the medicine.

In order to achieve the desired pharmacological response, a drug must first be available in a suitable form and be given by an appropriate route. The action may be local, but in many cases the drug must be absorbed and distributed, via the circulation, through the body to its site of action. For the effect to wear off, the drug must be metabolised and the metabolic products excreted from the body, although in certain instances the drug may be eliminated without being metabolised.

FIRST-PASS METABOLISM BY THE LIVER
(Fig. 6.1)

Orally and rectally administered drugs which are absorbed from the gastrointestinal tract are carried by the hepatic portal vein to the liver.

Those drugs which have a high hepatic extraction ratio exhibit marked first-pass effects, i.e. a large proportion of the drug is removed before it can enter the general circulation. For certain drugs, (e.g. glyceryl trinitrate if swallowed), the rate of hepatic metabolism is so rapid that the quantity of active compound reaching the systemic circulation after the first pass through the liver is only a small fraction of the dose. Some drugs which are extensively metabolised during the first pass through the liver may still be given orally if their metabolites are active, (e.g. propranolol).

SUBLINGUAL ADMINISTRATION

First-pass metabolism is avoided when drugs are given by the sublingual route (or by injection or transdermal administration) since the drug passes directly into the general blood circulation. The patient should be instructed to place the tablet under the tongue or between the gum and cheek and refrain from swallowing saliva for as long as possible as this will contain the drug which will be absorbed. As absorption through the oral mucosa is rapid,

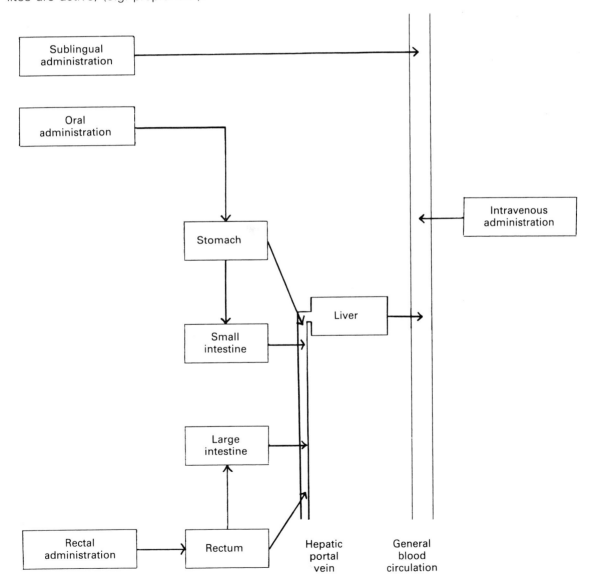

Fig. 6.1 First-pass metabolism

the effects of the drug become apparent within a minute or two.

The sublingual route is more convenient than the oral route. It is a simple method of administration requiring no water and demanding little effort from the patient. The co-operation of the patient is necessary, however, and a clear explanation of this method of administration should be given to him. Although no harm will ensue if the tablet is swallowed, he will benefit from the drug *only* if it is taken sublingually. The ease with which drugs can be given by this route can be used to advantage in post-operative patients and those who are terminally ill, where swallowing of tablets can be a problem. Buprenorphine, an analgesic, is commonly used in these situations. The sublingual route is also useful when there is risk of symptoms arising unexpectedly and when a rapid effect is wanted, such as in angina pectoris. Patients who have been prescribed glyceryl trinitrate tablets for prevention of anginal attacks should be advised to carry with them a small supply of the tablets at all times. The expiry date (8 weeks after dispensing.) should be carefully noted. Once the individual patient gets to know which activities tend to precipitate an attack, he should get into the habit of placing the tablet under his tongue just before embarking on any of these activities. When the tablet is used to alleviate an anginal attack, it should be taken immediately the pain is experienced and retained under the tongue until the pain is relieved, after which any of the tablet remaining is spat out. This may help prevent headache caused by cerebral vasodilation which often follows administration of this drug.

TRANSDERMAL ADMINISTRATION (Fig. 6.2)

Although most preparations are applied topically to give a local effect, topical medications are now also used because of their systemic action. Glyceryl trinitrate, a vasodilator used for relief of angina pectoris, can be applied as a 2% ointment (Percutol). Magnitude and duration of effect are directly related to the amount of ointment applied, consequently the dosage

is titrated against the clinical presentation of the patient. The usual dose, 25–50 mm (1–2 inches) squeezed from the tube, may be applied every 3–4 hours. The optimum dosage is best determined by starting with an application of 12 mm (0.5 inches) of ointment on the first day and increasing the dose by 12 mm (0.5 inches) increments on each successive day until headache (the outcome of cerebral vasodilation) occurs; this length is then reduced by 12 mm (0.5 inches)

Another novel drug delivery system is Transiderm-Nitro. This is a transdermal drug delivery system comprising a self-adhesive, pink-coloured patch containing a drug reservoir of glyceryl trinitrate. It is designed to achieve a prolonged and constant release of glyceryl trinitrate causing venous and arterial dilatation and redistribution of myocardial blood flow. One patch is applied to the lateral chest wall every 24 hours. Drugs administered in this way avoid first-pass metabolism by the liver (see Fig. 6.1).

ORAL ADMINISTRATION

For ease of administration, it is most convenient for patients to receive medication by mouth. Tablets, capsules and liquid preparations are generally easy to administer and are effective when taken by this route. To prevent tablets and capsules sticking in the oesophagus and causing irritation, patients ideally should sit up, take a draught of water and then swallow the preparation with another draught of water.

Some substances are destroyed in the stomach or in the intestine. For example, erythromycin base is destroyed by the acidity of gastric juice and compounds of a protein nature such as oxytocin, insulin and most vaccines are destroyed by digestive enzymes. Some of these limitations can be overcome by using a different route of administration (oxytocin is given by injection). Alternatively a drug can be protected from stomach acidity by surrounding the tablet or capsule with an enteric or acid-resisting coating. This passes through the acid contents of the stomach

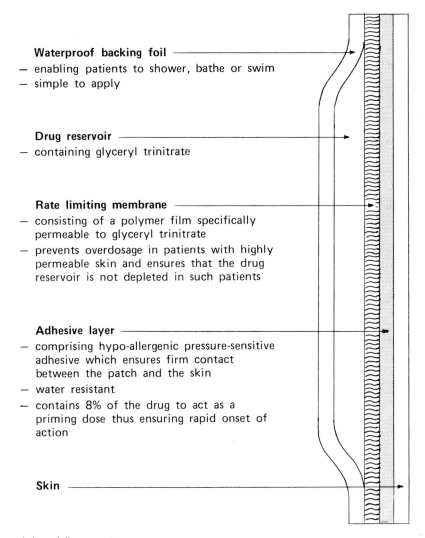

Waterproof backing foil
— enabling patients to shower, bathe or swim
— simple to apply

Drug reservoir
— containing glyceryl trinitrate

Rate limiting membrane
— consisting of a polymer film specifically
  permeable to glyceryl trinitrate
— prevents overdosage in patients with highly
  permeable skin and ensures that the drug
  reservoir is not depleted in such patients

Adhesive layer
— comprising hypo-allergenic pressure-sensitive
  adhesive which ensures firm contact
  between the patch and the skin
— water resistant
— contains 8% of the drug to act as a
  priming dose thus ensuring rapid onset of
  action

Skin

Fig. 6.2 Transdermal drug delivery system

intact and dissolves in the intestine where the pH is higher. This technique may also be used to protect the stomach from certain drugs such as aspirin, which is irritant and may cause gastric bleeding.

Erythromycin base may be administered as an enteric-coated tablet or alternatively given in the form of erythromycin stearate which is less readily destroyed in the stomach but dissociates in the duodenum liberating the active erythromycin which is absorbed.

Drug absorption following oral administration

When a medicine is taken by mouth, both the amount of drug absorbed and the rate of absorption are determined by many factors; in particular the physical nature of the dosage form, the presence of food in the stomach, the composition of the gastrointestinal contents, gastric or intestinal pH, gastrointestinal motility,. mesenteric blood flow and concurrent oral administration of other drugs. Gastrointestinal absorption following administration of tablets and capsules takes place only after the dosage form disintegrates and the released drug is dissolved in the gastrointestinal fluids. In liquid dosage forms, disintegration, and in many instances dissolution, of drugs is already accomplished, therefore these tend to be more

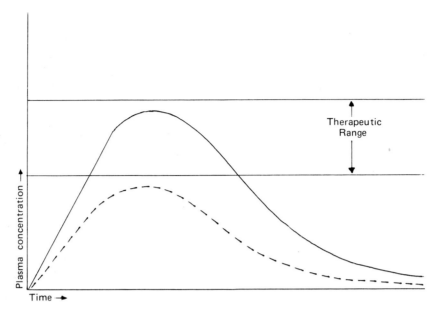

Fig. 6.3 Plasma concentrations of the same drug in two different formulations.
— bioavailability allows a therapeutic response
– – bioavailability lower due to a poorly formulated preparation.

rapidly absorbed. Gastrointestinal motility effects thorough mixing in the gastrointestinal tract and this increases the efficiency with which the drug is brought into contact with surfaces available for absorption. The level of the mesenteric blood flow will affect the rate of removal of the drug from the site of absorption.

BIOAVAILABILITY

To produce therapeutic effects, the drug, after release from the dosage form, must reach an adequate concentration in the blood. The amount and rate of appearance of the drug in the blood after administration of the dosage form are termed bioavailability. The bioavailability of drugs administered intravenously is 100% because of direct introduction into the bloodstream. The bioavailability of oral medications can vary greatly. Drugs which are poorly soluble in body fluids will have a low bioavailability. Furthermore tablets containing the same active principle but produced by different manufacturers may differ in bioavailability depending on the degree of compres-

sion, or the nature of added substances (excipients), which in turn affect disintegration and dissolution. Some years ago one manufacturer was able to improve a formulation of digoxin tablets to such an extent that the new tablets became twice as effective as the old ones, although drug content of the two was identical. Where doubts arise regarding bioavailability, it is recommended that individual patients stick to one brand once their treatment has been stabilised (Fig. 6.3).

Phenytoin is another example of this phenomenon where both the crystal size of the active ingredient and the excipients used have altered the bioavailability (Bochner et al, 1972). Stricter control of manufacturing processes in Britain now ensures that in the vast majority of instances, where the same drug is produced by a number of different companies, bioavailability is equivalent.

Effects of food

The bioavailability of a number of drugs (e.g. penicillins, erythromycin, rifampicin and thyroxine) is reduced by food. In such cases it is recommended that these preparations should be taken half an hour before meals.

Drugs may also require to be taken before meals for specific reasons — anthelmintics will have better contact with worms on an empty stomach and the local anaesthetic effect of oxethazaine, a constituent of the antacid Mucaine, will lessen oesophagitis as food passes through the oesophagus. Drugs including aspirin, nitrofurantoin, metformin, metronidazole, potassium chloride, spironolactone or triamterene cause gastric symptoms if taken on an empty stomach. When taken with or immediately after a meal, these substances will mix with the food which gives a degree of protection from the gastric side-effects.

It is often assumed that food will, in general, delay drug absorption. However, this is an oversimplification (Melander, 1978) since food may increase, decrease or have no consistent effect on the amount of drug absorbed. The absorption of preparations including aspirin, paracetamol, digoxin, bumetanide and frusemide, is delayed by food. This contrasts with an improvement in absorption of other drugs in the presence of food which may be due to an alteration in tablet disintegration and drug dissolution, or the variable effects of different types of meals on intestinal transit time.

The increase in bioavailability in the presence of food may be due to a number of factors:

1. First pass metabolism is reduced, e.g. metoprolol, propranolol.
2. Drug poorly soluble in water but readily soluble in fat, e.g. griseofulvin
3. Delayed gastric emptying increases the time available for dissolution of poorly soluble tablets, e.g. nitrofurantoin, spironolactone

It should be noted that if a patient is in a state of shock, stomach emptying may be delayed, sometimes for several hours, so that drugs given orally will not reach the small intestine and consequently will not be absorbed.

Mechanism of absorption of oral preparations

There are four possible mechanisms of absorption — pinocytosis, filtration through pores, active transport and passive diffusion.

Pinocytosis
Utilising this mechanism, microscopic particles of the drug are engulfed by the cell membrane but this is of minor importance.

Filtration through pores
These pores between cells are so small that only compounds with a molecular weight less than 100 (e.g. alcohol, lithium) can be absorbed in this way.

Active transport
In this type of transport energy is required to convey a drug across a cell. This highly specific method is used for the transport of naturally occurring substances such as amino acids, sugars and some vitamins, but rarely for drugs although methyldopa and levodopa are both absorbed by active transport.

Passive diffusion
This is by far the most important mechanism of absorption. No energy is required and the drug transfer across the cell membrane is directly proportional to the concentration gradient (i.e. it passes from an area of high concentration to one of low concentration). The drug must initially be present in aqueous solution at the surface of the cell membrane, then dissolve in the lipid membrane and finally pass into the aqueous phase on the other side of the membrane. Some compounds are absorbed only to a limited extent, usually because they lack the ability to dissolve in the lipid walls of the cells lining the intestines. Lack of this lipid solubility means that they cannot readily cross the cells of the mucous membrane to gain access to the bloodstream. Outstanding in this respect are some antibiotics such as streptomycin and gentamicin, and tubocurarine. These drugs have therefore to be given by injection.

Since drugs spend only a short time in the stomach and the surface area of the stomach is small compared with the intestine, most drugs are absorbed from the small intestine. The intestinal villi present a huge surface area for the absorption of food and drugs.

GUIDELINES FOR ADMINISTERING ORAL SOLIDS

Assisting patients who have difficulty swallowing tablets

1. A drink beforehand moistens the mouth and gets the swallowing process started.
2. Where the tablet is large and is scored, it may be split in two or even four. A specially designed tablet splitter (Fig. 6.4) may be found helpful. In certain instances the tablet may be crushed using a mortar and pestle or specially designed tablet crusher (Fig. 6.5). Enteric coated or sustained release formulations must not be split or crushed. Some patients find it helpful to place the tablet at the back of the tongue, take a draught of water and tilt the head back before swallowing. For those who cannot swallow tablets or capsules, there may be soluble or liquid forms of the medicine available from the pharmacy.

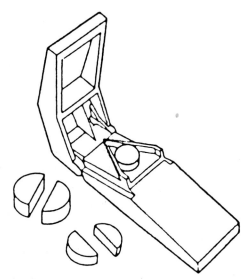

Fig. 6.4 Tablet splitter

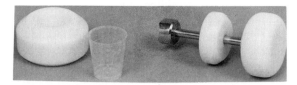

Fig. 6.5 Tablet crusher

The process of getting the medicine safely into the patient

Whenever possible, the patient should put the tablet or capsule into his mouth himself. By observing the patient attempting to take a tablet and assessing his capabilities generally, the nurse can decide how best to present further medicines to him. The various methods employed are taking directly from a spoon, medicine glass or palm of the hand, or picking up using the thumb and forefinger. Some difficulties are incurred by each of these methods. A spoon is not advisable for patients with any degree of tremor. Medicine glasses are not designed with the size of an adult's nose in mind and so access may be difficult! Unless the medicine glass is completely dry, tablets can adhere to the glass and go unnoticed. Tablets or capsules may be dropped or may stick to the hand if moist. Intention tremor and stiff joints may make picking up difficult or impossible.

Generally speaking, patients who are elderly, frail, poorly sighted or confused, are helped if the tablets are placed in a row on the medicine tray accompanied by a glass of water or a suitable beverage. In this way they are more likely to see what they are to take — the colour of the tablets and the number. They can then safely pick each one up themselves and so retain some degree of independence. Hemiplegic patients find this a helpful method especially when more than one tablet have to be taken. Using the unaffected hand, they require to break down the process, e.g.

1. pick up glass, take a drink, lay down glass
2. pick up first tablet and place in mouth
3. pick up glass, take a drink, lay down glass
4. pick up next tablet, . . . and so on.

Care must be taken, particularly where there is facial paralysis, to ensure that the tablets are swallowed and not retained in the side of the mouth. Patients who do not want to take their tablets are sometimes known to retain the tablet between the gum and the cheek until the staff are out of sight and then reject the tablet, often into the bed.

An adequate volume of fluid, e.g. at least 100 ml, ensures transport into the gastrointestinal tract. Apart from personal tastes and preferences, the choice and volume of liquid to be used will depend on a number of factors. Clearly, for patients on restricted fluids the volume may be critical. Milk may inhibit the absorption of some drugs and acidic fruit cordials tend to cause capsules to swell which may make swallowing more difficult. Improved formulations are a help in disguising the taste of many drugs but children of all ages may welcome the traditional 'spoonful of sugar'.

If a patient rejects part of a dose or vomits after swallowing a dose of a medicine, the doctor should be informed along with the time lapse between drug administration and emesis or rejection. Vomitus should be retained for examination of drug content.

GUIDELINES FOR THE ADMINISTRATION OF ORAL LIQUIDS

1. All liquid medicines should be thoroughly shaken before use and measured at eye level in a good light.
2. Viscous suspensions, syrups, etc. can be more completely administered if taken from a suitable spoon rather than from a medicine measure. A standard 5 ml spoon should normally be used. However medicine spoons of different designs are available, the choice depending mainly on patient acceptability. Care should be taken not to overfill a medicine spoon when administering a viscous preparation.
3. The formulation of liquid medicines presents many problems not least of which is to achieve an acceptable taste. If particular problems are experienced, the ward pharmacist should be consulted, as dilution or alternative formulation may be of assistance.
4. While it is necessary to ensure that soluble tablets are completely dissolved, it is unwise to use an excessive volume of water since an unpleasant taste may result in rejection by the patient.
5. Where the medicine is presented in powder form to be reconstituted, the date of reconstitution or expiry should be marked on the bottle.

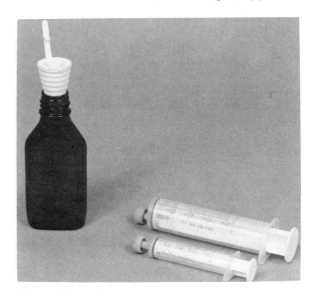

Fig. 6.6 Oral syringes

6. When liquids are being instilled in the mouth from a dropper, a separate bottle and dropper are used for each patient.
7. In some instances a specially designed oral syringe may be useful, e.g. in paediatrics or where specially potent oral liquid medicines are in use (Fig. 6.6).

RECTAL ADMINISTRATION

Drugs can be absorbed from the rectum if they are given in the form of suppositories. Alternatively a solution or suspension of the drug can be given as an enema and retained for a sufficient length of time in the rectum. The rectal route may be utilised when drugs cannot be swallowed (e.g. because of vomiting, coma, stricture), when drugs cause severe irritation of the upper gastrointestinal tract (e.g. sulphasalazine), when a prolonged nocturnal action is desired (anti-asthmatics, analgesics, hypnotics) or when a local action is required (laxatives, haemorrhoid treatments).

The absorptive surface area of the rectum is small but the blood supply is extremely efficient and absorption can be quite rapid. However, the presence of faeces may slow absorption, and irritation may cause early evacuation.

Given the option, perhaps more patients on

long-term drug therapy would choose this route of administration. It is debatable whether doctors in the UK will follow continental practice in the years ahead by more frequently prescribing drugs for rectal administration. Where this is the chosen method, patients should be encouraged to insert suppositories themselves and may be taught self-administration of a small disposable enema containing a soluble form of prednisolone (Predsol) in the treatment of colitis.

Although it is generally assumed that suppositories should be inserted narrow end first, the work of Walker (1982) has shown that it is more effective and causes less irritation to insert the blunt end first.

Procedure for administration of medications by the rectal route

1. Check details of the medication with the prescription. Identify the patient.
2. Explain to the patient what you intend doing and how he can co-operate.
3. Ensure warmth, privacy and comfort.
4. Assist patient into the left lateral position with the head on one or two pillows, buttocks in line with the edge of the bed and knees drawn up towards chin.
5. With clean hands place incontinence pad(s) under left buttock.

Suppositories	*Enemas*
6. Wearing disposable glove, apply lubricant (e.g. 'KY jelly') or melt tip of suppository in hot water as directed on the packet.	6. Expel air from enema nozzle and lubricate.

7. Encourage patient to relax.
8. Carefully locate anus avoiding external haemorrhoids where present.

9. Gently insert suppository as far as possible.	9. Gently insert nozzle for 4–6 cm and, slowly roll up enema pack to introduce contents

10. Withdraw finger smoothly.	10. Withdraw nozzle gently.

11. Wipe the anal region and remove gloves.
12. Make the patient comfortable.

Evacuant suppositories or enemas
— leave call bell within reach
— position commode at bedside
— encourage patient to hold in situ the medication if he can for approximately 20 minutes and to postpone the first few urges to defaecate, before finally expelling the contents of the rectum.

Retention suppositories or enemas
— administer the medication on retiring to bed so that it can be retained overnight.
— leave the incontinence pad(s) in position to help the patient to feel more secure.
— ensure the patient knows that it is to be retained.
(Elevating the foot of the bed may help the patient to retain the medication.)
13. Dispose of equipment.
14. Wash hands.
15. Record administration.

INJECTIONS

Drugs are given by injection for a number of reasons. They may not be absorbed when given by mouth (gentamicin) or may be destroyed in the stomach (insulin). Rapid first-pass metabolism may be extensive (lignocaine). A fast onset of action may be required or very precise control over dosage may be needed.

Subcutaneous and intramuscular injection

In clinical practice, the routes most commonly used for injections are subcutaneous and intramuscular despite the increased use of the intravenous route for antibiotic therapy.

The site of injection should be clean before being swabbed with a swab containing 70% alcohol and a disinfectant such as chlorhexidine.

The angles at which the needle is directed

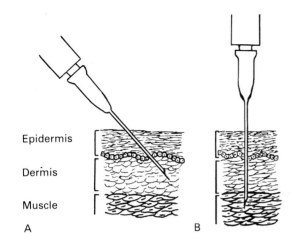

Fig. 6.7 Needle angles for (A) subcutaneous and (B) intramuscular injections

for these routes of administration of injection are illustrated (Fig. 6.7A & B).

Injection pain can be reduced in several ways:

1. Use sharp fine-bore needles
2. Inject a small volume of fluid
3. Cool the skin with a volatile spray such as ethyl chloride
4. Incorporate a local anaesthetic agent, normally procaine hydrochloride.

Subcutaneous administration may be carried out by high pressure jet injection which pushes the injection through a fine hole into the subcutaneous tissue without the aid of a needle. This technique is particularly useful in mass inoculation programmes.

The rates at which drugs are absorbed and take effect after subcutaneous or intramuscular injection depend on two factors:

1. the local blood circulation
2. the nature of the drug solution or suspension.

Subcutaneous absorption occurs chiefly through the capillaries and is much faster compared with absorption following oral medication but usually slower than intramuscular absorption because of muscle tissue's excellent blood supply. Absorption may be speeded up by massaging the area of injection. Drugs commonly given subcutaneously include insulin,

heparin, atropine and vaccines, and given intramuscularly, antibiotics and corticosteroids.

In states of shock, blood flow to the skin and superficial muscle may be greatly reduced thus reducing the absorption of drugs from these sites. In this case deep intramuscular or preferably intravenous injections should be used.

Administration of subcutaneous injection
The procedure is very similar to that of an intramuscular injection. For subcutaneous injections, however, a shorter needle of finer bore is used. For adults this is normally 5/8 inch, 25 gauge. The sites most commonly used are the middle outer aspect of the upper arms, middle anterior aspect of the thighs and the anterior abdominal wall below the umbilicus (Fig. 6.8). The back and lower loins may also be used. Diabetics are taught to rotate the use of these sites to reduce irritation and improve absorption. The usual angle at which the needle is directed is 45° although some physicians and manufacturers advocate pinching up the skin and injecting at 90° when a ½ inch 25 gauge needle is used for injecting the abdomen. No more than 2 ml should be injected at one site.

The needle with the bevel up is pushed through the skin and after checking that a blood vessel has not been entered (by withdrawing the plunger) the medication is slowly and steadily injected. The needle is carefully withdrawn and slight pressure is applied over the site until any oozing stops. Insulin-dependent diabetics are discouraged from massaging the site vigorously in an attempt to preserve the state of the capillaries.

Administration of intramuscular injection
The needle used for giving an intramuscular injection has to be sufficiently long to reach deep into the muscle so as to increase the speed of effect and to reduce the likelihood of the drug seeping back along the needle track. For adults a 1½ inch, 21 gauge is normally used. In severely emaciated adults and in small children a 1 inch, 23 gauge needle may be used. The choice of needle bore depends on how viscous the medication is. Oily preparations and other viscous injections require a wider

Epidermis

Dermis

Muscle

A   B

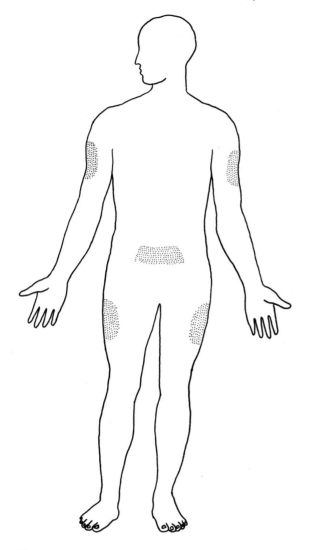

Fig. 6.8 Commonly used sites for administration of subcutaneous injections

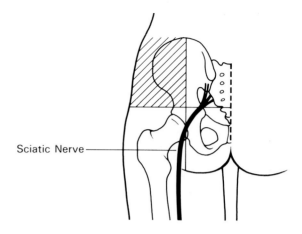

Fig. 6.9 Posterior view of left buttock showing upper outer quadrant

bore. The sites most often used are the upper outer quadrant of the buttock (Fig. 6.9) and the middle outer aspect of the thigh. It is vital that the injection is confined to one of these areas to avoid damage to the sciatic nerve. The administration of an intramuscular injection may be made less painful by encouraging the patient to relax and, when the buttock is the chosen site, asking the patient to adopt the prone position and point the feet inwards. Intramuscular injections are administered at an angle of 90° to the skin surface. The volume injected at any one site should normally be of the order of about 2–5 ml. Where a volume in excess of 5 ml is to be given, two separate sites should be used.

Requirements
On a clean tray:

> ampoule or vial containing drug
> ampoule of water for injections
> 2 alcohol swabs
> syringe of suitable size
> needles of suitable size
> disposable gloves
> prescription sheet.

Procedure
Preparing the equipment and the drug
1. Obtain keys from nurse-in-charge.
2. Wash hands.
3. Collect equipment and prescription.
4. Assemble syringe and guarded needle. Place in tray.
5. Check details on prescription sheet regarding
   (a) the patient, (b) the prescription.
6. Select medicine from cupboard and compare name, dose and route on ampoule with prescription. Ensure preparation has not passed expiry date.
7. Lock cupboard.
8. Make any necessary calculation.
Drawing up the injection
9. Flick ampoule with fingers so that contents are collected in body of ampoule.

10. Wipe neck of ampoule with swab.
11. Snap ampoule at neck holding same swab to protect the fingers and place in tray. (A plastic 'sleeve' may be used to protect the fingers.)
12. Remove needle guard.
13. Hold syringe and needle in one hand and ampoule in the other.
14. Insert needle into ampoule taking care to avoid touching anything en route.
15. Fill syringe to required amount by withdrawing plunger.
   (Make sure the needle is in contact with the liquid. Tilting the ampoule helps.)
16. Remove syringe and needle from ampoule.
17. Place ampoule in tray.
18. Replace guard on needle.
19. Expel air bubbles from the syringe by:
   (a) holding it perpendicular at eye level in a good light.
   (b) pulling the plunger back slightly.
   (c) tapping the syringe with the fingers to collect small bubbles into one.
   (d) pushing the plunger until liquid fills the needle.
20. Place syringe and needle in tray.
21. Recheck name of drug and dose on ampoule with prescription. Enter code letter on recording sheet.

Preparing the patient

22. Take tray and prescription to the patient.
23. Identify the patient.
24. Explain your intentions and tell the patient what you want him to do.
25. Ensure privacy, warmth, and comfort.
26. Position the patient suitably. He may:
   (a) do this unaided.
   (b) be assisted by the second nurse.
   (c) require two nurses.
27. Wash hands again if involved in positioning.

Administering the injection

28. Take care to expose a sufficiently large area to allow you to select the exact site for the injection while maintaining maximum privacy.
29. Clean the actual site to be used with the second swab and place on skin alongside proposed site.

30. Stretch or pinch up skin and tissue between thumb and fingers.
31. Insert needle *quickly* with other hand holding it as you would a pencil.
32. Release hand from tissues and transfer it to support barrel of syringe.
33. Withdraw plunger slightly to verify that the needle has not penetrated a blood vessel. [If blood appears, the needle is withdrawn and the injection repeated at another site using a fresh dose, syringe and needle].
34. Inject fluid *slowly* until plunger driven home.
35. Resume pencil grip.
36. Place swab against needle.
37. Withdraw needle *quickly*.
38. Compress site for a few seconds with swab.
39. Remove swab when minor seepage stops.
40. Replace needle and syringe in tray.
41. Restore patient to comfortable position.

Completing the procedure

42. Dispose of needle, syringe and ampoule carefully into disposal bin set aside for the purpose.
43. Wash tray with soap and warm water, dry and store
44. Wash hands.
45. Enter initials on recording sheet.
46. Return keys to the nurse-in-charge.

Further and special aspects of injection procedures

1. The medicine for injection may on some occasions be presented in a rubber-capped multi-dose vial, especially where the dose is variable. When this occurs, there are some important points to remember. The self-sealing rubber closure must be thoroughly cleaned with an alcohol swab and allowed to dry prior to puncturing it with a needle. Great care is essential in calculating what portion of the total volume is required. To facilitate withdrawal of fluid, the plunger of the syringe is first withdrawn and air injected, the volume of air being the same as the volume of fluid to be with-

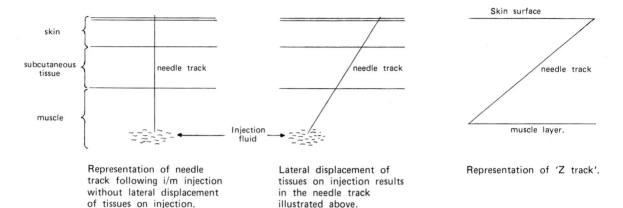

Representation of needle track following i/m injection without lateral displacement of tissues on injection.

Lateral displacement of tissues on injection results in the needle track illustrated above.

Representation of 'Z track'.

Fig. 6.10 Z-track technique

drawn. It is customary to change the needle after drawing up the injection and before injecting the patient.

2. The medicine may be presented in powder form and require reconstitution. Most often this is done using Water for Injections but in certain instances special diluents may be required. It should be recognised that the addition of 1 ml of diluent to 250 mg of a drug will produce a volume in excess of 1 ml. Normally this is of little consequence, but may be important if a fraction of the total content of the vial is to be administered. For emaciated patients the volume of reconstituting fluid used should be the minimum compatible with the physical and other properties of the drug, e.g. solubility, and any possible local irritancy should be taken into account. On occasions it may be desirable to combine two drugs in the same injection. This may present problems, e.g. physical/chemical incompatibility in the syringe and in the management of any subsequent drug reaction. The prime considerations here should be patient safety and comfort. Clearly, comfort for the patient should not be allowed to detract from safety in drug therapy. Advice of the prescriber and clinical pharmacist will often be helpful in resolving these difficult situations.

3. The injection may be known to stain the skin if its seepage along the needle track to the epidermis is allowed to take place (e.g. iron dextran injection). To prevent this, several precautions should be taken. After the syringe

is filled, the needle is changed so that the substance is contained in the syringe only and is less likely to drip from the tip of the needle as it penetrates the skin. The injection must be made deep into the muscle of the upper outer quadrant of the buttock — never into the arm or leg. A 21 gauge, 2 inch, needle should be used for the normal adult. The recommended technique is by Z-track, i.e. displacement of the skin laterally prior to injection (Fig. 6.10). The injection is made slowly and steadily. Before withdrawing the needle, a few seconds should be allowed to elapse so that the muscle mass may accommodate the volume of the injection. The injection site is not massaged.

4. When drawing up and injecting antibiotics, disposable gloves should be worn to prevent possible contact with the skin and the development of a sensitivity reaction. The special precautions which require to be taken when handling cytotoxic drugs are given on pages 167–170.

5. Glass syringes should be used for administering paraldehyde since it reacts with plastic and rubber on prolonged contact.

6. An inflamed or oedematous site should be avoided for the administration of intramuscular and subcutaneous injections to prevent a worsening of the inflammation and therefore, a delay in absorption.

7. Rotation of the sites used for intramuscular and subcutaneous injections helps to reduce the likelihood of irritation and improves absorption.

Intravenous injection

The intravenous route avoids all complications of drug absorption and as a result an effective blood level of the drug can be achieved in a matter of seconds. This route is used:

1. in emergency situations such as shock and status asthmaticus (hydrocortisone).
2. where subcutaneous or intramuscular injections would cause intolerable pain.
3. for intravenous anaesthetics (e.g. thiopentone sodium).
4. for larger volumes e.g. 5–20 ml.
5. where the preparation has irritant properties

Intravenous injections may be associated with a number of complications such as a haematoma from puncturing through, rather than into, the vein. Necrosis may result if a drug escapes into the surrounding tissues when the needle slips out of the vein. Phlebitis at the injection site results from a high concentration of an irritant agent, repeated injections or prolonged administration. Because of rapidity of action after intravenous injection, intoxication or death may result if an error is made in calculating or measuring the dose.

INTRAVENOUS INFUSION

Intravenous infusion is a method of administering large volumes of fluid (50 ml upwards) over a prolonged period of time in order to restore blood volume, supply electrolytes or nutrients, or to deliver drugs continuously. Irritant drugs such as certain cytotoxic agents are administered by this route. Intravenous infusions are packed in glass bottles which require an airway to vent the bottle as the fluid runs through the administration set, or in plastic containers which collapse as they empty and no airway is required.

Before assembling an intravenous line, it is important to read and check carefully the label on the infusion container against the fluid prescription. The container should also be inspected to ensure it has no flaws and that the fluid is clear and free from particulate matter. The rubber cap or entry port is pierced by the spike of the appropriate administration

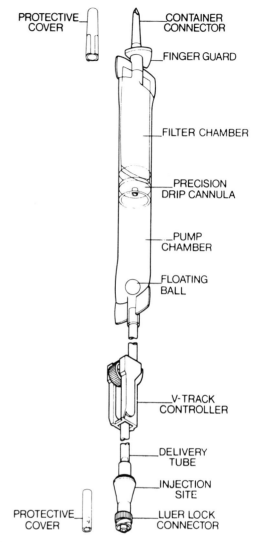

Fig. 6.11 Intravenous administration set

set, (Fig. 6.11) the filter chamber is squeezed to fill the set with fluid, air is removed from the tubing and the control clamp is closed. The free end of the administration set is covered by its sheath until required for use. The drip chamber contains a small diameter dropper tube to deliver a certain number of drops per ml. The flow rate, expressed as a number of drops per minute, is adjusted by means of a roll or screw clamp attached to the tubing. Where accurate control of flow rate is essential, an automatic infusion system is used which pumps solutions at a preset rate. Infusions are administered usually at a rate varying from 50–150 ml per hour in adults.

Adjuncts are sometimes used in conjunction with this system e.g. a calibrated burette may be incorporated in the system into which the infusion drips. One or more drugs can be added to the burette and this is very useful, particularly in intensive care, for intermittent infusion of potent drugs in precise volumes. Drugs may be slowly injected through an additive port in the administration set or can be added to minibottles or minibags usually containing either 5% w/v glucose in water or 0.9% w/v sodium chloride injection. These secondary containers are piggy-backed to the large volume primary container by inserting the needle from the minicontainer administration set into an injection port on the primary administration set (Fig. 6.12). Piggy-back containers

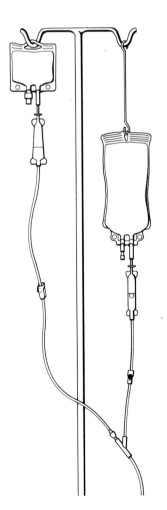

Fig. 6.12 Piggyback administration system

may be used to give a higher intermittent blood level of a particular drug than would be achieved if the drug were added to the larger primary container, or to avoid an incompatibility with a drug which may already be present in the primary container.

Drugs commonly given by intravenous infusion include antibiotics, lignocaine, heparin and potassium chloride. This infusion maintains a steady blood level of the drug over a prolonged period of time and the patient is spared the pain of frequent injections. The addition of drugs to intravenous infusion fluids presents a number of hazards (e.g. resulting from interaction between the drug and the infusion fluid). It is advisable to consult the information pharmacist where two or more drugs are to be added. Drugs should not be added to blood, plasma, lipid emulsions, saturated mannitol solutions, sodium bicarbonate solutions, amino acid solutions or dextran solutions because these infusion fluids are particularly likely to be degraded.

In addition to interactions, the fluid infused can be contaminated by micro-organisms if admixtures are not carried out under strict aseptic conditions. Ideally, these additions should be made by pharmacy staff in laminar air flow cabinets in aseptic rooms and administered within 12 to 24 hours. Complications such as thrombophlebitis may arise at, and spread beyond the site of cannula insertion. This results from physical or chemical irritation often related to the duration of the infusion or the type of fluid infused. Glucose is mildly acidic and on autoclaving a small quantity is broken down to hydroxymethylfurfural and these two factors appear to cause a higher incidence of thrombophlebitis when glucose infusions are given. Blood for transfusion should never be mixed with any drug or solution other than 0.9% sodium chloride because of the danger of interaction. If a unit of blood is preceded by a solution such as glucose agglutination may result. To avoid this, the administration set should be flushed with 0.9% sodium chloride solution or changed. All administration sets should be changed every 24 hours and care taken during this operation to avoid introducing micro-organisms into the container or at the cannula site.

ADMINISTRATION OF INTRAVENOUS DRUGS OR FLUIDS

Procedural aspects

Intravenous administration of drugs and fluids plays an important role in medical emergencies, surgical procedures and day-to-day care of patients. Because of the similarity in administering drugs and fluids intravenously, the section on these procedures which is common to both is given first, then each is discussed in turn.

The details on the drug or fluid container must be carefully compared with the prescription and the standard method of prescribing, administering and recording drugs followed. When a syringe or administration set has been filled ready for intravenous use, all air bubbles must be expelled in order to avoid causing an air embolism.

To reduce the risk of introducing microorganisms into the bloodstream, it is essential that the hands are washed prior to the procedure, sterile equipment is used and an aseptic technique is practised. It is important to explain to the patient, if possible, what you plan to do and why. Some pain is usually experienced with the insertion of a needle and many patients appreciate having the support and encouragement of a nurse at this time. The patient should be comfortable, with the site of introduction of the drug or fluid exposed and well lit. For intravenous infusion, the patient may require to change into a garment with wider sleeves. The commonest sites of introduction are the forearm, the back of the hand or the antecubital fossa at the elbow. In an emergency, a vein in the foot or the external jugular vein may have to be used. The venous outflow is blocked and the vein distended by applying pressure above the site with a tourniquet, sphygmomanometer cuff inflated to 100 mm of mercury, or with the help of an assistant, making sure not to apply too great a pressure as this may occlude the arterial supply. Asking the patient to open and close the fist, gently tapping the vein or immersing the hand in warm water will make the vein become more prominent. A large straight vein preferably at the junction of two veins and not running over a joint is the one of choice. The site of injection is swabbed with a suitable antiseptic. Finger contact with the vein should be avoided once the area has been cleaned.

Intravenous injection of a drug

A syringe with an eccentric nozzle and a 1 inch 20 gauge needle with an intravenous bevel are used for giving an intravenous injection. Holding the syringe in line with the vein, the needle with the bevel up is pushed through the skin into the vein in the direction of the heart (Fig. 6.13). Before injecting, the position of the needle must be verified by pulling the plunger. If blood is not aspirated the needle must be withdrawn and another attempt made. After releasing the tourniquet and making an initial injection of 0.1 ml, there should be a pause of at least 30 seconds to observe the response before the remainder is slowly injected (up to 10 minutes). It is dangerous to give a rapid intravenous injection as this exposes tissues and organs such as the heart and brain to high concentrations of a drug which has been poorly diluted with blood. A drug solution injected over 2 minutes will be 60 times more dilute than if injected over 2 seconds. After completing the injection, a sterile swab should be placed over the injection site, the needle slowly removed and gentle pressure maintained to avoid a haematoma.

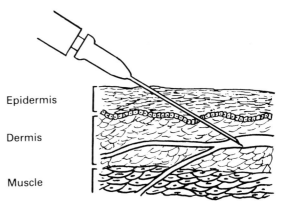

Epidermis

Dermis

Muscle

Fig. 6.13 Intravenous injection

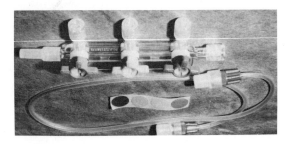

Fig. 6.14 Multiple inlet device

Alternatively, intravenous drugs may be administered intermittently via the side inlet of an indwelling intravenous cannula or into the administration set of an intravenous infusion by means of a three-way stopcock or multiple inlet device. (Fig. 6.14). If there is not a continuous fluid infusion to keep the cannula patent, a dilute heparin solution should be injected to prevent blood from clotting in its lumen.

Intravenous infusion of fluid

Intravenous cannulae of different gauges are obtainable. As large a gauge as possible should be used especially for administration of viscous fluids. The cannula is checked to ensure that it is patent and has no obvious defects. With the bevelled edge uppermost, the cannula is firmly entered under the skin a short distance away from the vein, always pointing the cannula proximally towards the heart. It is then gently pushed into the vein making sure to enter the plastic covering on the needle as well as the needle itself into the vein. Some types of cannula show a flash of blood at the hilt of the needle indicating that the needle, but not necessarily the plastic cannula, is in the vein. The tourniquet is then removed and simultaneously the needle is withdrawn and the plastic cannula is gently advanced into the vein. A well-sited cannula should introduce with little or no resistance. The tubing of the administration set is quickly attached. Gentle pressure on the vein proximal to the cannula tip prevents a leakage of blood through the cannula. When a small vein is used, the tubing may be attached earlier so that the cannula advances, whilst at the same time infusing fluid through it, thus displacing the walls of the vein. The cannula and adjacent tubing are

taped securely. A splint may be applied and is essential if the cannula has been positioned over a joint. The control clamp is released and the flow rate observed. Subcutaneous swelling around the cannula indicates that it is not in the vein and must be removed.

If the infusion is not running, there are several checks to be made;

1. The control clamp is open,
2. All connections have been made secure,
3. There are no kinks in the tubing,
4. The air inlet is patent in the case of a bottle,
5. The limb is in a relaxed position.

If there is any doubt about the infusion running satisfactorily, the cannula should be removed and replaced. The patient should be made comfortable with the arm supported on a pillow if required. A regimen of fluids to be infused is prescribed by the doctor in the standard way.

Alternative methods of introducing an intravenous line are either by surgically cutting down on a vein and introducing the cannula under direct vision (e.g. when no veins are visible or patent) or by means of a central venous line (e.g. for prolonged feeding or for central venous pressure measurement). Both of these techniques are specialised procedures which are undertaken by experienced medical staff.

Other routes of injection

Although parenteral administration is normally accomplished by subcutaneous, intramuscular or intravenous routes, occasionally other routes are used to deliver a drug to a particular tissue or organ.

Intra-arterial injections

This route is sometimes used to inject or infuse drugs into an artery supplying the affected organ if the drugs are rapidly metabolised or systemically toxic. Cytotoxic drugs for the treatment of local neoplasms or radio-opaque substances used in arteriography may be injected in this way.

Intra-articular injection

In inflammatory conditions of the joints,

particularly in rheumatoid arthritis, cortico-steroids are given by intra-articular injection to relieve inflammation and increase joint mobility. Insoluble, long-acting compounds such as triamcinolone hexacetonide are used. Cortico-steroids should not be injected into infected joints. Tissues or joints injected with cortico-steroids have an increased susceptibility to infections. It is therefore essential to observe full aseptic precautions when making these injections.

Intradermal (intracutaneous) injections
Intradermal injections are small volume injections, often of the order of 0.02 to 0.1 ml, given with a tuberculin syringe and a fine, 26 gauge needle. The injection is given *just* under the skin, holding the syringe about parallel to the skin. The technique is most commonly used for the administration of certain diagnostic agents such as tuberculin PPD and skin testing solutions in the diagnosis of allergy.

Intrathecal injections
It is necessary to administer some drugs intrathecally if they have poor lipid solubility and, as a result, do not pass the blood–brain barrier. In the treatment of meningitis, water-soluble antibiotics are administered by the intrathecal route to achieve adequate concentrations in the cerebrospinal fluid (CSF). Drugs administered by this route include penicillins, the choice of which will depend on the results of bacteriological examination of the CSF. Doses have to be very carefully calculated and are much smaller than would be given by intra-muscular or intravenous injection, since in effect, the antibiotic is being introduced into a closed system. Examples of drugs and adult doses administered intrathecally are as follows:

Ampicillin   20 mg   Cloxacillin 20 mg
Benzylpenicillin 6–12 mg Gentamicin1 mg
Carbenicillin   20 mg

Reduced doses are given to infants and children. Methotrexate is administered intrathecally (15 mg at weekly intervals) to treat meningeal leukaemia. In addition, antifungal agents, opioids, corticosteroids and radio-opaque substances, used in the diagnosis of spinal lesions, are sometimes administered by this route. A product specially prepared for the intrathecal route should be used. In many instances intrathecal therapy is supported by a course of the drug given by intramuscular or intravenous injection.

Technique. Drugs for intrathecal injection are normally injected between lumbar vertebrae 3 and 4 into the subarachnoid space of the spinal cord as part of the procedure of lumbar puncture. The role of the nurse is directed towards careful positioning of the patient, assisting the doctor in maintaining an aseptic technique and providing the patient with support and encouragement throughout the procedure.

It is vitally important to maintain full asepsis in this procedure because of the risk of infection being introduced into the CNS. Great care has to be taken with all the manipulations involved. Any diluent (in some instances CSF) used for the drug must of course be sterile and must be free from any bacteriostatic agent or preservative which would damage the delicate tissues of the CNS. The injection as well as being sterile, must not contain particulate matter. A sterile, disposable bacterial filter (0.22 micron) must be used between the syringe and needle as a final safeguard for the patient.

INHALATION THERAPY

Drugs can be introduced into the pulmonary system as aerosols or gases and have a fast onset of action. Absorption of drugs from the lungs is rapid because of the very large surface area of the alveoli, the single layer of epithelial cells and the rich blood supply. In this way high concentrations of drugs can be obtained in the bronchial mucosa and smooth muscle with minimal systemic side-effects.

Within the last 10 years there has been a great increase in the number and in the selectivity of drugs available to treat obstructive airways disease. Methods of administering these drugs for both prophylaxis and treatment of an acute attack have also improved greatly. Inhalation of drugs can be accomplished by a number of inhalation devices such as the aerosol inhaler, the dry powder inhaler and the wet nebuliser.

Aerosol inhaler. Most commonly, drugs are delivered to the lungs as sprays from pressurised aerosol dispensers. The drug and its inert propellant, such as freon, are maintained under pressure in a small canister. When the valve is activated, a measured quantity of propellant carrying the drug is released through the mouthpiece. Maximum benefit is obtained by the patient only when the proper technique of inhalation is used. The inhaler should first be shaken. The mouthpiece of the inhaler can be positioned 3–4 cm from the open mouth or held by the lips. The patient breathes out fully, one puff of the inhaler is taken at the start of a long slow breath in through the mouth, then the breath is held for 8–10 seconds. People whose hands are not strong may find it easier to use both hands to depress the canister.

Many patients have difficulty in using an aerosol and it helps if oral instructions are backed up with a written explanation. The dose delivered from the inhaler can be seen as a fine white mist. If any can be seen escaping from the mouth or nose then the inhaler is not being used correctly. For patients with an ideal technique only about 10% of the dose enters the lungs. Even although this is only a tiny fraction of the oral dose it is enough to be effective. The remainder of the dose lands on the tongue or the back of the throat and is swallowed, but in such a small quantity that it has no systemic effect. A spacer device attached to the inhaler improves the dose delivery to 15%.

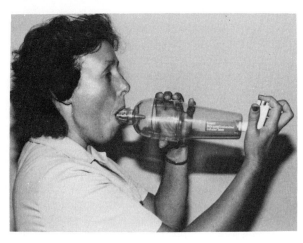

Fig. 6.15 Using the Nebuhaler

The Nebuhaler, a plastic cone of 750 ml capacity increases efficiency to about 20%. (Fig. 6.15). A pressurised aerosol is fitted at one end and the patient inspires through a one way valve at the other. On expiration the valve returns to the closed position and a hole in the mouthpiece allows the escape of gas which prevents rebreathing and build up of carbon dioxide. The Nebuhaler is designed in a cone shape to minimise deposition of bronchodilator on the walls and the patient can inhale when ready. There is no need to co-ordinate firing of the canister with inhalation. Another aid which is reported to help some patients is the breath-activated Pulmadil Auto. When used correctly the inhaler is automatically activated and a click is heard so that the patient knows medication is being received.

Aerosol inhalers are widely used to administer bronchodilators such as selective beta 2 agonists, e.g. salbutamol, terbutaline, fenoterol, or anticholinergic drugs, e.g. ipratropium. (See modes of drug action p. 78.) These drugs give quick relief and act for a number of hours. One or two puffs can be given at one time up to a maximum of 12 puffs per 24 hours. Corticosteroids such as beclomethasone dipropionate can be administered by aerosol and have a very potent topical anti-inflammatory activity without the side-effects associated with oral therapy. Beclomethasone dipropionate has a preventative action and should therefore be taken at regular intervals, e.g. 2 puffs 4 times daily. If a patient is having concurrent bronchodilator therapy and corticosteroid therapy, the bronchodilator should be taken first, as the dilator effect will increase the effectiveness of the corticosteroid therapy. *Candida albicans* infection of the mouth, pharynx and larynx is the most common side-effect associated with continuous use of beclomethasone dipropionate aerosol. The incidence is dose-related occurring more often in patients on higher doses. The infection may spontaneously resolve, may clear on dosage reduction with or without combined treatment with topical nystatin or amphotericin B. Huskiness of the voice is a common side-effect.

Sodium cromoglycate is also available in aerosol form. This drug acts prophylactically by preventing the release of mediators which cause allergic or asthmatic attacks. It should be given when the patient's condition is stable, and should *not* be given to treat an attack since it is not a bronchodilator. Sodium cromoglycate has very few side-effects.

With the exception of the 'Nebuhaler', aerosol inhalers are easily carried in the pocket or handbag, helping the patient to be independent. Nurses supervising patients using this type of device should observe discreetly the patient's inhaling technique but avoid giving any impression of hurrying him in the process. The patient requires to concentrate on what he is doing at this time and so cannot engage in conversation. The same advice applies to the dry powder inhaler.

Dry powder inhaler. For those who cannot co-ordinate aerosol inhalation, alternative methods of administration include a dry powder inhaler (e.g. Rotahaler — salbutamol or beclomethasone dipropionate, Spinhaler — sodium cromoglycate). Gelatine capsules containing the active drug, diluted with a suitable inert powder such as lactose, are placed in this small hand-held device which is twisted to break the capsule. With the mouth placed on the mouthpiece, the patient inhales through the device causing drug particles to be entrained and drawn into the respiratory system. No co-ordination of hand movement and breathing is required. Young children can be trained to use these dry powder systems but they should be encouraged to use aerosols as soon as they are old enough to do so. It should be remembered that twice as much drug from a dry powder inhaler is needed for the same effect compared with an aerosol. For the chronic asthmatic or bronchitic who is very breathless, a dry powder inhaler may be easier to use than a pressurised aerosol but it is particularly in these patients that wet nebulisers should be considered.

Wet nebuliser (Fig. 6.16). A high-pressure gas source (air or oxygen) is used to suck up the bronchodilator from a reservoir. In order to produce particles of the correct size, a flow-rate of 8 litres per minute is required. Nurses may find that this rate has to be reduced slightly if it cannot be tolerated by the patient.

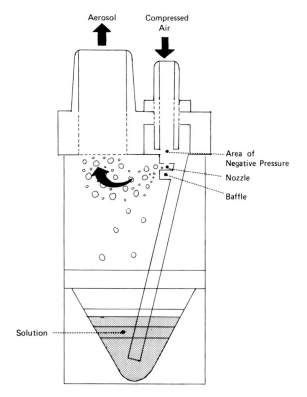

Fig. 6.16 Wet nebuliser

The particles produced impinge on a baffle. Particles of the correct size pass on and are breathed in by the patient, while larger particles fall back to be nebulised again.

After the respirator solution has been nebulised, a proportion remains in the nebuliser chamber. This is because a nebuliser has a 'dead space' i.e. a quantity of the respirator solution has to be nebulised to fill this space before the particles start to leave the nebuliser and achieve a therapeutic effect. Depending on the design of the nebuliser this volume of solution may be 1–2 ml and for the nebuliser to function efficiently it must have a starting volume of fluid of not less than 4 ml. In order to achieve this volume, sufficient sterile 0.9% w/v sodium chloride solution must be added to the bronchodilator solution(s). 0.9% w/v sodium chloride solution is chosen since it is isotonic, non-irritant and compatible with commercially available bronchodilator solutions.

Examples of regimens are as follows:

Sympathomimetics
(see p. 77)

Terbutaline respirator solution 0.5–1 ml made up to 4 ml with 0.9% sodium chloride solution
or
Salbutamol respirator solution 1–2 ml made up to 4 ml with 0.9% sodium chloride solution
or

Anticholinergics
(see p. 77)

Ipratropium solution 0.5–2 ml made up to 4 ml with 0.9% sodium chloride solution
or
a combination of sympathomimetic and anticholinergic solutions.

These regimens are normally for 4 hourly administration but this may be varied depending on the patient's condition. Some drugs, e.g. ipratropium, are given hourly in severe chronic obstructive airways disease. Each patient should be allocated his own nebuliser and mask for use on repeated occasions. The mask may be wiped at intervals and the nebuliser should be rinsed and dried after use to maintain efficiency. Both mask and nebuliser are disposed of completely when treatment is finally discontinued.

Compliance

Compliance is more likely to be achieved if the patient is well informed. As well as knowing how to use the inhaler, the dose to be taken, the time interval and the maximum number of inhalations which should be taken in 24 hours, the patient is more likely to co-operate if he knows something about the disease, the purpose of therapy, how to recognise deterioration in his condition and what to do if deterioration is suspected. It is the responsibility of doctors, nurses and pharmacists to promote understanding of the technique involved by teaching, demonstrating with the aid of a placebo inhaler and checking the patient's performance at intervals (Fig. 6.17). On this basis, alterations in the choice of device may be made so that the patient derives maximum benefit.

Administration of steam and medicated inhalations

Decongestants such as steam and menthol may be helpful when breathed in from a Nelson-type inhaler. The greatest care must be taken to prevent the patient from scalding himself while receiving an inhalation. Some health authorities stipulate that all patients must be supervised throughout the procedure. In any situation, nurses must make a careful

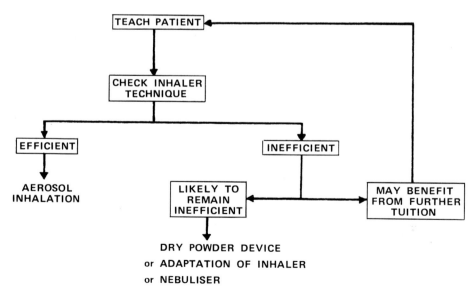

Fig. 6.17 System for checking inhaler technique

assessment of the patient's capabilities and take every possible precaution to avoid such an accident. Psychiatric and mentally handicapped patients, the elderly and children, must be closely supervised, as should any patient who is weak, fevered or suffering from cerebral hypoxia.

Requirements
Nelson's inhaler complete with protective cover and bowl
Sterilised mouthpiece (glass or disposable)
Gauze swab and $\frac{1}{2}$ inch adhesive
Medication as prescribed, e.g. tincture of benzoin compound, menthol crystals.
Hot, not boiling water.
Sputum carton, paper tissues and disposal bag
Prescription sheet.

Preparation of the equipment. It is important to check that the mouthpiece is not chipped or cracked before neatly wrapping round it a gauze swab which is then secured with tape. Before use, the inhaler is preheated with hot water.

Preparation of the patient. The patient is told what is involved. He is then assisted into an upright position leaning forward, well supported with a backrest and pillows, or better still, if his condition permits, assisted into a supporting chair. His shoulders should be kept warm. A bed table is placed in front of him at a suitable height with a sputum carton, paper tissues and disposal bag within reach.

Preparation of the inhalation. The warmed inhaler is refilled with hot water to below the level of the air inlet. The details of the prescription are checked. For medicated inhalations, 5 ml tincture of benzoin compound is put into the warmed inhaler before the hot water is added. When menthol is used, one medium-sized crystal is added to the already prepared inhalation at the bedside. The gauze-covered mouthpiece is firmly secured to face in the opposite direction to the air inlet.

Administration of the inhalation. The inhaler complete with protective cover is placed in a bowl on the bed table with the air inlet away from the patient. Instructions are given to the patient to apply the lips to the covered

mouthpiece, to breathe in through the mouth and breathe out through the nose. It is important to encourage and assist the patient to expectorate as required. After 5–10 minutes when the inhalation is no longer effective the patient is made comfortable and the equipment cleared away.

Completing the procedure. The inhaler is washed and dried using soap and water. Stains from tincture of benzoin compound can be removed with industrial methylated spirit. Care should be taken to clean and pack the mouthpiece carefully for re-autoclaving. A record is made of the administration of the inhalation.

MEDICAL GASES

Medical gases are used extensively in acute hospitals and to a limited extent in the community. Because of their physical characteristics, gases require to be stored under pressure. This demands the use of special apparatus and techniques. Medical gases are supplied from either cylinders or bulk tanks.

Cylinders
In order to maintain safety standards, cylinders must be manufactured to British Standards Institution and Home Office specifications which cover all aspects of design, type of metal, thickness of wall etc. In addition, specifications are laid down for cylinder valves. Three types are commonly used — bull-nose valves, handwheel valves and pin-index or flush-type valves.

Medical gas cylinders are painted in colours which serve to identify the gas contents. A general classifying colour is used for the cylinder body whereas colours on the cylinder shoulders give an exact identification. The shoulder painting may be in quadrants of different colours to indicate gas mixtures.

Medical gas pipelines and outlets are identified by using bands of the same colours as for cylinders.

Gases are stored in cylinders either as compressed gases (oxygen, helium) or in liquid form (nitrous oxide, carbon dioxide). Any gas can be liquefied by cooling it to a sufficiently

Medical gas cylinder colour code

Gas	Body colour	Shoulder colour
Oxygen	black	white
Nitrogen	grey	black
Oxygen + Carbon dioxide	black	white/grey
Oxygen + Helium	black	white/brown
Carbon dioxide	grey	grey
Air	grey	white/black
Nitrous oxide	blue	blue
Nitrous oxide 50% + Oxygen 50 %	blue	blue/white
Cyclopropane	orange	orange
Helium	brown	brown

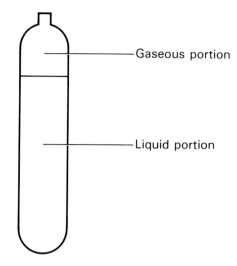

Fig. 6.18 Cylinder containing liquefied gas

low temperature. Alternatively it can be liquefied by compression provided the ambient temperature is below the critical temperature for the gas. The critical temperature is the temperature at which the gas changes to liquid as a result of compression. In filling cylinders, those containing compressed gas are filled from a gas main until the pressure in the cylinder reaches that of the main whereas the quantity of liquefied gas is determined by weighing.

In a cylinder containing liquefied gas (Fig. 6.18), the upper part of the cylinder above the liquefied gas contains compressed gas. When the valve is opened and this discharges, the gas pressure within the cylinder starts to fall. The liquid phase then evaporates into gas and this maintains a continuous supply.

Cylinder manifolds

To obtain high gas flows, a number of cylinders are connected up so that the emissions are combined. This is commonly referred to as a cylinder manifold. The gas can be piped to theatres or wards where it is required and this eliminates the need to have cylinders at the location.

The normal arrangement with cylinder banks is to have a two-armed manifold, each arm carrying the same number of cylinders, e.g. six. One arm is utilised while the other is in reserve. When cylinders on the supply arm are

exhausted, the reserve arm automatically comes into use. The empty cylinders are then replaced. Outlets from pipeline systems are located at convenient positions near beds or in operating theatres. The terminals are identified by gas name and colour which corresponds to the colour coding of the cylinder shoulders.

Bulk tanks

In addition to carrying gas from cylinder banks, pipelines are often used as a means of supplying oxygen from a central storage tank. This greatly reduces cylinder handling. The oxygen is stored in liquefied form at low temperature (between −150°C and −175°C) in a vacuum-insulated tank fitted with a vapouriser. The vapouriser changes the oxygen from liquid to gas which then passes along the pipeline. The storage tank is topped up as required from a bulk tanker.

Safety

Care must be taken in handling equipment under high pressure and in correctly identifying gases in containers which are similar in many respects. Correct identification is aided by the fact that fittings on equipment such as anaesthetic machines and resuscitators will only marry up with valves from cylinders containing the correct gas. This is achieved by methods such as pin- indexing where the valve face has locating holes which will only receive projecting pins corresponding to a particular pattern.

Cylinders should be stored in a clean, dry, well-ventilated location not exposed to extremes of heat or cold. A 50:50 mixture of nitrous oxide and oxygen (Entonox) separates if stored at a temperature below −7°C. Large cylinders should be stored upright on a hard floor and held in position with chains or straps to ensure that they cannot fall over. Smaller, easily portable cylinders are usually stored horizontally on suitable shelving. Because of its highly inflammable nature, a separate storage area is required for cyclopropane.

Cylinders must be handled with care and not dropped or violently struck. When a new cylinder is required, the plastic seal or valve cap is removed and the valve opened slowly and only momentarily in order to blow out any dust or grit which may be situated in the valve port. Index-locating pins on the equipment to be connected should seat easily into the cylinder holes if the fitment is of the correct type. Excessive force should not be used to tighten union nuts or yoke screws. On no account should cylinder valves or fittings be lubricated with oil or grease because of the danger of explosion. In order to measure gas pressure, cylinders are fitted with pressure regulators. Only the correct regulator designated for a particular gas should be used.

A hissing sound indicates a gas leak. A very slow leak, which is inaudible, may be suspected because of loss in pressure when equipment is not in use. In either case the main valve should be shut off and an engineer called as soon as possible. Where inflammable (cyclopropane) or oxidising gases (oxygen, nitrous oxide) are used separately or in combination great care must be taken to avoid ignition. In addition to open flames, hot surfaces, lighted cigarettes, static electrical charges or arcs in running electric motors will initiate combustion.

Commonly used medical gases
The range of gases commonly having medical applications is listed, on page 72.

Compressed air is used extensively to drive ventilators. *Nitrous oxide* is asphyxiating when inhaled in the pure form. When administered with about 20% oxygen, which prevents hypoxia, nitrous oxide induces a rapid but rather shallow anaesthesia. Nitrous oxide/oxygen mixtures containing between 25% and 50% nitrous oxide are useful for analgesia and sedation. For short duration therapy nitrous oxide/oxygen is non-toxic and without any permanent effect on the body since the danger of administration without enough oxygen to avoid hypoxia is well recognised. Nitrous oxide/oxygen should not be administered for periods longer than 24 hours to patients maintained in mechanical ventilators as intensive exposure over long periods may cause bone marrow depression. Nitrous oxide supports combustion and care must be taken in its use.

The discovery that a 50:50 mixture of nitrous oxide and oxygen (Entonox) can be compressed without liquefying the nitrous oxide has greatly increased its use in analgesia, particularly when self-administered, using a demand valve, in obstetrics. This standard mixture can be administered from cylinders with no risk of anoxia or nitrous oxide overdosage.

In air 0.03% carbon dioxide is present. *Carbon dioxide* mixed with air or oxygen in a proportion between 3% and 7% will cause the respiration rate and depth to increase. (Above 50% carbon dioxide the mixture is lethal after inhalation for a short time). Absorbers are used for removing carbon dioxide from recycled gas for rebreathing in anaesthetic or other apparatus. The commonly used absorbing medium is soda lime granules. This usually contains an indicator which changes colour when the soda lime is spent.

Cyclopropane is a potent anaesthetic. In air 15%–25% cyclopropane, or other mixtures, gives deep anaesthesia with muscle relaxation; 7%–10% maintains light anaesthesia. It is a useful induction agent in paediatric and obstetric practice but has lost popularity as a maintenance agent in major surgery because of its explosive properties.

Helium and *nitrogen* are inert medical gases used as diluents for gases such as oxygen. Helium and oxygen mixtures are also used as gases for breathing in deep-water diving to avoid nitrogen narcosis caused by breathing ordinary air at high pressure. Liquid nitrogen causes 'cold burns' when in contact with the skin and is utilised in the treatment of skin warts.

Oxygen which comprises approximately 21% of air, is essential to all forms of animal life. Medical uses of oxygen include:

1. maintaining tissue oxygenation during anaesthesia
2. treatment of diseases including chronic lung disease, myocardial infarction and pulmonary embolism
3. treatment of cardiopulmonary arrest
4. treatment of newborn babies with respiratory distress

Medical oxygen is used outwith hospitals, e.g. in ambulances and in the home. A register is maintained of community pharmacists who stock oxygen cylinders and administration sets. These are supplied on prescription to patients who require to use or have oxygen on standby. Consideration is being given to supplying the more cost-effective oxygen concentrators for domiciliary use to those patients who would otherwise require many cylinders. Clearly, education of the patient and family in the safe use of oxygen in the home is an important aspect of the work of community nurse, doctor and pharmacist.

Administration of oxygen

Oxygen administration is a potentially dangerous procedure and every precaution must be taken to ensure that standards of safety are maintained. All nurses must be able to identify a cylinder of oxygen correctly, i.e. black with a white shoulder and marked with the word OXYGEN. Since the oxygen in cylinders is in compressed form, valves or flowmeters should only be removed by those trained to do so and in accordance with local policy. This noisy procedure should take place outwith patient areas. At all times, cylinders should be supported in a stand so that they cannot be knocked over and stored away from direct heat to prevent explosion. Nurses require to anticipate when a replacement cylinder will be needed, taking into account that there will be a rapid decrease in pressure as the gauge

reaches the empty mark. Sufficient time also needs to be allowed for a new supply to be delivered to the ward. Emergency oxygen equipment should be checked each day.

Oxygen may only be administered on a nurse's own initiative in a life-threatening situation as it has potentially harmful effects on some patients. It should normally be prescribed by a doctor giving its name, the type of appliance to be used (e.g. face mask, nasal cannulae, tent or hood), the choice of mask for delivering the appropriate percentage of oxygen, the flow rate of oxygen (e.g. 4 litres per minute), and the frequency of administration.

Face masks are the commonest method used for administering oxygen. Improvements in materials and design have led to a variety of masks which are lightweight, efficient and for most patients, comfortable, and which allow for easier observation of lip colour. Care must be taken to ensure that the mask fits snugly and that its position is maintained for effective delivery. Redness and sores can result from pressure and chafing from the mask over the bridge of the nose and from the elastic strap over the temporal region and above the ears. When discomfort persists after adjusting the tension of the elastic, this may be relieved by inserting a neat layer of cotton wool between the appliance and the skin. In the course of time, the mask can become moist and sticky and patients appreciate having it removed for a few moments to allow the face and the mask to be wiped clean and dry.

Nasal cannulae have an advantage over face masks in that they do not interfere with feeding and communication. In addition, those patients who experience feelings of claustrophobia with a mask, may find nasal cannulae acceptable. Before inserting nasal cannulae, the patient is asked to blow his nose, or the nostrils should be cleaned with moist cotton-tipped applicators.

Oxygen tents and hoods are used in paediatric wards as very young children do not tolerate oxygen masks. A nurse can do much to help a child overcome feelings of isolation by staying close by and making physical contact with him through the appropriate openings in the apparatus.

Since oxygen supports combustion and can convert a spark into a flame, precautions must be taken in the immediate area of its use. The patient involved, the surrounding patients and any visitors should have these precautions explained to them. *Printed warnings should be in evidence.* Items likely to be of danger should be removed, i.e. matches and cigarette lighters, electric shavers, battery-operated or friction-driven toys. Care should be exercised when bedmaking and combing hair to reduce the risk of sparks created by static electricity.

Periodic observations must be made by the nurse as long as the patient is receiving oxygen. At least every 15 minutes, a check should be made of the patient's colour and respirations, the flow rate of oxygen, the volume of oxygen remaining in the cylinder and the general environment to ensure that safety is being maintained. The patient should be assisted and encouraged to increase his fluid intake to counteract the drying effect of oxygen. For the same reason, the frequency of oral and nasal hygiene should be increased. Clinical signs associated with hypoxia should be noted. These are alterations in the rate and depth of respiration, bounding pulse, high blood pressure, warm clammy skin, lethargy and confusion.

Unless being given at a concentration greater than 40%, oxygen taken through a mask does not require to be humidified, as the air with which it mixes on inspiration contains sufficient water vapour.

Administration of oxygen

Requirements
Oxygen source
Oxygen tubing
Oxygen mask, cannulae, tent or hood
Prescription sheet.

Procedure
1. Check details of prescription. Identify patient.
2. Select appropriate mask or cannulae.
3. If cylinder in use, ensure adequate amount of oxygen.
4. Explain to patient what is involved including necessary precautions.
5. Remove potential hazards from immediate environment.
6. Connect tubing to source and mask or cannulae.
7. Turn the flow meter control knob until top of bobbin or middle of sphere correspond with prescribed rate.
8. Test flow of oxygen on palm of hand.
9. *Mask.* Place mask to fit neatly around nose and mouth, and adjust elastic for patient's comfort.
   Cannulae. Insert cannulae into anterior nares, hook cannulae tubing round patient's ears and adjust toggle to secure tubing.
10. Ensure patient is relaxed and comfortable.
11. Record administration.

REFERENCES

Bochner F, Hooper W D, Tyrer J H, and Edie M J 1972 Factors involving an outbreak of phenytoin intoxication. Journal of Neurological Sciences 16:481
Melander A 1978 Influence of food on the bioavailability of drugs. Clinical pharmacokinetics 3:337
Walker R 1982 The correct insertion of rectal suppositories. British Journal of Pharmaceutical Practice 5: 8–9

FURTHER READING

Peck N 1985 Perfecting your IV therapy techniques. Nursing 85. Part I May p 38–43, Part II June p 48–51, Part III July p 32–35
McMillan E 1984 Oxygen therapy. Nursing Add-on Journal of Clinical Nursing August 2 (28): 822–825
The Royal Marsden Hospital 1984 Manual of clinical nursing policies and procedures. Harper and Row, London
Scholes M E, Wilson J L, Macrae S 1982 Handbook of nursing procedures. Blackwell, Oxford

7 PRINCIPLES OF DRUG ACTION

DISTRIBUTION OF DRUGS AND THEIR BINDING TO PLASMA PROTEINS

When a drug enters the bloodstream it is rapidly diluted and transported throughout the body. Movement from the blood to tissues is influenced by a number of factors which can greatly affect the resultant drug action. Plasma proteins, particularly albumin, can bind many drugs. Only the *unbound* fraction of the drug is free to move from the bloodstream into tissues to exert a pharmacological effect. The bound drug is pharmacologically inactive because the drug–protein complex is unable to cross cell membranes. It provides a reserve of drug since the complex can dissociate and quickly replenish the unbound drug as it is removed from the plasma. The degree of protein binding will thus affect the intensity and duration of a drug's action.

In addition, if a patient suffers from a disease in which plasma proteins are deficient (e.g. liver disease, malnutrition, nephrotic syndrome), more of the drug is free to enter the tissue. A normal dose of a drug could then be dangerous because so little is bound by available protein, thus increasing the transfer of unbound drug to the tissue.

Different drugs may share the same protein-binding site. If two drugs are administered concurrently, the one with higher affinity will be preferentially bound and will displace the drug with lower affinity from the protein-binding site. For example, clofibrate will displace warfarin from protein-binding sites thus increasing the level of free warfarin and potentiating its pharmacological action. This may result in haemorrhage.

Other factors which affect the rate and extent of distribution are cardiac output and regional bloodflow. If the patient is nursed in a warm environment this will help to maintain a better blood circulation and improve drug distribution, an important factor in patients receiving antibiotics. Similarly, inflamed tissues have increased vascularity and permeability which leads to an increased rate of passage of drugs, especially antibiotics.

Should pus build up in the course of an infection to form an abscess, antibiotics may be unable to penetrate this and surgery may be required.

DRUG TRANSFER

Unbound drug is transported in circulating blood to body tissues. To diffuse into these tissues and exert its action, a drug must cross a lipid i.e. fat layer. If the drug is highly fat-soluble, it will pass across and be taken up rapidly by the tissues. The rapid distribution of lipophilic drugs is especially pronounced in the CNS which has the most efficient bloodflow in relation to tissue mass. Because of this, there is an almost immediate onset of general anaesthesia once an anaesthetic agent (e.g. thiopentone sodium) enters the systemic circulation. However, because of its great lipid solubility compared to its solubility in water, thiopentone sodium is also rapidly taken up in fat cells. This transfer is so marked that some hours after administration of the drug, little remains in the bloodstream yet quite a large amount may still be present in the fat. The fat store thus helps to remove the drug from the bloodstream and shortens its action. This will also influence the effect of a second dose of the drug. If the fat stores are already saturated, the drug will not be removed from the bloodstream into the fat and a greater proportion will be free to exert its pharmacological action. This may have a toxic effect.

TRANSFER BARRIERS

Most of the CNS is surrounded by a specialised membrane, that is the blood-brain and blood–cerebrospinal fluid barriers. This membrane is highly selective for lipid-soluble drugs: e.g. the penicillins diffuse well into body tissues and fluids but penetration into the cerebrospinal fluid is poor, except when the meninges are inflamed. Chloramphenicol, because of its lipid solubility, is one of the few antibiotics which reaches the cerebrospinal fluid in appreciable concentrations.

During pregnancy the placenta provides a barrier between mother and fetus. Some drugs cross it relatively easily (e.g. ethanol, chlorpromazine, and morphine), while others (e.g. decamethonium and succinyl choline) are not transferred. Since fetal liver and kidney are unable to metabolise or excrete drugs and the fetus is likely to be more sensitive to them, drugs must be used with caution in pregnancy and in general, few are used.

MODES OF DRUG ACTION

Drugs act by affecting biochemical or physiological processes in the body or by controlling changes in these processes brought about by disease. Some drugs exert an effect because of a specific chemical property; e.g. antacids neutralise gastric acid, ferrous iron is chelated by desferrioxamine in the treatment of iron poisoning, potassium citrate mixture makes the urine alkaline and relieves discomfort in urinary tract infection, docusate softens the faecal mass and relieves constipation. However, in the majority of cases drugs act at specific cell receptors. The magnitude of the response depends on the concentration of the drug at the site of action which in turn depends on dosage, absorption, metabolism and elimination. The drug and receptor form a reversible drug–receptor complex, the response being directly proportional to the amount of complex formed.

A *specific drug* forms a complex with only one type of receptor but may produce multiple effects due to the location of this receptor in cells of different organs or tissues, e.g. atropine causes paralysis of ocular accommodation, dilatation of the pupil, increase in heart rate, decreased production of saliva, sweat and gastrointestinal secretions and decreased intestinal motility.

A *selective drug* acts at a receptor in a particular tissue at concentrations which produce little effect on similar receptors in other organs. Selective beta 2 adrenoceptor agonist bronchodilators such as salbutamol and terbutaline show specific selectivity for beta 2 receptors in bronchial smooth muscle and at therapeutic doses cause little or no stimulation to the beta 1 adrenoceptors in the heart. This selectivity is greater when these drugs are inhaled into the lungs than when given orally or by injection. Isoprenaline is less selective. It causes bronchodilatation by stimulating the beta 2 adrenoceptors but also causes cardiac stimulation due to its effect on the beta 1 adrenoceptor. The effects of chemical transmitters are summarised in Tables 7.1 and 7.2.

METABOLISM OF DRUGS

As has been previously noted, drugs dissolve in gastric fluid and in order to diffuse across membranes they must be lipid-soluble. The higher solubility in lipid compared to its aqueous solubility (lipid/water coefficient), the more rapidly the drug diffuses into the tissues. When drugs pass through the kidney, lipid-soluble drugs are reabsorbed at the distal tubule and return to the plasma. To get rid of these drugs the body must metabolise them into compounds which are less lipid-soluble and more water-soluble. These metabolites are not reabsorbed at the distal tubule and are excreted in the urine (Fig. 7.1).

The rate of metabolism will determine the duration of action of the drug. Metabolites formed are usually, but not always, less active than the parent compound. A few drugs are made active by metabolism, e.g. talampicillin is the pro-drug for ampicillin and the cytotoxic agent cyclophosphamide is the pro-drug for several metabolites which produce the phar-

Table 7.1A Specific actions of sympathetic nervous system chemical transmitters: noradrenaline + adrenaline from adrenal medulla (main actions only are given; adrenaline only active when given by injection)

Adrenaline

alpha effects	beta 1 effects	beta 2 effects
Vasoconstriction of arterioles — blood pressure rises Dilation of pupil Relaxation of gut	Acceleration of heart rate Increased force of contraction of heart	Dilation of blood vessels in muscle Bronchodilation Muscle glucose release
Bronchoconstriction		
Sphincter constriction in gastrointestinal tract and bladder		

Table 7.1B Drugs affecting the sympathetic nervous system

Drug groups	Drug	Actions
Sympathomimetics (mimic action of sympathetic system)	adrenaline	alpha beta 1 beta 2
Range of activity will vary. Drugs with more selective action now available	isoprenaline salbutamol, terbutaline, fenoterol etc.	beta 1 beta 2 beta 2
Alpha adrenoceptor blocking drugs	prazosin	Blocks alpha effects of adrenaline causing vasodilation
Beta-adrenoceptor blocking drugs (Beta-blockers)	propranolol	Blocks the beta 1 and beta 2 actions of adrenaline
This group of drugs has been introduced for the treatment of hypertension. They relieve the symptoms of angina pectoris and are beneficial in the secondary prevention of myocardial infarction	oxprenolol, pindolol, acebutolol metoprolol, atenolol	More selective. Act to block beta 1 effects of adrenaline — less bradycardia More selective — less effect on airway resistance

macological effect. Many drugs including imipramine, propranolol, and diazepam are themselves active but also have active metabolites which contribute to the overall effects of the drug. Diamorphine is an active narcotic which is converted to morphine which has approximately half the narcotic activity of its parent compound. Morphine is further metabolised to inactive products.

The main site of drug metabolism is the liver but other tissues may also metabolise drugs, e.g. lungs, kidneys, blood, and intestine. Isoprenaline is metabolised in the gut wall, therefore it must be given sublingually or by injection. In order to make them more water-soluble, some drugs undergo a variety of

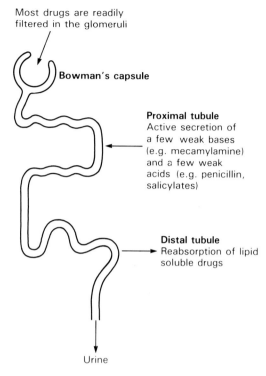

Fig. 7.1 Filtration of drugs through the kidney tubule

Table 7.2A Specific actions of parasympathetic nervous system chemical transmitter: acetylcholine (destroyed by the enzyme cholinesterase)

Muscarinic effects	Nicotinic effects
Depression of cardiac activity, bradycardia Vasodilation Tonic action on smooth muscle Lachrymal, salivary, sweating, gastric secretions increased	Stimulant of skeletal muscle Stimulant of autonomic ganglia and adrenal medulla

Table 7.2B Drugs affecting the parasympathetic nervous system

Drug groups	Drug	Actions
Parasympathomimetics (mimic action of the parasympathetic system)	carbachol	Muscarinic and nicotinic Lowers intra-ocular pressure by opening the inefficient drainage channels resulting from contraction or spasm of the ciliary muscle Increases muscle contraction of bladder and may relieve urinary retention Side-effects — sweating, bradycardia, intestinal colic
	pilocarpine	Muscarinic Relieves glaucoma as for carbachol
	bethanechol	Muscarinic Relieves urinary retention
Anticholinesterase drugs (block the action of cholinesterase thus prolonging the action of acetylcholine in the body)	neostigmine	Muscarinic and nicotinic Used to treat myasthenia gravis
	distigmine	Muscarinic and nicotinic but more prolonged than neostigmine
Anticholinergic drugs	atropine	Blocks all actions of acetylcholine secretions, dilates pupils
	glycopyrronium bromide	Side-effects — tachycardia, constipation, unable to micturate

chemical reactions, e.g. oxidation, reduction, or hydrolysis, of which oxidation is by far the most important. Other drugs are conjugated with naturally occurring substances such as glucuronic acid, sulphate, or glycine. A number of drugs undergo chemical reaction and conjugation.

The metabolism of drugs in the liver is influenced by enzymes, whose activity can be increased, giving more rapid metabolism, or decreased, slowing metabolism, by a wide variety of drugs and chemicals. Barbiturates, phenytoin, and rifampicin increase the amount of enzyme that increases metabolism of corticosteroids. Thus larger doses of corticosteroids require to be administered. This process, known as enzyme induction, is responsible for much of the tolerance which develops with chronic drug administration. Should a patient be on concurrent therapy of an enzyme inducer and warfarin, he will need a higher than normal dose of warfarin to give the desired degree of anticoagulation. Cessation of the inducer drug without a corresponding lowering of the warfarin dose could result in haemorrhage. If a patient is taking oral contraceptives, the oestrogen and progestogen may be rapidly degraded when there is enzyme induction and the level of steroids may be insufficient to give a contraceptive effect. Patients who are taking oral contraceptives and are prescribed enzyme inducing drugs should be warned of the consequences and advised to use barrier methods of contraception.

Heavy cigarette smoking causes enzyme induction that results in faster metabolism of theophylline. (Ogilvie, 1978). Heavy smokers therefore require a higher dose of theophylline.

Conversely, drugs such as isoniazid and chloramphenicol inhibit the enzymes involved in the metabolism of phenytoin. Concurrent therapy would result in phenytoin toxicity if the dose of phenytoin is not lowered to take this factor into account. Patients in a state of malnutrition, or who have liver disease, suffer from a reduced rate of drug metabolism because their enzyme function is inadequate. The ability to metabolise drugs is reduced in the very young and for some drugs in the elderly.

The rate of metabolism for the same drug may vary between individuals because of genetic or racial factors. Isoniazid undergoes conjugation with acetyl coenzyme A to form acetylated isoniazid. This proceeds at different rates in different individuals, over half the population being slow acetylators and the remainder fast acetylators. The fast acetylators will require a higher dose than the slow acetylators in order to give an equivalent therapeutic effect. Other drugs which are acetylated such as procainamide, phenelzine and hydrallazine will be affected similarly.

DRUG EXCRETION

Most drugs are excreted by the kidney, either unchanged or after metabolism. Most drugs are lipid-soluble and will be reabsorbed at the distal tubule when they pass through the kidney. They must therefore be metabolised before elimination. Examples of drugs eliminated unchanged by active secretion at the proximal tubule include penicillin, digoxin, and salicylates (see Fig. 7.1).

The rate of excretion varies greatly between drugs, some being excreted within an hour or two and others taking days or weeks. The elimination of penicillin can be delayed with probenecid, which inhibits the active secretion of penicillin at the proximal tubule thus prolonging its antibacterial action. It should be noted that if renal function is impaired, drugs which are primarily excreted unchanged or as active metabolites will be eliminated more slowly. This will have important consequences if the usual dosage is not reduced, since the plasma level of the drug will rise and may produce toxic effects, e.g. high plasma levels of gentamicin are nephrotoxic and ototoxic.

In some cases the rate of excretion can be increased (e.g. by altering urinary pH.) Aspirin excretion can be increased by the administration of sodium bicarbonate which raises the urinary pH. Advantage is taken of this in the treatment of salicylate poisoning.

Although the kidney is the major pathway for excretion of drugs and their metabolites, other organs will excrete drugs too. Neomycin which

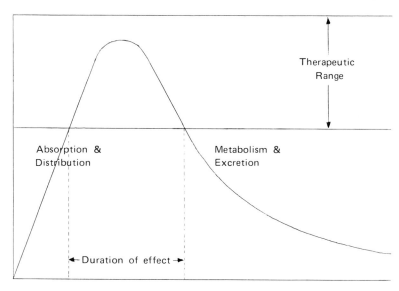

Therapeutic
Range

Absorption &
Distribution

Metabolism &
Excretion

←Duration of effect→

Fig. 7.2 Effects of absorption, distribution, metabolism and excretion on the plasma concentration of an administered drug

is used for sterilisation of the large intestine when taken orally, is not absorbed and is eliminated in the faeces. General anaesthetics such as nitrous oxide and halothane are eliminated from the lungs. Some drugs and drug metabolites are excreted into the bile. Ampicillin and rifampicin are excreted in high concentrations in the bile, so they may be utilised in a biliary tract infection. Certain drugs, undergo enterohepatic circulation. (e.g. indomethacin and oestrogens). They are excreted in the bile, enter the gastrointestinal tract, and are subsequently absorbed from the intestine before returning to the circulation.

DOSE/EFFECT RELATIONSHIP

Safe and effective therapy can be achieved only with doses which produce optimal concentrations of a drug in the plasma and target tissues. Smaller doses will be ineffective and larger doses will not increase the benefits and may have toxic effects. Between the minimal dose which gives the required therapeutic response and the dose at which toxic symptoms appear is a dose range called the therapeutic dose range. Some drugs have a narrow range whereas others have a wide therapeutic range.

After administration of a drug, its plasma

level rises; the more rapidly the drug is absorbed, the faster its plasma level rises (Fig. 7.2).

As drug absorption decreases, and distribution, metabolism, and excretion rates increase, the curve reaches a peak. It then descends as elimination occurs more rapidly than absorption. As we have previously noted, the route of administration influences the time taken for the drug to reach maximal concentration. This is fastest with an intravenous injection, and slower with intramuscular and subcutaneous injections and oral doses.

As the dose of a drug is increased, its therapeutic effect increases as more receptors are occupied. Eventually the dose is reached that produces a maximal effect when all the receptors of the target organs are occupied by drug molecules. Increasing the dose further will therefore not increase the therapeutic effect.

HALF-LIFE OF DRUGS

The rate at which drugs are eliminated from plasma is commonly expressed in terms of the drug's half-life ($t\frac{1}{2}$). This is the time required for the concentration of the drug in the plasma to decrease to one half of its initial value. The half life of gentamicin is two hours. If the plasma concentration is measured and found to be 8

μg per ml, 2 hours later (one half-life) the level will be half, i.e. 4 μg per ml.

The plasma concentration of a drug at one half-life is 50% of its initial value, at two half-lives 25%, at three half-lives 12.5%, at four half-lives 6.25% and at five half-lives is just over 3%. If we take our original gentamicin concentration of 8 μg per ml, after one half-life (2 hours) the concentration will be 4 μg per ml, after two half-lives (4 hours) 2 μg per ml, after three half-lives (6 hours) 1 μg per ml, after four half-lives (8 hours) 0.5 μg per ml and after five half-lives (10 hours) 0.25 μg per ml. Thus most of a drug (almost 97%) is eliminated in five half-lives regardless of the dose or route of administration.

This rule of thumb can be applied in calculating the time required to elapse when discontinuing one drug and starting another which may interact if given in conjunction with the first. It is also useful in estimating how long it will take a toxic plasma concentration (after overdosing) to clear from the body.

Half-lives of different drugs vary widely, e.g. the $t\frac{1}{2}$ of theophylline is 3 hours, $t\frac{1}{2}$ of aspirin is 6 hours, $t\frac{1}{2}$ of metronidazole is 9 hours, $t\frac{1}{2}$ of digoxin is about 36 hours and $t\frac{1}{2}$ of phenobarbitone is about 5 days. A short half-life may result from extensive tissue uptake, rapid metabolism, or rapid excretion and a long half-life may be the consequence of extensive plasma protein binding, slow metabolism, or poor excretion. The knowledge of half-lives of drugs is essential in determining the intervals between drug doses.

Certain conditions can be treated with a single dose of medication (e.g. analgesics for a headache). Many conditions, however, require continuous drug action (e.g. diabetes mellitus, infections, arthritis). This can be achieved through the administration of repeated doses at regular intervals. In such therapy the second, third and subsequent doses will add to whatever remains of the previous dose causing gradual accumulation until stable concentrations are maintained (Fig. 7.3.).

The level of drug in the plasma rises after absorption, reaches a peak, then falls to minimal effective concentration. Administration of the next dose raises the drug concentration to a peak. The concentration falls as the drug is metabolised and excreted, then rises again after the next dose. If the interval between doses is too long or the dose too small the plasma concentration will have fallen below the therapeutic range before the next dose is given. As a result the drug concentration is within the therapeutic range only for short intervals.

If a drug is administered too frequently or in too high a dose the plasma concentration will rise above the therapeutic range and may give

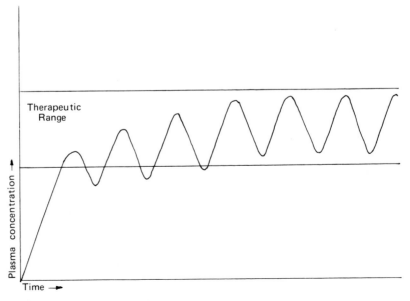

Fig. 7.3 Concentration of drug at appropriate time intervals

rise to toxic effects. In theory, the optimal dosage interval between drug administrations is equal to the half-life of the drug. Initially the drug accumulates in the body. If 100 mg of drug is given with a half-life of 6 hours, when the second dose of 100 mg is given 6 hours later, 50 mg of the original dose will still be present in the body giving a total of 150 mg. After a further 6 hours, 75 mg will remain when the third dose of 100 mg is administered, giving a total of 175 mg. At the next dose, 88 mg remains giving a total of 188 mg. As can be seen, the rate of accumulation becomes less between doses, i.e. 50 mg after second dose, 25 mg after third dose, 13 mg after fourth dose and, in practical terms, a steady state maximal concentration is reached after approximately five doses. In the steady state the plasma level rises and falls between doses but remains within the therapeutic range — the quantity of drug supplied by each dose is equal to the amount eliminated between doses.

The time required to reach a steady concentration depends on the half-life of the drug. The shorter the half-life the faster the steady state is reached, irrespective of the route of administration. Aspirin, with a half-life of 6 hours, will reach equilibrium in five half-lives, i.e. 30 hours.

A dosing interval equal to the half-life of a drug may be impractical for drugs with very short half-lives. Penicillin would have to be given every 30 minutes. This would be inconvenient (if not impossible) for the patient and would lead to poor compliance. Penicillin, however, has a wide therapeutic range and high doses are relatively non-toxic, so that much higher doses can be given every 6–8 to hours compared with the dose that would be given every 30 minutes. This ensures that the therapeutic level in the blood is maintained until the next dose. Short half-life drugs, such as lignocaine, which have a narrow therapeutic range must be given by intravenous infusion since larger doses given infrequently would cause toxic effects.

Most drugs obey a simple relationship between steady state concentration and dose. Usually the dose and steady state concentration are directly proportional; if the dose is doubled, the steady state concentration doubles. For some drugs however, the rate of clearance decreases with increasing serum concentrations (e.g. phenytoin, aspirin). When dosages of these drugs are increased, steady state concentrations increase more than expected. There are also drugs with the opposite effect, i.e. clearance increases with increasing concentration (e.g. disopyramide, valproic acid). In these cases, increased dosages will produce a smaller than expected increase in steady state concentration.

LOADING DOSE

In certain conditions it is desirable to reach an effective level of drug in the blood without waiting for accumulation to take place (e.g. if a patient has an infection and requires antibiotic treatment). This can be achieved by giving the patient an initial dose which is twice the maintenance dose. The effective blood concentration is reached after the first dose (e.g. 500 mg) and maintained during subsequent dosing intervals by giving appropriate doses (e.g. 250 mg). With a drug which has a long half-life this regimen is impractical and may be dangerous. It is usually better to allow gradual accumulation following the usual dose and dosage intervals. The patient will then reach his individual steady state concentration in due course.

APPLICATION OF PHARMACOKINETICS

Pharmacokinetics is defined as the study of the absorption, distribution, metabolism and elimination of drugs in humans. Knowledge of how much of the dose is absorbed and bound to proteins and how fast the drug is cleared from the body is helpful in establishing dosage schedules that are likely to produce the desired plasma concentrations, thus minimising the risk of ineffectiveness due to underdosing, or toxicity due to overdosing. For a number of drugs effectiveness can be measured by clinical response. The measurement of blood pressure will indicate the therapeutic response to an antihypertensive drug, the effect of an analgesic can be subjectively measured, and response to a hypoglycaemic drug can be calculated from blood sugar levels. However, the response to many other drugs is difficult to assess quickly by clinical methods. An approach utilising pharmacokinetics can be followed. This is especially important for drugs which have a narrow therapeutic range, in other words where a small variation from the optimal dose is either ineffective or causes toxicity. Such drugs include digoxin, lithium, phenytoin, theophylline, gentamicin, lignocaine.

The total quantity of drug appearing in the body after administration depends on the dose and the route of administration. When a drug is given intravenously, the total dose will appear in the circulation. If A_b is the amount of drug in the circulation and D is the dose injected intravenously then $A_b = D$.

When drugs are given by other routes, the amount reaching the circulation will be less than the total dose since, depending on its bioavailability, only some of it will be absorbed and part of this may be broken down by first-pass metabolism in the liver. In these cases only a proportion of the dose (F) will be available systemically. To calculate the amount available to exert a therapeutic effect the dose (D) is multiplied by F.

From the literature F for digoxin is 0.62, therefore if 250 μg digoxin tablets are given then the amount in the body (A_b) which will give a clinical response can be calculated.

$A_b = F \times D$
   $= (0.62 \times 250)\ \mu g$
   $= 155\ \mu g$

Volume of distribution
The volume of distribution (V) of a drug is a term which relates the plasma concentration of a drug to the amount of drug in the body. V is determined by the lipid and water solubilities of the drug, plasma protein and tissue protein binding,and the degree and rate of perfusion of tissues. Factors that tend to keep the drug in plasma, such as low lipid solubility, extensive binding to plasma protein, or decreased tissue binding, reduce the apparent volume of distribution (e.g. that of penicillins and warfarin). Factors that tend to keep the

drug outside the vascular space such as decreased plasma protein binding, increased lipid solubility and increased tissue binding, increase the apparent volume of distribution (e.g. that of digoxin and antihistamines).

The concept of the volume of distribution (V) is useful in calculating loading doses or in predicting the initial plasma concentration after the administration of a given dose.

Examples
1. What dose of aminophylline should be given by intravenous bolus injection to achieve a plasma concentration of 15 mg/litre in a 50 kg person?
85% of aminophylline is metabolised to the active theophylline.
From the literature V for theophylline = 0.45 litres/kg
Therefore for this patient V = 0.45 × 50 = 22.5 litres
To achieve a level of 15 mg/litre in 22.5 litres a dose of 15 × 22.5 mg, i.e. 337.5 mg of theophylline. Since only 85% of aminophylline is converted to theophylline then the dose of aminophylline required is $\frac{100}{85} \times \frac{337.5}{1}$ mg = 397 mg (i.e. approx. 400 mg).

2. What peak plasma concentration would be obtained after administering a single dose of 160 mg gentamicin intravenously to a 80 kg person?
Since the drug is given by intravenous injection the amount in the body (A_b) will equal the dose.
The concentration in the plasma (C_p) will be equal to the dose divided by the volume of distribution, i.e. $C_p = \frac{A_b}{V}$

From the literature V for gentamicin = 0.25 litres/kg
Therefore for this patient
V = 80 × 0.25 = 20 litres
$C_p = \frac{A_b}{V}$
   $= \frac{160}{20}$ mg/litre
   $= 8$ mg/litre

Drug elimination
After administration of a drug the body will begin to eliminate it. If the level of drug in the plasma is measured at intervals after administration, it will be found to decrease as it is eliminated from the body. From this information can be calculated the rate (k) at which the drug is eliminated. This rate will be related to the drug's half-life ($t\frac{1}{2}$). Drugs which have a longer half-life will have a slower rate of elimination and vice versa, i.e. a drug with a half-life of 4 hours will be eliminated twice as quickly as a drug with a half-life of 8 hours. Using this information the plasma concentration (C_p) can be calculated at any given time after drug administration using the equation:

C_p = Original concentration $\times$ e^{-kt}

where

k = elimination rate constant
e = base of natural logarithms = 2.72
t = time during drug elimination

Multiple dosing

When medications are given on a continuous basis e.g. by infusion or by the oral route, after approximately five half-lives of the drug an average steady state plasma concentration is reached. The doses required to give the optimal steady state concentration can be calculated using pharmacokinetic principles. The process is monitored by measuring drug levels in blood samples.

Blood sampling

In order to interpret plasma levels of a drug properly, it is necessary to take blood samples at appropriate times in relation to the dosage schedule. Ideally these samples should be taken under the following conditions:

1. The patient has received the drug for a duration of time equal to five half-lives in order that a steady state concentration has been achieved. Each time the dosage is altered a steady state concentration will be achieved after five half-lives.
2. In the case of a drug which is eliminated slowly, (e.g. digoxin), blood samples, if taken too soon after a dose, tend to give high readings since it is rapidly absorbed and reaches high concentrations in the blood, before distributing more slowly into various tissues. Digoxin readings should be taken 7–8 hours after administration.
3. If the drug is rapidly eliminated (e.g. gentamicin, theophylline) two blood samples may be required in order to measure the peak and trough concentrations. This is advisable for drugs which have a narrow therapeutic range as a slightly low dose will be ineffective and a slightly high dose will be toxic. Plasma concentrations of gentamicin are measured approximately 1 hour after an intramuscular injection or 20 minutes after an intravenous injection and also just before the next dose. In order to avoid toxic effects peak levels of gentamicin should not be greater than 12 μg/ml and trough levels should not be greater than 2 μg/ml.

THE EFFECT OF PATHOLOGICAL STATE AND BIOLOGICAL VARIABILITY

Prediction of dosage can be greatly aided by the use of pharmacokinetic parameters. It should be emphasised that these parameters can vary when drug absorption, distribution, metabolism or elimination are abnormal because of age, genetic factors, functional state of the kidney, heart or liver, or the severity of the disease process affected by other drugs taken concurrently. Consequently, in some individuals the average or usual dose of a drug may result in plasma levels that are either too low and cannot produce the desired therapeutic effect, or are too high and produce toxic effects.

Liver disease

The liver is the main organ of metabolism for many drugs and any disease process that results in damage of liver cells, slowing of hepatic blood flow, or decrease in plasma protein may raise plasma concentrations of many drugs. Toxicity of most drugs is related to their elevated concentration in plasma resulting from a decrease in the rate of metabolism. This occurs in hepatic disease. It may therefore be necessary to avoid certain drugs (e.g. lignocaine) or to reduce doses (e.g. of propranolol, aminophylline, chlormethiazole) and monitor plasma concentrations. Severe liver disease results in a low level of albumin in blood. Drugs which have a high degree of protein binding, such as phenytoin and prednisone, will be bound to a smaller extent and consequently there will be more free drug available which may give rise to toxic effects. There will also be a reduction in the hepatic synthesis of blood clotting factors and this is indicated by a prolonged prothrombin time. Anticoagulants (e.g. warfarin) should therefore be avoided.

Chronic alcoholism induces microsomal oxidation enzymes which participate in the metabolism of certain drugs (e.g. theophylline). When these drugs are given in normal doses there will be a more rapid metabolism due to a higher level of enzymes. This will result in inadequate plasma concentrations. The opposite effect will occur in advanced *cirrhosis of the liver*, since the flow of blood through the liver will be impaired. Drugs such as propranolol, pentazocine and pethidine which are extensively metabolised by first-pass metabolism, will therefore reach the tissues in higher concentrations. Dosage should be altered accordingly. Monitoring of plasma concentrations of the drugs may be necessary to prevent overdosage and consequent toxic effects.

Renal disease

Renal disease has the potential to reduce the rate of elimination of drugs. The greater effect will be produced on drugs which are eliminated by the kidney entirely or partially in an unmetabolised form, or where the metabolites are pharmacologically active. As a result, the half-lives of such drugs may be considerably lengthened and plasma concentrations will rise, which will increase the potential for toxicity. Dosage adjustment must take account of the extent of renal impairment and the relative toxicity of increased plasma concentrations. However, if only a small percentage of the drug is excreted by the kidney and the metabolites are not toxic, there will be little risk of accumulation in renal failure.

Based on these considerations no action would be required on drugs such as erythromycin and lignocaine which are eliminated principally after metabolism by the liver. A second group (e.g. benzylpenicillin, ampicillin), have a wide therapeutic range and only in severe renal impairment would dosages require lowering. Certain drugs (e.g. nitrofurantoin, allopurinol) should be avoided as toxicity is caused by their metabolites which accumulate to high concentrations in the plasma of patients with impaired renal function. Drugs with a narrow therapeutic range and which can cause problems of toxicity at plasma concentrations only slightly above those required for a therapeutic effect, must be monitored carefully and require lower dosages in all degrees of renal failure e.g. gentamicin, kanamycin, digoxin, procainamide. The total maintenance dose of a drug can be reduced either by reducing the size of the individual dose or increasing the interval between doses. For some drugs, if the size of the maintenance dose is reduced, it will be important to give a loading dose if an immediate effect is required, since it takes five half-lives to achieve steady state plasma concentrations, otherwise, it may take many days to achieve therapeutic plasma concentrations. Nephrotoxic drugs (e.g. amphotericin, cephaloridine) should be avoided where possible in patients with renal disease.

Altered doses

Since renal impairment results in a decreased capacity of the kidney to eliminate drugs, dosages must be adjusted to achieve drug therapeutic plasma levels.

Severity of renal impairment is expressed in terms of glomerular filtration rate (GFR) also known as creatinine clearance. Creatinine is an end-product of muscle metabolism and is eliminated from the body by the kidney. Creatinine clearance is obtained by measuring the plasma creatinine concentration in a 24 hour collection of urine. Where this is difficult to obtain, the serum creatinine concentration is used. Normal creatinine clearance is 100–120 ml/minute for both men and women. Renal impairment is divided into three grades:

Grade	Glomerular filtration rate (Creatinine clearance)
Mild	20–50 ml/min
Moderate	10–20 ml/min
Severe	< 10 ml/min

Renal function declines with age, and many elderly patients have a glomerular filtration rate less than 50 ml/minute.

If the glomerular filtration rate is only 50% of normal, the half-life of a drug, eliminated in an unchanged form by the kidney, will be doubled. The dose can be adjusted either by being halved or by giving the normal dose at double the time intervals.

For drugs with a narrow therapeutic range, the predicted dosage schedule should be regarded only as a guide to initial treatment. The recommended intramuscular dose for gentamicin is 2–5 mg/kg daily in divided doses every 8 hours. In renal impairment the interval between successive doses should be increased to 12 hours when the creatinine clearance is 30–70 ml/min, to 24 hours when 10–30 ml/minute and to 48 hours when 5–10 ml/min. Predicted dosage schedules should be regarded only as a guide to initial treatment and subsequent treatment must be adjusted according to the clinical response and the serum levels achieved.

SIDE-EFFECTS OF DRUGS

In addition to having a main therapeutic effect, most drugs produce one or more unwanted effects, some of which occur to some degree in all patients; others may occur in some patients and not in others. Side-effects may be short-lived, or can be overcome by reducing dosage, by using alternative drugs, or where severe, by stopping the treatment.

A side-effect occasionally arises secondary to the therapeutic action of a drug. Guanethidine, an antihypertensive drug, is a ganglion-blocking agent preventing the release of adrenaline and noradrenaline. However, it also causes a reduction in cardiac output and reduces the vasoconstriction which normally results from standing up. This results in postural hypotension which causes patients to feel faint. It is more pronounced in the elderly.

Antihistamines, used to treat motion sickness and hay fever, often cause drowsiness. This can be dangerous if the patient has to drive or operate machinery. Newer antihistamines such as terfenadine are much less sedative, probably because they do not cross the blood–brain barrier.

Both magnesium salts and aluminium salts are used as antacids. Magnesium salts also have a laxative action and aluminium salts cause constipation. When an aluminium salt is formulated with a magnesium salt to form a compound mixture or tablet, these opposite effects are overcome. Aspirin, a very useful analgesic, anti-inflammatory and antipyretic drug, may cause bleeding in the stomach. To overcome this it can be taken with or after a meal, as the presence of food in the stomach will accelerate gastric emptying and lower the incidence of this side-effect. Alternatively it can be manufactured with an enteric coating. This will ensure that the aspirin is released in the alkaline medium of the small intestine following passage through the stomach. Diamorphine and morphine are most effective in the treatment of severe pain. However they constrict the pupils, cause sweating and constipation, are addictive and in larger doses cause respiratory depression.

Dosage reduction may be effective in reducing side-effects. Modern oral contraceptives contain lower doses of oestrogen than formerly. This has resulted in lowering the incidence of side-effects. Similarly, corticosteroids are administered by inhaler to treat respiratory problems in much smaller doses than would be required systemically to produce an equivalent therapeutic effect. This has obviated side-effects which would occur with larger doses. Ensuring plasma levels of aminoglycosides are within the therapeutic range, particularly where there is renal impairment, minimises the risk of ototoxicity.

Many older and well-established drugs have well known side-effects such as rashes (penicillins) or dry mouth (atropine). More modern drugs used in cancer chemotherapy are notorious for most unpleasant side-effects such as nausea and alopecia. However, the pharmaceutical industry constantly tries to improve formulations to minimise these effects and in conjunction with academic research, new effective drugs with minimal adverse effects are being sought.

DRUG TOLERANCE

This term refers to a diminished response to the same dose of a drug which is taken regularly. In order to achieve a satisfactory therapeutic effect the dose must be increased. Diamorphine and morphine, for example, induce tolerance to such an extent that the doses must be continuously increased to many times their initial level in order to control pain The exact mechanism of tolerance is not known but it may be due to a blocking action of a chemical which triggers drug receptors, or induces synthesis of liver microsomal enzymes involved in drug biotransformation.

ALLERGY (HYPERSENSITIVITY)

Drug allergy is becoming more common with increasing multiple drug therapy and is responsible for a large proportion of adverse drug reactions. A proportion of the population is more susceptible to allergic reactions. Almost any drug can produce hypersensitivity but in practice the penicillins are most commonly involved. This allergic reaction requires previous exposure to the drug itself, or to a closely related drug, which results in the formation of antibodies in the blood. On subsequent occasions when the drug is given, it reacts with these antibodies and chemicals, such as histamine, are released and cause an allergic reaction.

ANAPHYLACTIC SHOCK

This term describes several different clinical syndromes, all severe, life-threatening, and of rapid onset. The patient who may feel faint, cold, and clammy, is pale and cyanosed with weakening pulse; to this may be added bronchospasm, (sometimes extremely severe), while other less serious features include flushing, nasal congestion, rhinorrhoea, urticaria, and hoarseness. The incidence of these serious reactions is low but in their rarity lies danger. It is most likely to occur after parenteral, rather than oral, administration of certain drugs such as antibiotics, iron injections, anti-inflammatory analgesics, heparin, hyposensitising preparations and neuromuscular blocking drugs. Other agents capable of precipitating anaphylactic shock include blood products, vaccines and insect stings.

In order to avoid possible interaction the patient should be asked if he is currently taking any other drugs. A history of the patient may reveal previous allergies such as occur in asthma, hay fever, eczema or adverse reactions to other drug injections.

First-line treatment includes restoration of blood pressure, laying the patient flat, raising the feet and administering intramuscularly 0.5–1 ml of adrenaline injection 1 in 1000 (0.5–1 mg), repeated every 15 minutes until improvement occurs. Following the adrenaline injection, antihistamines such as chlorpheniramine are given by slow intravenous injection and continued for 24–48 hours to prevent relapse. Since the onset of action of corticosteroids takes several hours they are only used to prevent further deterioration in severely affected patients. Some patients with severe allergy to insect stings may be advised to carry adrenaline inhalations or syringes prefilled with adrenaline solution.

IDIOSYNCRASY

Idiosyncrasy is an abnormal reaction which occurs due to a genetic abnormality. It may alter the normal metabolic pathways of drugs and produce serious adverse reactions in certain individuals. Unlike drug allergy, this response does not require previous sensitisation. Two examples illustrate this condition. Patients with a deficiency of a red blood cell enzyme, glycose-6-phosphate dehydrogenase, suffer haemolytic anaemia when administered e.g. sulphonamides or nitrofurantoin. A deficiency in the enzyme cholinesterase greatly prolongs the action of the muscle relaxant suxamethonium.

PROLONGATION OF DRUG ACTION

Because most drugs are absorbed, then cleared from the body fairly quickly, therapeutic effects are maintained for a relatively short time. In order to prolong the therapeutic effect, the drug must be administered frequently or by constant infusion. It may be desirable to reduce the frequency of dosage (e.g. where compliance is poor) or to simplify regimens where a number of drugs are being administered. This may be achieved by regu-

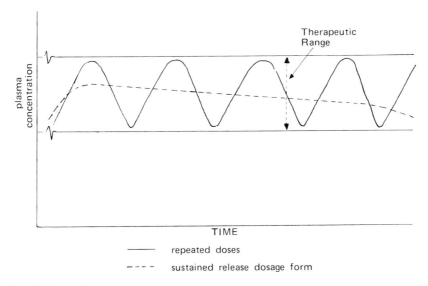

Fig. 7.4 Prolongation of drug action

lating the release of the active drug from the dosage form in order to maintain therapeutic plasma concentrations (Fig. 7.4).

Absorption can be delayed and the drug's action correspondingly prolonged in a number of different ways. In local anaesthesia with lignocaine, the addition of adrenaline causes constriction of local blood vessels, thus delaying absorption of the anaesthetic into the bloodstream and prolonging its local effect. Delay can also be achieved by giving the drug as an insoluble suspension (e.g. insulin zinc suspension) which dissolves and is absorbed slowly.

In certain instances, extremely slow absorption may be desirable. In psychiatric practice, long-acting preparations can be used to avoid frequent drug administration to patients who find it difficult to remember, or refuse to take their tablets. The introduction of oily injections of fluphenazine ensures that non-compliant chronic schizophrenic patients can be treated satisfactorily by single intramuscular injections at four or six-weekly intervals. Similarly, long lasting contraception can be achieved with depot injection of progestogen. Single depot injections of 15 mg of vitamin D have proved successful in combating nutritional osteomalacia in elderly women in whom compliance with oral medication is often a problem (Burns & Paterson, 1985).

Longer acting oral preparations

A sustained release can be achieved in a number of ways.

Coated granules. The active drug is contained in small granules packed in a gelatin capsule. Some granules have no coating and dissolve immediately. Other granules have coatings of varying thickness of different materials such as waxes. The granules with thin coatings will dissolve and release the drug faster than those with thicker coatings. In this way the active drug can be released over a length of time and a steady plasma level maintained by one dose instead of three or four individual doses of the conventional preparation.

Multilayer tablets. Sustained action can be achieved by manufacturing tablets consisting of a number of layers or several coats. The drug is dissolved immediately from one layer or the outer coat and more slowly from succeeding layers or coats.

Matrix preparations. The active ingredient is distributed throughout an inert wax or plastic matrix. The drug is slowly leached out of this network and its action may be sustained for up to 24 hours. A variation of this involves the active substance being embedded in a tablet which is surrounded by a porous coating. The pores are filled with water-soluble crystals, which are dissolved on contact with aqueous liquids and the active ingredient is released in a controlled manner by diffusion through the pores.

Controlled-release oral dosage forms may be more convenient than conventional preparations because they require less frequent administration, thus improving patient compliance. In addition, the gastric mucosa is exposed to a lesser concentration of drug than would be the case with immediately released products. This may be important when the drug causes irritation or bleeding of the gastrointestinal tract.

However, in practice, the results obtained from controlled-release dosage forms may be far from ideal and may vary between patients. The contents of sustained-release preparations may not be released completely and may tail off, giving therapeutic concentrations initially, but only sub-therapeutic concentrations prior to the next dose.

Implants. Gentamicin impregnated copolymer beads for the treatment of chronic bone infections are left in situ in the bone cavity for 10–30 days, providing higher concentrations of the drug than would be attained by standard systemic therapy. Implants of other drugs, such as testosterone, have been used to achieve a very long-acting systemic effect (4–8 months).

Ophthalmic prolonged release. Continuous application of drugs to the eye is necessary both to achieve an intense local action and to avoid systemic complications. If therapy is not regularly maintained, optimal therapy may not be achieved. A unit has been developed which can be placed comfortably in the conjunctival sac and will allow slow diffusion of pilocarpine over several days. The system consists of a core reservoir of pilocarpine surrounded by a membrane which controls the drug's diffusion from the system into the tear fluid. The dose is lower than that required in eye drops, resulting in a marked reduction in side effects. The device does not interfere with the use of other ophthalmic drugs.

Intra-uterine medication for long term contraception. An intra-uterine device was developed which had a contraceptive action through controlled release, over 18 months, of small doses of progesterone but this has been subsequently withdrawn from use.

Infusion systems. Miniaturised infusion systems are being developed suitable for implantation under the skin to administer insulin or heparin. A new method for treating hepatic metastases involves the implantation of a pump to infuse continuously a cytotoxic drug.

DRUG INTERACTIONS

When two or more drugs are administered at the same time, they may exert their effects independently or they may interact. This may result in the action of one drug being more potent or being reduced due to an effect by the other drug. Many drug interactions are harmless and a particular drug combination may only cause harm to a small proportion of individuals who receive it. The drugs most often involved in serious interactions are those with a narrow therapeutic range (e.g. aminoglycosides, phenytoin) and those where the dose must be closely monitored according to the response (e.g. anticoagulants, hypoglycaemics). Patients at increased risk from drug interactions include those with impaired renal and liver function and the elderly because of changes in physiology due to ageing and also because the elderly are prescribed proportionately more drugs than the young.

Drug interactions can be considered under three main headings — chemical interactions, pharmacokinetic interactions and pharmacodynamic interactions.

Chemical interactions

These may occur when incompatible drugs are mixed in syringes or added to infusion fluids prior to administration, or when the vehicle may be incompatible with the drug. Amphotericin B must be diluted in glucose 5% injection with a pH greater than 4.2. Care must be taken when calcium salts and phosphate are added to an intravenous infusion since above certain concentrations a precipitate is formed (Downie, 1979).

Pharmacokinetic interactions

These occur when one drug alters the absorption, distribution, protein binding, metabolism or excretion of another, thus reducing the amount of drug available to produce its pharmacological effects.

Interactions affecting drug absorption
When iron and tetracycline are required, they should be administered separately, as absorption is diminished when both are administered at the same time. The absorption of iron, tetracycline and several other drugs is affected by antacids.

Interactions due to changes in protein binding of drugs
The extent of effect of a drug depends on its level in the plasma since the higher the level the more will diffuse from the plasma to its site of action. A proportion of the drug after absorption will be free in the plasma and the remainder will be bound to plasma protein. Should a drug (e.g. warfarin) be displaced from plasma protein by another which has a stronger binding action (e.g. tolbutamide) there will be an increased concentration of unbound warfarin in the plasma which will result in a greater therapeutic effect and may lead to haemorrhage. This is exacerbated since in this particular reaction warfarin metabolism is inhibited.

Interactions affecting drug metabolism
Many drugs are inactivated by metabolism in the liver. One drug may inhibit the metabolism of another due to competition by both drugs for a particular drug-metabolising enzyme. Inhibition leads to lengthening of the plasma half-life of the inhibited drug, elevated plasma concentrations and an enhanced pharmacological effect which may cause toxicity. The potentiation of warfarin by co-trimoxazole and dextropropoxyphene is due partly to this mechanism in addition to changes in plasma protein binding. Similarly cimetidine affects phenytoin and diazepam metabolism.

Interactions affecting the renal excretion of drugs
Drugs are eliminated through the kidney both by glomerular filtration and by active tubular excretion. Competition can occur when drugs share the active transport mechanisms in the proximal tubule. Probenecid delays the excretion of all penicillins and some cephalosporins which leads to their increased plasma levels. A combination of aspirin and methotrexate leads to a risk of toxicity from increased levels of methotrexate due to competition for tubular secretion.

Pharmacodynamic interactions
These occur between drugs which have similar or antagonistic pharmacological effects or side-effects.

Interaction at receptor sites
Increased anticholinergic side-effects such as dry mouth, constipation and urinary retention occur when antihistamines and antidepressants interact with anticholinergics such as propantheline or benzhexol. Aminoglycosides potentiate the action of competitive neuromuscular drugs such as tubocurarine resulting in prolonged paralysis.

Interactions between drugs affecting the same system
Acetazolamide, carbenoxolone, corticosteroids and corticotrophin interact with thiazide diuretics, frusemide, bumetanide and ethacrynic acid, causing increased urinary potassium loss resulting in hypokalaemia. Antihypertensive drugs are potentiated by hypnotics, tranquillisers and levodopa which produce hypotension as a side-effect.

Interactions due to alterations of physiological factors
This can occur in a number of ways, e.g. carbenoxolone and corticosteroids antagonise the effect of antihypertensive drugs due to fluid retention. Potassium-losing diuretics may give rise to digoxin toxicity due to increased potassium loss.

Drug interactions with alcohol
Alcohol can interact with many drugs. It has a depressant effect on the nervous system and when administered concurrently with CNS

depressants the effect is additive. Alcohol increases the risk of death from an overdose of these drugs. The vasodilator effect of alcohol increases the postural hypotension of antihypertensive drugs. It can cause postural hypotension with peripheral vasodilators (e.g. oxpentifylline) and anti-anginal drugs (e.g. nitrates, verapamil). This interaction can also occur with metronidazole and procarbazine. Some alcoholic drinks contain tyramine. If this is taken along with mono-amine oxidase inhibitors such as phenelzine or tranylcypromine there is a risk of a hypertensive crisis.

REFERENCES

Burns J, Paterson C R 1985 Single dose vitamin D treatment for osteomalacia in the elderly. British Medical Journal 290: 280–281
Downie G 1979 Pharmaceutical aspects of parenteral nutrition. Proceedings of the Guild of Hospital Pharmacists 9: 23–25
Ogilvie R I 1978 Clinical pharmacokinetics of theophylline. Clinical Pharmacokinetics 3: 267

FURTHER READING

Smith S 1984/85 How drugs act. 12 part series. Nursing Times. Nov. 28–Feb. 20

8 LOCAL DRUG THERAPY

TOPICAL THERAPY IN DERMATOLOGICAL CONDITIONS

Although patients with specific skin diseases may be nursed in dermatological wards with specially trained and experienced staff to care for them, many patients in other wards and in the community, will, at some time, require nursing care for skin conditions. Consequently the subject of skin care is of concern to all practising nurses.

In the past nurses may have tended to place particular emphasis on the need for washing patients and caring for their pressure areas with minimal concern for the skin as an organ. Many systemic diseases manifest at least one of their diagnostic features in the skin. In congestive cardiac failure the skin may be cyanosed, sweating and oedematous. Hypertensive patients are often highly coloured; in contrast, patients with obstructive airways disease have a dusky hue. The patient with obstructive jaundice has a deep yellow colour and may complain of itching due to a deposition of bile salts in the skin. During a hypoglycaemic episode the patient sweats profusely. Diabetic coma is characterised by a dry skin which may have the smell of acetone due to the accumulation of ketone bodies. The high metabolic rate in thyrotoxicosis results in the skin becoming warm and moist, whereas the low metabolic rate of myxoedema causes the skin to become dry and coarse. Renal failure, iron deficiency anaemia and pernicious anaemia all cause changes in skin colour. Viral diseases of childhood display their own characteristic rashes and accompanying itch. The skin is indeed a barometer of health generally and this should not be forgotten when treating skin diseases as such.

Treatment selection

Advertising pressures both in the professional and lay press should be resisted when selecting a product for the treatment of a particular condition. Going for the quick results that may be claimed for a product will often be counter-productive. There is no substitute for identifying the cause of the problem and tackling it at source. Since two people suffering from the same condition will rarely present in an identical way it is essential that a thorough assessment is made by examination and questioning. Both visual (often using a hand lens) and tactile examination will be required. Temperature, tension and sensitivity of the skin may be ascertained by careful touching of the affected part(s) using a disposable plastic glove as appropriate. Where it is suspected that a skin condition is due to a reaction to an irritant or allergen, systematic questioning may help to identify the cause, as will carefully managed patch testing. Selection of a product by either doctor or nurse requires care, since the choice is very wide indeed. The BNF alone contains some 500 different topical applications. In addition, specially formulated products can be prescribed for patients whose needs cannot be met by either an 'off the shelf' proprietary or non-proprietary formulation. In this case the range of products available is as wide as the prescriber's imagination.

Many skin conditions will require the attention of a consultant dermatologist (or other clinician), who will prescribe the treatment. In most primary care, nurses will use their own professional expertise to determine how best to care for a patient's skin problem. The question of where the dividing line lies between the action that it is appropriate for the nurse or doctor to take may create problems. These can be avoided in two ways. Within a particular ward there may be a local agreement that nurses have delegated authority to use certain topical preparations in accordance with a defined treatment schedule. Another approach, developed in the Grampian Health Board Area, is to define, in a formulary of nursing care products, those preparations which are routinely available, without medical prescription, for use by nurses. (Tables 8.1 and 8.2).

Table 8.1 Contents of Nursing Formulary

The following items can be obtained from the Pharmacy Department:

Hair	Malathion Lotion 0.5%
	Malathion Shampoo 1%
Nose and mouth	Hydrogen Peroxide 20 volumes (6%)
	Mouth Wash Solution Tablets
	Paraffin White Soft
	Sodium Bicarbonate 1–160 aqueous solution
Topical applications Skin care	Benzalkonium Cream
	Benzoin Compound Tincture
	Calamine Lotion
	Chlorhexidine Hand Scrub
	Chlorhexidine 0.5% in 70% industrial methylated spirit
	E.45 Cream
	Hexachlorophane Powder
	Solution of Iodine
	Kaolin Poultice (Unit Pack)
	Lubcricating Jelly
	Opsite Spray
	Paraffin White Soft
	Plaster Remover
	Povidone Iodine Solution
	Talc
	Thovaline
	Uvistat
	Zinc and Castor Oil Ointment
Wound cleaning & care	Chlorhexidine/Cetrimide/Sterile Solution (Sachets)
	Normal Saline Sterile Solution (Sachets)
Bowel clearance	Medical advice to be sought
Bladder preparations	"G" Solution
	Lignocaine Gel (1% or 2%)

The formulary does not include products containing antibiotic, corticosteroid or other potent drugs, since the uncontrolled use of these agents is fraught with many dangers. Symptoms may be masked by the use of corticosteroids, and the use of certain antibiotics is associated with sensitisation reactions (see also Table 8.3).

Prescribing of topical therapy

All topical preparations which contain a specific drug should be regarded in exactly the same way as any other medicine. It follows therefore that prescribing, recording and administration of such products should be in accordance with those established for systemic therapy.

Table 8.2 Monograph from Nursing formulary

NURSING CARE FORMULARY — SKIN CARE

Povidone Iodine Solution (Betadine Antiseptic Solution)

Actions
Betadine Antiseptic Solution is an aqueous, red brown solution containing Povidone Iodine 10%. Povidone Iodine is an antiseptic which is effective against a wide range of organisms.

Applications
Betadine antiseptic solution can be used where a mild antiseptic is required, especially in the presence of broken skin. The dark coloured stain caused by the Betadine clearly delineates the treated area. Typical indications include the general cleansing and disinfection of skin and contaminated wounds especially where more irritant products are unsuitable.

Precautions
Betadine antiseptic solution should be used undiluted then be allowed to dry. Care should be taken when using Betadine antiseptic solution on patients known to be allergic to Iodine, as the product may cause skin reactions in these patients.
Betadine antiseptic solution is for external use only. If accidentally swallowed medical advice should be sought immediately.

Availability
Betadine antiseptic solution is available in containers of 500 ml.

Storage
Store in a cool place away from light and in a locked cupboard set aside for external preparations.

Cost

Special prescription sheets (Fig. 8.1) are required for the prescribing of topical preparations in hospital as it is necessary to incorporate a greater amount of information than a standard in-patient prescription allows. The prescription should include:

date of the prescription
name of the preparation
- a specially made up formula may contain several different substances which should be listed.

formulation and its strength
- where necessary, details such as aqueous or oily should be given.
- it is better where possible to describe the strength as a percentage. Ratios (e.g. 1:9) can be misleading.

quantity to be applied
- this may be difficult to describe. Sparingly, liberally, 1 cm or a 'worm' are expressions which may be used. The most commonly used instruction given is 'as sparingly as possible'.

site(s) for application
- these should be described specifically (e.g. 'all active areas', 'wherever the skin is dry'). Vague expressions such as 'all over' should be avoided.

dressings and bandages to be used
- the size of each should be appropriate to the size of the patient's lesion.

number of times of administration
- this should span a 24 hour period and should be divided evenly throughout the patient's waking day.

doctor's signature;

Prescribing systemic therapy for dermatological conditions is carried out in the same way as other systemic prescribing.

Nursing care aspects

Topical applications should not be applied to normal skin as this wastes time, wastes the product and may do harm. Generally speaking, if the condition is acute then the frequency of the treatment and the strength of the active ingredient(s) may be increased rather than the amount applied. It is only the active ingredient(s) in contact with the affected skin which is going to aid healing — not the layers on top. 'A little can do a lot of good, a lot can do a lot of harm' is a maxim worth remembering.

Irrespective of the treatment being followed, patients with skin conditions need to be cared for with real sensitivity. Feelings of shame, disgust and fear have for long troubled patients with skin diseases forcing them to hide from the gaze of others. To some extent, this situation has been perpetuated by the attitude of health professionals towards these patients. Sadly, staff may make patients with skin conditions feel 'unclean' by isolating them unnecessarily in single rooms and adopting overprotective measures while treating them. In time, the patient may respond with antisocial behaviour which in turn may affect the

	DATE COMMENCED	MEDICINES (Block Letters)	METHOD / SITE OF APPLICATION	TIMES PER DAY				SIGNATURE	DISCONTINUED	
									DATE	INITIALS
R										
S										
T										
U										
V										
W										
X										
Y										
Z										

WARD	HOSPITAL	SURNAME	FORENAME	AGE	UNIT NUMBER	CONSULTANT	KNOWN DRUG / MEDICINE SENSITIVITY	SHEET NO.
							1	
							2	

Fig. 8.1 Prescription sheet for topical medicines

attitude of others until what can only be described as a 'leper complex' develops. Unless it is absolutely necessary to do otherwise, these patients should be shown the same consideration afforded to all other patients. Trust and confidence need to be restored by adopting an open and optimistic outlook. This in itself has a beneficial 'therapeutic' effect.

Skin conditions are frequently of a chronic or recurring nature which often necessitates teaching patients and/or relatives how to continue treatment. Advice given may include appropriate skin cleansing, the method of application as well as any special precautions such as skin protection and protection of personal linen. Teaching should be realistic and helpful if a reasonable degree of compliance is to be assured. There would be little point in asking a patient to apply a tar preparation before going out in an evening because of its antisocial effect. To most patients, a large unsightly dressing would be equally unacceptable. For the application of an ointment, some disabled patients may find a long-handled ointment applicator of assistance in reaching inaccessible parts of the body (e.g. see Fig. 8.2). Where there is a degree of difficulty in applying skin preparations, in the absence of a capable family member it is essential to arrange for the treatment to be carried out by the district nurse.

In hospitals topical applications should be kept in a locked cupboard set aside for external preparations, careful attention being paid to expiry dates. Disposable gloves should be worn by staff when applying skin preparations as protection from absorbing any of the drug. To prevent cross-infection, patients should be supplied with individually dispensed skin applications. Where this is not possible, a quantity of the preparation should be removed from its container with a spatula. If more of the preparation is required, a new spatula should be used. Since rolling up a collapsible tube to expel the contents may obliterate the label it is preferable to squeeze the tube progressively along its entire length.

Procedural aspects

Skin cleansing
Before applying a topical preparation the skin should be clean. To prevent accumulation, previous applications to the skin should be removed. This is especially important where drugs such as corticosteroids are involved. In order to remove creams, paints, powders or lotions, the patient, or the site, should be bathed using simple soaps and warm water. (Perfumed toilet soap should be avoided.) Pastes, ointments and certain paints are best removed with cotton wool soaked in liquid paraffin or olive oil.

Bathing
Often nurses are not completely satisfied with

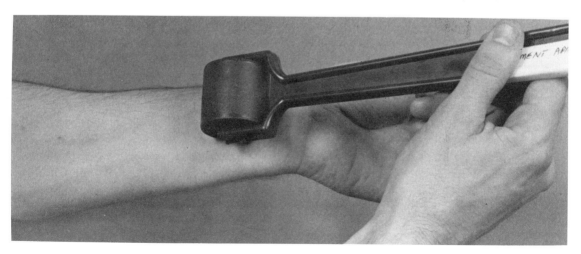

Fig. 8.2 Ointment applicator

their work unless all their patients have been bathed. With increasing changes in the skin towards dryness after about the age of 35, the tendency should be towards a reduction in the frequency in bathing. Soaking in a hot bath makes the skin dry due to loss of natural oils and causes epidermal cells to shrink on drying. Any itching of the skin is increased. A conscious effort should be made to adjust routine and not to overwash patients, particularly elderly people and those patients whose skin is noticeably dry. With the shift of emphasis towards individualised nursing care, nurses are better placed to make an assessment of the patient's skin condition and decide on the care required.

Patients with skin conditions should be advised to resist the temptation to use any cosmetic bath additives. Detergents or antiseptics may cause the patient further problems and should be avoided. To occlude the skin and thus prevent drying by evaporation, liquid paraffin or olive oil may be used. An emollient such as emulsifying ointment may be added to the bath water. This also acts as a mild occlusive and helps to retain moisture in the skin. An oily bath is obviously exceedingly dangerous and therefore it is vitally important that the patient is forewarned of the risk of falling. The nurse should make a careful judgment as to whether the patient can be safely left to get out of the bath unaided. In any case, the bath should be emptied before the patient rises out of the bath. A secure bath mat should be made available. After using an emollient, the bath needs careful cleaning. It should be filled full with hot water and have a suitable detergent added having first ensured that there are no patients in the vicinity who may mistakenly think that the bath has been filled for their use. The bath is then allowed to empty and as it does so, the water should be agitated and the sides cleaned to remove all traces of the emollient.

Scalp treatment

Shampoos may be used for cleaning or for treatment purposes. Triethanolamine lauryl sulphate 40% forms the basis of shampoos. It has no additives and is the least irritant. It is therefore useful as a simple cleansing agent for the scalp. Psoriasis of the scalp may be treated with either a tar-based or a desquamative shampoo. Antiseptic shampoos are available for the infected scalp.

Precautions have to be taken to protect the neck and face from contact with shampoos used as treatment. The patient should be warned to keep his eyes closed throughout the procedure. With gloved hands, two applications are made — the first a thorough wash to cleanse the scalp, the second, active treatment. Between applications and at the finish, the shampoo should be rinsed out of the hair. The hair is dried with a hair drier as soon as possible. Some scalp applications are flammable and when using such products patients should be warned not to dry the hair near naked flame.

Formulation aspects of topical preparations

Several different pharmaceutical preparations (ointment, lotions etc.) are available, each of which has distinctive physical characteristics quite apart from the nature of the active ingredient. In some instances products are used solely for their physical properties, e.g. emollients, barrier preparations and sunscreens. Although a detailed discussion of formulation aspects is outside the scope of this book, certain important principles are emphasised below since they have practical implications for the nurse. Typically a pharmaceutical product intended for topical application will have some, or all, of the following components:

- *Active ingredient(s)*
  The concentration of the active ingredient(s) will normally be expressed as a percentage.
- *Vehicle*
  The overall characteristics of the product will depend on the vehicle chosen. The vehicle may be aqueous, non-aqueous, liquid or semi-solid depending on the properties required and nature of the active ingredient. Penetration of the active ingredient into the skin will also be influenced by the properties of the vehicle.

- *Antimicrobial preservative agent*
  The risk of microbial contamination of topical products during their use is significant, so it is essential, unless the product is a single-use pack, to include an antimicrobial agent.
- *Emulsifying/suspending agent*
  These are required to give a product physical stability, e.g. an emulsifying agent provides stable oil-in-water preparations, and a suspending agent is necessary when insoluble powders of high density are included in a liquid preparation.
- *Other additives*
  E.g. a buffering agent may be included to give a preparation with a pH approximating to that of normal skin.

Features and method of use of topical preparations

A brief description is now given of the main features and method of use of topical pharmaceutical preparations used in dermatological conditions and skin care.

The terms cream, ointment and lotion etc, are fairly precise but may not always be used in a totally consistent way. Care should always be taken to determine the actual properties of the product which, like other pharmaceuticals, may not always be conveyed by the name.

Creams

Creams are normally oil-in-water emulsions which, since water is the continuous phase, are easily removed, even from hairy areas, by normal cleansing procedures. The evaporation of the water present in the cream produces a useful cooling effect. Drainage from a lesion is facilitated because creams absorb exudates. Drugs normally incorporated into creams include corticosteroids, antibacterial and antifungal agents. Good penetration of the active ingredient into the skin is achieved and may be enhanced due to the presence of a surfactant (emulsifying agent) in the cream. Creams have also a softening effect on thickened lesions.

Although creams normally contain an antimicrobial preservative they should be used with

great care to avoid microbial contamination since the antimicrobial agents available for incorporation into creams have a limited spectrum of activity. The antimicrobial agent (and/or active ingredient) may cause skin sensitivity in some patients.

Ointments

It is very important to distinguish between ointments and creams because the properties of the two products are generally very different. Ointments are normally greasy anhydrous preparations which do not mix with water and therefore should not be applied to exuding lesions. Ointments are more difficult to remove from the skin than creams. Soft paraffins are widely used as ointment bases, incorporating liquid paraffin to achieve the required consistency. Ointments soften crusts but are generally not suitable for application to hairy areas.

Being non-aqueous, antimicrobial agents are only occasionally required to be included in ointments and so there is less risk of sensitisation from this source than with creams. However, lanolin (wool fat) and derivatives are sometimes included in ointments and may cause contact sensitivity.

It should be noted that water-miscible ointment bases are now available when this property is required.

Application of creams and ointments. As already stated, ointments and creams generally have different properties and the indications for their use relate to these. However the guidance given above is not inflexible. A most important aspect is to use a preparation which is acceptable to the patient. These products should be applied as sparingly as possible to the affected part(s). If applying a prescribed product the prescriber's instructions must be complied with. Creams and ointments are best applied in the same way as make-up. Small dots of the product are placed at suitable intervals over the area to be treated. Using the tip of the index finger and/or second finger for small areas and the palm of the hand for larger areas, the cream should be spread evenly as far as it will go within the area to be treated. Plain lint or gauze dressings may be required to cover areas to which creams and ointments have been applied.

Pastes

These preparations are essentially similar to ointments but contain a high proportion of powders, have a very stiff consistency, and will adhere to lesions at body temperature. Pastes also have protective properties. Compound zinc paste for example contains 25% by weight of zinc oxide and 20% by weight of starch with 50% white soft paraffin.

Application of pastes. Pastes should only be applied to specific lesions, e.g. in psoriasis, and not to the surrounding skin. Where a paste contains a highly active ingredient (e.g. dithranol), it will be necessary to protect the skin adjacent to the lesion with a bland product such as yellow soft paraffin. If the paste is soft enough (temperature will obviously influence the consistency of the product), it may be applied with the finger(s) of a gloved hand. Pastes which cannot be applied in this way may be applied with a wooden spatula. Pastes will seldom be required to be covered with a dressing, except where it is necessary to protect the patient's linen from staining by the active ingredient.

Dusting powders

Dusting powders are of two main types, medicated and unmedicated. All dusting powders normally have a basis of starch (absorbent) and talc (lubricant). Unmedicated powders are used in general nursing care to reduce friction and absorb moisture between skin folds. Excessive use should be avoided since 'caking' in these folds may result, causing local irritation.

Medicated powders have a limited place in the active treatment of skin diseases since it is generally not possible to achieve a satisfactory concentration of active ingredient at the site of the lesion for any length of time. Dusting powders containing suitable active ingredients are mainly used in prophylaxis (e.g. the prevention of athlete's foot, or the prevention of neonatal staphylococcal cross-infection). Dusting powders containing antibiotics are occasionally used in the treatment of superficial bacterial infections such as impetigo

when the powder will tend to stick to the lesions.

Collodions

A collodion is a non-aqueous solution containing a film-forming agent. On application the volatile solvent in the collodion evaporates leaving a film which holds the dissolved drug in prolonged contact with the lesion. Collodions have also been used to seal minor wounds providing physical protection and reducing the likelihood of infection. Collodions are highly flammable and should *never* be used near naked flame. Collodions can be applied to the lesion using a small camel-haired brush or cotton-tipped applicator.

Lotions

Lotions are normally simple formulations containing active ingredients in an aqueous solution or suspension. Occasionally oily lotions are used, but such preparations have very different properties to a lotion with an aqueous base, and are more akin to ointments. In very acute conditions lotions are used to relieve superficial inflammation and assist in the removal of crusts. When the presence of fine solid particles cannot even be tolerated by the patient, lotions which are simple solutions are used until the most acute phase of the condition has passed. Then lotions containing powders in suspension can be used. The cooling properties of a lotion may be enhanced by the addition of alcohol to the vehicle, but this may cause stinging. (Excessive cooling due to the use of lotions must be avoided especially in the elderly.)

Lotions may be useful for the application of a drug to a hairy area of the body where the use of a greasy ointment or stiff paste would be inappropriate or impracticable. In very acute conditions lotions may be applied as wet dressings using lint or other closely-woven fabric. As with all dressings, care should be taken on removal so as to avoid damaging the epithelium. Any dressings that have dried out should be thoroughly wetted with the lotion before being carefully removed. Lotions may also be applied to small lesions using cotton wool or to larger areas using a suitable flat brush.

Paints

Paints are solutions of the active drug in a suitable solvent, such as water, alcohol or a mixture of solvents, depending on the nature of the active ingredient. Application to the skin is normally by means of a brush. Antiseptic agents are often applied in the form of a paint.

Pressurised aerosols

Pressurised aerosols are widely available for the application of drugs to the skin in such conditions as superficial bacterial infections. Protective applications can also be applied in this way. It is important to use the product in accordance with the manufacturer's recommendations, and to ensure safe disposal of the empty canister. Pressurised aerosols are convenient to use, and confer the advantages of 'no touch' technique, but are relatively expensive.

Medicated dressings

Ointments and pastes (and other topical products) are often used in association with some form of surgical dressing such as gauze or lint. Products are available which have the main properties of a dermatological preparation and some of the properties of a surgical dressing. Two main types of these combined products are in use. Tulle gauze dressings impregnated with soft paraffin and an antibiotic such as framycetin or sodium fusidate, are used to prevent and treat infections in a variety of lesions. As an alternative to the use of antibiotic-containing preparations a tulle impregnated with soft paraffin and chlorhexidine is available. These products are essentially gauzes impregnated with an ointment and are presented in a sterile form ready for immediate use.

The second type of combined product is the paste bandage. A range of bandages is available impregnated with a zinc oxide paste combined with either coal tar, calamine, ichthammol or hydrocortisone. Paste bandages are used for the treatment of such conditions as eczema, leg ulcers and chronic dermatitis.

Another type of medicated dressing of interest combines the antiseptic properties of povidone-iodine with those of a non-adherent dressing.

Table 8.3 indicates some potential problems that may occur following the use of dermatological preparations.

Table 8.3 Potential problems following use of topical dermatological preparations

Potential Problem	Ingredients of dermatological products which require particular precautions.
Absorption — systemic	Corticosteroids Neomycin Dithranol Salicylic acid Avoid contact as far as possible, use gloves, wash hands after use
Eye irritancy	Crotamiton Sulphur Dithranol Podophyllum resin Should never be used on the face Patients should be warned not to rub the eyes
Infection risks	All dermatological preparations should be used with care to avoid microbial contamination.
Inflammable products	Alcohol (high percentage) Collodions Should never be used near naked flame
Skin/fair hair discolouration	Dithranol Coal tar products Clioquinol
Skin irritancy	Dithranol Formaldehyde Podophyllum resin Normal skin should be protected by a bland agent, e.g. soft paraffin
Staining of personal linen, and the patient's bath	Dithranol Potassium permanganate Coal tar products
Sensitisation reactions	Local anaesthetics Antihistamines Neomycin
Photosensitivity	Antihistamines Coal tar Tretinoin
Radiation	**No** dermatological preparations should be applied to the area being treated either during or immediately after a course of radiation except on the advice of the doctor or radiotherapy staff. Cosmetics or perfumed talcum powder should not be used on the treatment area although a bland purified talc such as baby powder is permissible.

Topical corticosteroid therapy

In view of the major impact on dermatological therapy and of the considerable dangers and benefits inherent in the use of topical corticosteroids, particular emphasis is placed on this therapeutic group. Modern steroid chemistry has produced a wide range of compounds each having particular properties and potency. It is usual to classify topical corticosteroids according to potency. A rough guide is as follows:

Potency	Examples
Mild	Dexamethasone 0.01%
	Hydrocortisone 1%
Moderately potent	Clobetasone butyrate 0.05%
	Fluocinolone acetonide 0.01%
Potent	Betamethasone valerate 0.1%
	Beclomethasone dipropionate 0.025%
Very potent	Clobetasol propionate 0.05%
	Fluocinolone acetonide 0.2%

Mode of action
The anti-inflammatory action of corticosteroids is valuable in a wide range of inflammatory conditions as is their immunosuppressive action. Corticosteroids also have an antimitotic action which may be the source of the beneficial effect sometimes achieved in psoriasis. Where there is a risk of secondary infection it may sometimes be necessary to use an antimicrobial agent in combination with the corticosteroid. Neomycin should be avoided because of the risk of sensitisation. A non-antibiotic antibacterial agent such as clioquinol is often preferred.

Therapeutic indications and adverse effects
When originally introduced topical corticosteroids were used extensively for a wide range of conditions. Although many patients benefited in the short term, many suffered later from adverse effects. One of the main indications for the use of corticosteroids today is in the treatment of various forms of eczema.
    Adverse effects of topical corticosteroid therapy include:

- atrophy of the skin (especially the face) with thinning of the epidermis and dermis
- telangiectasiae, localised fine hair growth and striae
- delayed wound healing.

Absorption of the corticosteroid can occur, (with adrenal axis suppression), if the choice of preparation, dosage, duration, and method of use are inappropriate. It follows that the potent and very potent preparations are reserved for conditions unresponsive to milder preparations, and even then only short courses of treatment are given. A number of factors influence the extent of percutaneous penetration, including the site of application, (the groin and axillae can be penetrated more easily than the knees or palms), and formulation used. If the area being treated is occluded, increased penetration occurs. The technique of applying corticosteroids in conjunction with an occlusive dressing is now seldom used because of adverse effects which include infection and systemic absorption. Children are especially at risk from increased absorption owing to their greater proportion of surface area relative to weight and a thinner skin. Prescriptions for children are generally for mild or moderately potent agents, short courses of treatment being the norm. The use of topical corticosteroids on the face is fraught with dangers and is only very rarely indicated.

Practical aspects
- skin preparations should be applied sparingly with a gentle action
- polythene gloves should be worn when applying corticosteroid preparations to avoid the possibility of skin damage
- creams, especially those prepared by dilution of a proprietary product, may support bacterial growth and should be used with care to avoid contamination. All creams will bear an expiry date after which the preparation should not be used
- patients, relatives and carers should be counselled as appropriate on the correct use of topical corticosteroids
- topical corticosteroid preparations should only be used in accordance with a prescription, and never to treat a minor skin problem.

WOUND CARE

A wound can be described as any break in the

continuity of the skin resulting from surgical incision, puncture, laceration or ulceration. Irrespective of the type of wound being treated, the over-riding objective is to prevent infection. The risk to the patient of developing infection is far greater in hospital than at home because of exposure to pathogenic micro-organisms many of which have become resistant to antibiotics. While it is not possible to eliminate this risk totally, it can be kept to a minimum. Broad principles of wound care are applicable in many settings although the precise management of wounds is often based on the preferences of the individual clinician. The consensus of opinion today is that the more interference, albeit well intentioned, with a wound, the greater the likelihood of infection being introduced. Consequently, the routine changing of dressings has greatly diminished. With the development of the nursing process, nurses are giving greater thought to the needs of patients and their wounds on an individual basis. As a result, dressing rounds in hospital wards have become much less common.

However, this changing pattern of care has made the control of the ward environment less straightforward. For example, the timing of dressings in relation to ward cleaning is less easy to define and so both nursing and domestic staff have to strive for the best possible compromise in the patients' interests. Rooms set aside for aseptic procedures overcome this difficulty. Wherever possible, whether a single dressing is to be done or several dressings are being done consecutively, a working principle of 'clean to dirty' should be adopted. There is fairly conclusive evidence to show that the main source of infection generally, and in wounds in particular, is the hands of personnel especially those in close contact with the patient. Handwashing helps to prevent this transfer and contributes substantially to the overall control of hospital infection. A non-touch technique for aseptic procedures therefore must be adopted and correct handwashing technique practised.

Handwashing procedure
There are three forms of handwashing used in patient care — social, surgical and antiseptic

— each indicated when a different degree of skin disinfection is required. The hands should be socially clean before caring for any patient, following a visit to the lavatory and before administering medicines or serving food. Surgical handwashing is performed prior to surgery. Any procedure requiring an aseptic technique, such as the dressing of a wound, involves an antiseptic handwash. Specially formulated preparations containing chlorhexidine or povidone-iodine are suitable as they combine the cleansing action of a detergent with antiseptic properties. They remove and kill transient organisms on the skin and also have some effect on bacteria in deeper layers of the skin. Organisms on the skin include Gram positive ones such as *Staphylococcus aureus* and Gram negative ones such as *Escherichia coli* both of which are common causes of hospital infection. Regular use of an antiseptic handwash has a cumulative effect and an extremely low level of resident organisms can be achieved.

While working with patients, nurses should have short clean nails free of nail varnish and should not wear jewellery or a wrist watch. For each handwash, the hands should be wetted first before the handwashing agent is applied using an elbow dispenser. All surfaces are lathered including the wrists. Particular attention should be paid to the backs of the hands and fingers as well as between the fingers. Both hands should be cleaned thoroughly; right-handed people tend to clean the left hand more thoroughly and vice versa. Scrubbing the hands is no longer advocated as this action would seem to create disturbance of the resident flora of the skin. The hands and wrists are rinsed under running water to remove lather and the taps turned off with the elbows or if necessary holding a paper towel. Careful drying of the hands with a paper towel is essential to protect the skin from possible breakdown, to make it harder for micro-organisms to thrive and to facilitate the application of gloves. The exact timing of handwashing during an aseptic procedure must be left to the discretion of the nurse. Much will depend on the nature of the wound and whether assistance is given with the procedure.

Preparation of the environment

Wound contaminants in the environment take the form of dust and droplets. A few minutes spent in preparing the environment prior to an aseptic procedure is time well spent in helping to reduce these modes of spread. Before setting up the dressing trolley, an explanation should be given to the patient as to what is involved and he should be given the opportunity to eliminate at this time. Screens should be pulled gently as far in advance of the procedure as possible to allow particulate matter to settle. Sufficient space is essential so that the procedure can take place safely and efficiently. For example, the floor where the nurse is to be working should be clear, furniture may have to be moved to make way for the dressing trolley, and flowers should be removed from the immediate vicinity. Where the preferred technique involves the wearing of gloves, a flat surface such as the bedtable which later can be cleaned, should first be cleared. Traffic around the patient's bed should be reduced to a minimum.

The spread of droplet infection is another potential hazard for the patient with a wound. The wearing of masks was believed at one time to protect the patient from droplets from the nurse's upper respiratory tract. It is now thought that masks in themselves provide a warm, moist breeding ground for organisms and have gone out of favour for simple procedures such as removing sutures or dressing a sealed wound. Only in the case of extensive tissue damage (e.g. burns, skin grafts or deep wounds) or where the patient is immunosuppressed, are masks of high-filter performance used.

Nurses with colds and sore throats should never participate in aseptic procedures. While the wound is exposed and dressing packs are open, conversation should be restricted, the patient having had the reason for this explained at the time of preparation.

Preparation of the trolley

Trolleys for aseptic procedures should be set aside for the purpose. Before proceeding, the nurse washes her hands and dons a disposable cap and apron. The trolley is cleaned using a small amount of a suitable detergent and a damp paper towel. Trolley cleaning includes legs and bars as well as the shelves. It is then dried with a paper towel prior to the application of an alcoholic solution of a disinfectant in the form of a disposable swab, spray or liquid. Alcohol enhances the bactericidal effect of the active agent and is quick drying. A dry surface is less conducive to the growth of micro-organisms than a damp one. The top shelf is kept clear until the start of the dressing while the necessary requirements for the procedure are placed on the lower shelf. Going through the procedure mentally at this stage ensures that no essential item is omitted.

Packs of sterile equipment and materials should be inspected before use to ensure that they are intact. Further means of determining whether packs are safe for use vary. Satisfactory autoclaving may be confirmed by the indicator on some packs whereas the expiry date or known shelf-life for a specific pack indicates whether it may be safely used.

Single-use packs of sterile antiseptic solutions (normally containing chlorhexidine) are ideal for wound care. Where stability of the product permits, the solution should be warmed to body temperature before use, preferably in a solution warming cabinet. Desloughing agents, such as hydrogen peroxide are also used, but care must be taken because of possible irritant effects. Wounds are often irrigated with a solution of hydrogen peroxide drawn into a syringe. Its use should be restricted to the sloughy areas of the wound and, on completion of the irrigation, the surrounding skin should be mopped with a bland solution such as sterile 0.9% sodium chloride solution. Often, depending on its size, a cavity is packed with a wick, soak or pack which has been immersed in dilute sodium hypochlorite solution (containing 0.3–0.4% available chlorine). The packing serves to keep the cavity from closing over before granulation from its base has taken place.

Care of the wound

Having prepared the environment, herself and the trolley for redressing a wound, the nurse assists the patient into a suitable position which, as well as allowing ease of access, is as acceptable to the patient as is possible. Conventional analgesia may have been given in advance although sometimes for very painful procedures such as the removal of a large pack, Entonox, a gaseous mixture of 50% oxygen and 50% nitrous oxide, may be given to the patient to inhale at the time. Some patients prefer not to look at the wound. All patients require to be kept warm and have privacy.

Removal of a dressing from a wound requires great care to avoid damage to new epithelium. Where difficulty is encountered in removing a dressing, it may be soaked off with sterile sodium chloride 0.9% solution or the sterile antiseptic solution used in the procedure. Depending on circumstances the solution used is applied with a swab or a syringe. The nature of any soakage should be ascertained along with the ease with which the dressing separated from the wound. Undue difficulty in removing a dressing may be an indication for using an alternative dressing (see Table 8.4).

Special care must be taken when placing soiled dressings into a disposal bag. An examination of the wound should be made for signs of redness, swelling, bruising, haematoma or dehiscence. Any undue tenderness is noted. If there are signs of infection and a swab is to be obtained for bacteriological culture, this should be done before antiseptic solution is applied. A firm but gentle approach is essential in the vicinity of the wound. By bearing in mind the purpose of the procedure, e.g. to cleanse, to soothe, to deslough, to protect, the nurse can estimate whether the desired effect is being achieved. Whatever the purpose of the procedure and irrespective of the technique used, the care of the wound should be methodical. Recent research has shown that swabbing from the stitch line outwards is the most satisfactory method. The rim of an ulcerated area is usually swabbed first before swabbing methodically within the crater itself. The procedure is completed with the application of a surgical dressing where this is indicated. After making the patient comfortable and restoring the immediate clinical area to normal, care should be taken to place all used disposable materials in a polythene bag which is

Table 8.4 Dressings used in wound care

Type of dressing	Some advantages/disadvantages

Simple absorbent pads
  lint
  gauze
  gauze and cotton tissue
	Good absorbency, keep wounds warm, but may adhere to wound surface. Limited microbiological protection. May shed fibres into the wound.

Structured dressing pads	Dressing pads with an outer sleeve of non-adherent material have similar properties to the simple absorbent pads, but are generally easier to remove.
Laminated dressings	In such dressings a non-adherent film layer is bonded to an absorbent layer. Such a dressing has good general properties.
Semipermeable film dressings	Such films have a variety of uses including the management of superficial wounds and certain types of burns. Other uses for this versatile dressing include the prevention and treatment of pressure sores.
Newer products	Skin substitutes such as lyophilised porcine skin is now available. Specially treated foams and other novel materials such as 'Geliperm' are now finding a place in wound management.

then sealed ready for disposal. The trolley is thoroughly cleaned with the recommended disinfectant. Any necessary amendment is made to the patient's nursing care plan.

Prevention of wound infection
Apart from achieving high standards of asepsis during actual wound care procedures, certain pre-operative medicines are often taken to prevent (or reduce the likelihood) of post-operative wound infection. Intensive pre-operative skin preparation using a well-defined regime may be commenced three days prior to orthopaedic, cardiac, or other forms of surgery, where the infection risk is great and/or where the consequences of infection are especially dangerous for the patient. Such measures will

also reduce the possibility of infection becoming established in underlying tissues.

Apart from this topical approach, irrigation with an antibacterial agent during operative procedures may be carried out. Tetracycline, in the form of a sterile irrigation solution, has been found very effective in reducing infection following abdominal surgery.

Various forms of systemic therapy may also be used to prevent post-operative wound infection. A course of antibiotic or other form of antimicrobial therapy may be given. Gut irrigation procedures with a solution of anti-biotics have also been used pre-operatively.

Patients who are poor risks for good wound healing include the obese, the debilitated, the heavy smoker and those receiving cytotoxic therapy in combination with surgery. Some of these patients may need additional supportive therapy such as parenteral nutrition. Clearly any wound infection must be guarded against by all possible means.

Surgical dressings

Where it is necessary to apply a surgical dressing, the choice is governed by a number of factors, such as the degree of absorbency required. In many situations a very simple dressing only will be required. Indeed wounds are often left exposed to the air for varying periods of time. A detailed discussion of these factors is beyond the scope of this book but a brief summary of the desirable properties of surgical dressings is included since it is felt that a discussion of wound care would be incomplete without this. (A brief discussion of some medicated dressings is given on p. 101.) Ideally a surgical dressing (excluding adhesive tapes) should be:

- comfortable for the patient, providing a feeling of confidence and sense of security
- able to provide protection, both physical and microbiological, to the wound
- able to maintain optimal conditions for wound healing, including high humidity at wound surface, warmth, and gaseous exchange
- non-adherent to wound surface

- in a sterile presentation, preferably unit pack
- of good absorbency
- non-allergenic
- conveniently packaged for ease of removal in aseptic procedures
- free from toxic and particulate matter
- compatible with commonly used medicaments
- able to allow observation of wound and be radiotranslucent
- economical in use
- easy to dispose of.

No one dressing has all the above properties, although dressings developed in the last 25 years do, in a number of instances, combine many of the highly desirable properties listed. However, in some situations it may be necessary to use a combination of dressings to achieve the desired effect. Surgical dressings can be classified under a number of headings according to their structure and properties as indicated in Table 8.4.

PRESSURE SORES

Few topics in nursing have been written about and discussed to the same extent as the vexed question of pressure sores. The apparently endless list of topical applications which have been used in the prevention and treatment of pressure sores is evidence of the concern and even desperation felt by many nurses. For too long, nurses have battled against seemingly impossible odds to keep patients' skin in good condition. There is now a greater under-standing of the aetiology and pathology of pressure sore formation, and advances have taken place in the design of nursing aids and in the treatment of sores. Alongside these changes, however, advances in geriatric medicine and the treatment of progressive diseases, plus the growth of early discharge and out-patient treatment, have led to an increased concentration of 'at risk' patients in hospital wards (Norton, 1973). Fortunately, the view that pressure sores result only from a failure of nursing care is beginning to lose support. Regrettably, in spite of all the research and the improvement in aids and appliances, still not enough money is spent on the prevention of pressure sores. Wider promotion of nursing aids in conjunction with the provision of adequate numbers of staff to ensure the maintenance of turning regimes is all important.

Intact pressure areas, like clean mouths, seldom provoke comment; it is often only when things go wrong that interest mounts and there is feverish activity to implement vigorous nursing action. The risk of pressure sores will always be present and so cannot be overlooked. Their cost is almost incalculable not only in monetary terms but also in additional suffering for patients. Unfortunately, there is no satisfactory general term which describes the lesions in question. Terms used in the past have incorrectly implied that there was inevitably a loss of continuity of the skin surface and that sores were phenomena of bedfast patients only. The term 'pressure sore' has become something of a misnomer since factors other than pressure are now incriminated in their predisposition. These include shearing forces, friction, moisture, poor general nutrition, old age and diminished blood circulation. Nonetheless, the primary cause of pressure sore formation is continuous direct pressure.

Effects of pressure

Any pressure which occludes capillary circulation diminishes blood supply to the area and leads to ischaemia. If this pressure is maintained for more than a few hours the capillary endothelium is damaged resulting in sludging and thrombosis leading to necrosis and ulceration. Localised infection and protein loss may follow and in severe cases anaemia and systemic infection may also. The compression of tissues between two hard surfaces, (such as the bony skeleton and the unyielding surface of a bed or chair), is the commonest situation giving rise to pressure sores. Pressure generated sufficient to cause pressure sores depends on the weight of the patient and the surface carrying the weight. Any substantial deviation from ideal body weight

increases the risk of pressure sores developing. Thin patients lack subcutaneous fat and possibly nutritional reserve to combat the effect of pressure. Obese patients are well padded with fat but any benefit is likely to be offset by the increase in pressure caused by the extra weight. When a patient is lying down a greater number of pressure areas are involved than when he is in a sitting position but the wide distribution of weight reduces pressure being borne. Depending on the patient's position, bony prominences covered only by fat and skin bear the brunt of pressure. These are listed in Table 8.5.

Table 8.5 Pressure areas according to position

Recumbent	Lateral	Upright	Prone
Occiput	Ear	Scapulae	Ear
Scapulae	Shoulder	Thoracic	Elbows
Thoracic	Wrist	vertebrae	
vertebrae		Sacrum	Sternum
Elbows	Greater	Ischial	Iliac crests
	trochanter	tuberosities	
Sacrum	Knees	Heels	Knees
Heels	External	Toes	Toes
	malleolus		
Toes	Heel		
	Outer aspect		
	of foot		

Other factors

Further factors contribute to skin breakdown. Shearing force has been identified as a cause of pressure sores in semi-recumbent patients. This means simply that the skin over the sacrum or the heels stays put while the bony skeleton slides forward causing stretching and ultimate severing of the blood vessels of the deep fascia which unites the skin and the underlying tissues.

Friction can be the cause of superficial sores mainly as the result of two skin surfaces rubbing together or the skin being scraped across hard sheets at the time of lifting or turning a patient, especially if the skin is wet. Frictional damage is more common in obese patients because of the difficulty in lifting them clear of bed or chair surfaces.

Incontinence of urine and/or faeces and perspiration may contribute to the development of pressure sores as the result of maceration of the skin with the further likelihood of infection developing.

Vulnerability to pressure is increased where there is inadequate nutrition causing loss of subcutaneous fat and atrophy of muscle and skin. Established sores will be delayed in their healing in the absence of an adequate intake of protein and vitamin C.

With ageing the skin becomes more friable, there is loss of subcutaneous fat and circulation to the periphery decreases. At any age however, disruption of the flow of blood can lower the skin's resistance to breakdown. Vascular factors due to peripheral vascular disease, shock and cigarette smoking are therefore important.

Prevention of pressure sores

Pressure sores are harder to treat than to prevent.

Now that factors which increase a patient's susceptibility to pressure effects are recognised, 'at risk' patients are more readily identifiable. Obvious categories of patient are the elderly and incontinent. Less obvious groups include shocked patients, patients with lowered resistance to infection and those with impaired mobility or sensory loss. The simple scoring system devised by Norton et al (1975) highlighted the 'at risk' patient through an assessment of his general physical condition, mental state, degree of activity, mobility and level of continence.

The one major factor in the prevention of pressure sores is pressure relief which may be intermittent or continuous as long as adequate capillary circulation can be maintained. Manual turning of the patient is effective but it does represent a considerable nursing load and can be difficult to maintain at the required intervals. Two hours in one position seems to be about the maximum which can be allowed if pressure problems are to be avoided. Really high-risk patients may require to be turned more often. It may be helpful to compile a written schedule of turning which may be kept at the bedside for easy reference. A variety of beds have been designed to turn the patient automatically or to assist the process of turning. Manually operated turning beds include the Stryker frame and the net suspension bed. Numerous beds are also available to minimise or vary pressure distribution over the surface of the entire body. These include ripple beds, water beds and low air loss beds. Continuous reduction in pressure over bony prominences and protection can be provided through the use of such devices as foam wedges, gel pads, sheepskin rugs, bootees and elbow protectors. Foam rings are now thought more likely to endanger the blood supply to the area they are supposed to protect. None of the methods mentioned eliminates the need for turning.

Careful consideration should be given to the need for adequate hygiene in the prevention of pressure sores. Washing with soap undoubtedly reduces the bacterial population of the surface of the skin and is essential for the removal of debris and following an episode of incontinence. The skin however is naturally acid and therefore soap which raises the skin pH may interfere with its effect as a barrier to infection. Unless well rinsed off, soap leaves irritant deposits. The rubbing of soap into the skin is no longer accepted practice, vigorous massage being understood to damage the micro-circulation.

Some topical preparations have a place in the prevention of sores. For example, silicone creams may be helpful in preventing maceration of the skin by acting as a barrier against moisture. Excessively dry skin may benefit from sparing applications of a moisturiser. The vasoconstrictive effects of alcohol and alcohol/oil mixtures have not proved beneficial. The practice, popular at one time, of rubbing in applications containing spirit involves friction and therefore may actually damage tissues.

Attention to diet is important to prevent the development of pressure sores in any susceptible patient. Anaemia, hypoproteinaemia and deficiences of vitamin C or zinc can be made good by supplementing the diet.

Proper management of incontinence and the use of successful techniques of lifting such as the Australian lift for raising the patient clear of the bed make an essential contribution to the prevention of pressure sores.

Probably no other aspect of patient care calls

for the support of so many members of the hospital team as the prevention of pressure sores. They include dietitians, porters, operating department assistants, radiographers, physiotherapists, laundry managers, supplies officers and engineers.

Treatment of pressure sores

Preventative measures must always be continued in spite of the development of a pressure sore. If a sore is to heal it must be relieved of pressure as much as possible but the consequent risk of causing sores to develop elsewhere must be kept in mind. Turning schedules may have to be amended. As with any wound, precise treatment will depend on the extent of the sore and whether infection is present. If, following the culture of any exudate, local therapy is indicated, a non-antibiotic preparation is generally preferred since topical antibiotics may cause sensitisation and encourage the development of resistant organisms. Topical antibiotic preparations should always be medically prescribed. Systemic antibiotics should only be used where patients have developed a more generalised infection. Systemic therapy of a sore seems to be of limited value due to its compromised vasculature.

Local treatment of a sore. This involves an aseptic procedure whatever agent is used and for whatever purpose. Mechanical cleansing is done to remove organisms, pus and exudate. Sterile aqueous sodium chloride 0.9% w/v, povidone-iodine 10% w/v or sodium hypochlorite solutions at a suitable dilution may be used. Cell debris may be loosened using hydrogen peroxide solution (3–6%) for example. The removal of necrotic or devitalised tissue from the wound is known as debridement and allows the development of granulating tissue. The removal of tissue can be done by the nurse using sterile scissors in the ward (or at home), or it may be done under general anaesthetic, or by the use of enzymatic agents. The latter is a controversial method as there is no evidence that these agents are measurably better than hypochlorite solution. Certain products are available which promote granulation essential for the healing process to take place.

Benzoyl peroxide lotion and dextranomer beads (Debrisan) have both cleansing and granulation-promoting properties. All products which are prescription-only medicines must be prescribed by the doctor using the medicine prescription sheet. Those products listed in a nursing formulary may be applied without prescription.

After cleansing with an antiseptic solution superficial sores may be left exposed and pressure free or an occlusive film dressing may be applied. Deeper wounds require dressings not only to provide mechanical protection and prevent the introduction of infection but, by incorporating the agents previously mentioned, to stimulate healing. When a deeply penetrating sore involves muscle or even bone, surgical intervention is the only possible treatment likely to succeed. This may involve skin grafting or reconstruction using adjacent tissue, a tube pedicle or rotation flap.

Summary

The role of the nurse with respect to pressure sores is central to the comfort of a very large percentage of patients under her care. Early recognition of pressure sore potential and the implementation of appropriate preventative measures are fundamentally important. Where sores have developed, prompt and effective treatment must be instigated. Continuing involvement of coworkers and a united effort to protect patients from further suffering are of high priority. Further research is undoubtedly needed in this field but sufficient is now known for the majority of sores never to arise. It could be said that the prevention of pressure sores often directly results from the Hawthorne effect. That is to say, irrespective of the method used, the associated energy and enthusiasm put into practice result in a beneficial outcome.

STOMA CARE

Stoma care involves the active participation of a number of health carers, with the nurse taking a central part, not only in giving nursing care but also in the co-ordination of care which

others provide. The overall aim, is to rehabili-
tate the patient so that he may care for himself
within the framework of a near normal way of
life. There will, however, be situations where
self-care alone is inadequate, not because of
any failing on the part of the patient, but
because the patient's needs make it so. Obviously special care is required for new stoma
patients and the terminally ill. Some older
patients may become wholly dependent on the
nurse for the care of their stoma due to the
ravages of the ageing process. On the other
hand, many patients will manage very well
from day to day providing they have continual
general support and access to specialist help
and advice when they require it.

The medical knowledge and practical expertise of stoma care are included in every basic
nursing course, and the advent of the stoma
therapist provides the nurse with the opportunity to enhance her skills and knowledge.
This will help to build confidence in the nurse
which must be evident to the patient if the
care is to succeed.

Types of stoma

A stoma is usually created when it has been
necessary to form a surgical diversion of
faeces or urinary flow. There are three main
types.

(a) An operation which necessitates removal
of the rectum and sigmoid colon results in the
formation of a *colostomy*. At this advanced
point in the intestinal tract, the faeces are
generally well formed and evacuation fairly
predictable.

(b) When the large intestine has been
entirely removed, or diverted, the stoma is
made at the lower end of the small intestine
and is known as an *ileostomy*. With this type
of stoma, waste is looser because more of the
intestine has been removed, or diverted, at an
earlier stage in the process of disposal.

(c) In the treatment of certain bladder disorders, the ureters may be transplanted into a
short segment taken from the ileum to form
an ileal conduit or they may have been brought
to the skin surface in the formation of a *ureterostomy*. Waste in these cases is urine. In all
forms of stoma, since no voluntary muscles

are involved, the excretory flow cannot be
controlled at will. Management therefore is
directed towards modifying waste where this
is possible and applying some form of device
for its collection.

The newly formed stoma

Post-operative recovery as well as successful
management and acceptance of the stoma are
influenced by what happens pre-operatively.
Time must be found by both medical and
nursing staff to explain to the patient (the
ostomist) the operation and its implications.
More than one discussion is needed as
patients understandably do not always retain
all the information given on one occasion.
Opportunities should also be given to an
immediate relative of the patient to ask questions. Privacy is essential when selecting the
site of the stoma and when allowing the
patient to try various appliances. The patient
may be glad to meet with an ostomist and is
usually appreciative of being given some literature to peruse at his own pace.

During the immediate post-operative period,
in addition to the standard care and support
given, the nurse should make regular and
frequent checks of the stoma itself. It is
important to observe its colour so that early
signs of strangulation of its blood supply may
be noted and reported. Excessive bleeding or
sinking of the stoma must be reported also, as
a return to theatre may be indicated. From the
start the nurse's attitude to the patient should
be positive, being gentle yet firm. Nurses will
have to come to terms with any feelings of
revulsion which they may have when dealing
with the stoma. The thought of having to face
such operations is, at first, repugnant to many
patients although given the right psychological
support, most patients will find a stoma preferable to the discomfort of the illness they
previously suffered. Acceptance of the stoma
is the first and greatest hurdle to be overcome.
One of the hardest moments for the patient is
looking at the stoma for the first time and
nurses can be of great support during this
difficult period. 'Ready to leave hospital' for the
ostomist should mean that he is ready to care
for the stoma, no longer being regarded as a

patient but as an individual who happens to eliminate in a different way. Each person, naturally, will have his own particular problems and individual methods of overcoming them.

Diet

For those who have a colostomy or ileostomy, correct diet comes before anything else. The aim is to produce faeces which are as well formed as possible without causing constipation. Sensible eating can help to achieve this aim and can minimise other problems for the ostomist, (e.g. odour, flatus and excoriation of the skin). Dietetic advice is always available and aims to help the person find a diet which is as near normal as he can possibly manage. At first, a certain amount of experimentation may be required with food combinations. In time, the person usually finds that most foodstuffs can be taken in moderation with a few exceptions. Wind-producing foods are soon identified. Highly spiced foods and onions are to be avoided as they can produce loose and odorous faeces, and much flatus. Pulse foods and Brussels sprouts can cause flatus and noise although not so much odour. The timing of liquid in relation to food is important. It is safer not to drink immediately before, during or until about half an hour after a meal, so as to avoid loosening the faeces. Fizzy drinks are to be avoided and advice on which alcoholic drinks may be safely taken should be sought.

Odour

Odour is caused by either faeces or flatus and therefore good dietary management helps to keep it to a minimum. Very careful hygiene is essential of course, although deodorants also may be used. Chewing one or two sprigs of raw parsley has a deodorant effect. Deodorant solutions, gels and powders are available for placing in the stoma appliance although care should be taken not to allow liquid deodorants to touch the stoma or surrounding skin otherwise they may cause severe irritation. Some ostomy bags have a small vent at the top for inserting deodorant liquid or have a charcoal filter incorporated. A deodorising spray may be used at the time of emptying the appliance and a deodorising air device may be placed as appropriate.

Appliances

No single appliance is suitable for all those who have a stoma and this is reflected in the wide range of products currently available. The aim is to find a device which not only serves the purpose of satisfactorily collecting the waste but is discreet, rustle-free and acceptable. A detailed description of all the different appliances is beyond the scope of this book but there are several aspects which should be understood when considering appliances generally. Stoma bags may or may not be disposable and/or drainable. They are available either as one- or two-piece systems. One-piece appliances consist of a disposable collection bag complete with its own seal. Two-piece appliances comprise an adhesive face plate to which a disposable collection bag may be fitted. The face plate may be left attached for several days while the bag is replaced as often as necessary. Ureterostomy patients generally wear reusable appliances often made of rubber to support the weight of urine and to reduce the likelihood of puncture. Reusable apparatus should be removed for cleaning in soap and water then thoroughly rinsed and dried, so at least two sets are needed. The type and site of the stoma, manual dexterity and skin sensitivity all influence the choice of appliance.

Adhesives

Adhesives for stoma bags must be gentle and yet effective since any type of skin can tolerate only a certain amount of irritation from the fairly frequent changes of appliance. Many appliances involve the use of karaya gum which provides protection for the skin by absorbing moisture. Because of its malleability it moulds readily to the contours of the skin thus providing a good seal. In cold weather, the karaya piece may be warmed in the palm of the hand or placed near a heater to soften slightly for neater application. Microporous adhesives may also be used and are mostly well tolerated. A belt may be attached to different types of appliance for added support. Many permutations of apparatus have been produced and ostomists themselves make adaptations to suit their own needs.

Skin protection

In the same way as a person who is paraplegic lives with the threat of pressure sores, the ostomist must constantly take care to prevent irritation and breakdown of the skin which surrounds the stoma. A routine of changing the appliance right to the skin will be followed by each individual. Care must be taken to remove plasters without tearing the skin. The area around the stoma is washed using cotton wool, for example, and warm, soapy water, taking care to remove all traces of faeces, mucus, and skin applications. It is important to rinse off all soap to reduce irritation and to pat the skin dry. Any traces of adhesive should be removed using an adhesive solvent. Additional applications of barrier cream and skin gel may be used for protection of the skin. Creams should be applied sparingly to a radius of about 10 cm from the stoma but not on the stoma itself.

Skin breakdown. In the event of the skin becoming red and weepy, adhesives may have to be temporarily replaced with some form of dressing. This may be left in position for several days with the appliance being placed on top of the dressing. Efforts should then be made to identify the cause of the excoriation. It may be that the motions are too loose, calling for a change in diet or a bulking agent. Changing the bag more promptly helps to reduce faecal contact with exposed skin. The size of the aperture may be too big causing a similar problem and may have to be reduced. Ideally there should only be about 0.5 cm of a gap between the stoma and the appliance. Antiseptic solutions tend to be painful when applied to sore skin, causing further irritation, and are best avoided in preference to soap and water, thorough rinsing with cool water, and careful drying.

Disposal of appliances

Ostomists should be encouraged not to allow the care of the stoma to 'take over'. Bearing in mind that he is likely to be one of a family with others in the home to consider, stoma equipment should be kept together preferably out of sight. A travelling kit may be kept at the ready. The question of disposal of appliances and their contents is an important one for all concerned. Today, many patients dispose of the contents of the bag down the lavatory and as it is flushed they 'sluice' the bag. The empty bag is then wrapped in newspaper and sealed with tape to make a small package. If this is disposed of amongst ordinary domestic waste in the usual way there will be no problem. All ostomists are entitled to free prescriptions for all their stoma needs.

Medicines and ostomists

Certain precautions have to be taken by doctors prescribing medicines for patients with an ileostomy or colostomy. Nurses should also be aware of these and other problems relating to medicines that may arise for the ostomist.

Patients with an ileostomy

Diarrhoea with subsequent loss of water and potassium is a very real threat to the ileostomist at any time, and may be exacerbated by taking medicines.

Digoxin. The improvement in renal perfusion which results from digoxin therapy may cause additional potassium depletion. Potassium supplements may be needed when digoxin therapy is indicated.

Diuretics. These should be avoided whenever possible owing to the risk of dehydration and potassium loss. If diuretic therapy is essential a potassium-sparing diuretic should be used.

Bowel washouts. Any form of washout is contra-indicated because of the severe risk of dehydration rapidly occurring.

Tablets. Those with slow release properties are unsuitable. Such preparations are designed to release the drug from the tablet during its passage through the digestive tract over a period of 3–6 hours. In ileostomy patients this period is shortened, with the result that drug release may be incomplete leading to under dosage. For this reason, if potassium replacement therapy is required, a liquid form is used to ensure full absorption of potassium.

Patients with a colostomy

Constipation may be a problem for many colostomy patients and should always be borne in mind in their management. For the *treatment of constipation*, colostomy patients should increase their fluid intake or make some dietary adjustments in preference to taking medication. If this approach does not help then bulk-forming laxatives such as ispaghula husk or methylcellulose may be used. These act by increasing faecal mass which stimulates peristalsis and effects expulsion of faeces provided sufficient fluid intake is maintained. These medicines are supplied in tablet and granule form. Tablets may be broken up and should be chewed with a little water half an hour before a meal. Liquids are then withheld until about half and hour after the meal. Because these preparations have a hygroscopic action, the timing of fluid is important otherwise the medication absorbs fluid recently taken instead of the fluid content of the faeces. Not all patients find the granular form of these agents manageable as there is a tendency for the granules to swell in the mouth and thus be difficult to swallow.

Antacids. Those containing aluminium salts may cause the colostomy patient to become constipated.

Antidepressants. The anticholinergic effects of some antidepressants can lead to a number of troublesome side-effects including constipation.

Narcotic analgesics. Analgesics such as dihydrocodeine are especially constipating. Other narcotic analgesics such as codeine and morphine may also be troublesome.

Patients with ileostomy or colostomy

For any patient with an ileostomy or colostomy, oral antibiotics, oral iron preparations, and antacids containing magnesium salts, should be avoided whenever possible because of the likelihood of diarrhoea. If necessary, concurrent intestinal sedatives such as codeine phosphate may be given.

Conclusion

There can be no doubt that the formation of a stoma brings change to the individual's way of life. The prospect of such an operation for the individual and his family is a daunting one.

With the practical and psychological support of a team of staff through the peri-operative, rehabilitative and independent phases of stoma management, the individual has a very real chance of being able to pursue a career, raise a family, and resume many previously enjoyed activities. The ostomist has to acquire and maintain confidence in his ability to cope in order to lead a full life. Membership of associations and clubs for ostomists can generally help by providing an opportunity to offer and accept support against the background of a common, shared experience. In time, the need for such participation may diminish, but for many, the benefits of membership will continue to be enjoyed over the years.

BLADDER IRRIGATION

Special responsibility lies with nurses involved in the care of patients with a urinary catheter. Even when technical skills have been mastered and confidence gained, the potential harm which may be inflicted unwittingly on such patients must always be borne in mind. Infection is the commonest complicating problem. However, post-operative continuous bladder irrigation carries with it added risks. For example, sodium in the irrigating fluid may be absorbed through the operation site resulting in a raised blood pressure. Perforation of the bladder is another serious complication which can occur after operation, and its early detection calls for great vigilance by nursing staff.

Indwelling catheters, even when introduced into the bladder under the most rigorous aseptic conditions, are still an important source of urinary tract infection. In the course of time, crystallisation around and within the lumen of the catheter, increases the risk of infection further, by obstructing the flow and causing stasis of urine. By-passing of urine follows, leading to discomfort, embarrassment and skin breakdown. Patients who produce haematuric urine can develop severe drainage problems and discomfort, especially when the catheter is blocked by blood clots. The indications for washing out the bladder are to reduce and treat urinary tract infections and to prevent and clear obstruction of the eye(s) and lumen of the catheter by debris, crystals or blood clot. The three methods most commonly used for introducing fluid into the bladder are by instillation from an irrigation device, based on a plastic bag such as the Uro-Tainer; mechanical irrigation using a form of suction; and continuous bladder irrigation. The method used will depend on the reason for carrying out the irrigation.

The Uro-Tainer system

This system has greatly improved the management of indwelling urinary catheters in hospital and at home. The simple technique involved saves nursing time and can be mastered by patients or their relatives for use at home. Solution G and chlorhexidine solution are available in the form of a ready-to-use irrigation device. Solution G is weakly acidic and is used for flushing-out and for preventing crystal formation, or for dissolving crystals already formed in the catheter. Aqueous chlorhexidine solution (0.02% w/v) has a bacteriostatic action against many of the common urinary tract pathogens. Some clinicians recommend routine use of chlorhexidine solution immediately prior to the removal of all urinary catheters. The solution is left in the bladder until such time as the patient wishes to void.

Clot retention is usually treated by irrigation with sterile 0.9% w/v sodium chloride solution although where clots prove to be obstinate alternative methods of irrigation may have to be employed. Sterile sodium citrate solution 3% may also be used to break up blood clots. The volume of solution in each Uro-Tainer is 100 ml but the amount instilled into the bladder is not critical, rather the time the solution is left in the bladder, which may be up to half an hour. Gloves are not necessary when this method of irrigation is used. Thorough handwashing is essential and care must be taken to join the catheter and irrigation tubing without contaminating either of these. A regime in current use for patients with long-term catheters involves alternate use of a urinary antiseptic, such as chlorhexidine (0.02% w/v), with a decrystallising solution, such as solution G. A suitable regime would be

to use chlorhexidine solution every Tuesday, the other solution every Friday.

Mechanical irrigation using suction

In the event of a catheter becoming completely blocked by blood clots, the catheter may be washed out in an effort to break down the clots by a form of suction using a catheter-tipped syringe and irrigating solution from a bottle. Where blood clots are especially troublesome a large volume of sterile 0.9% w/v sodium chloride solution will be required. This method is based on first introducing approximately 50 ml of solution which is left in the bladder. This acts as a physical buffer to allow further volumes of fluid to be instilled under pressure then withdrawn by suction through the catheter, depending on the severity of the blockage. The nurse wears gloves for this procedure because of the many manipulative processes involved. It may take a considerable time until the catheter drains freely. The patient, who may already be in pain and be losing blood into the bladder, can find this a tedious and uncomfortable experience. He should therefore be kept warm and as comfortable as possible. As with all such procedures the encouragement and support of the nurse are vital throughout.

Continuous irrigation

Continuous irrigation of the bladder is commonly employed following prostatic surgery to rid the bladder of blood clots and prostatic debris. A three-way catheter, or alternative combination of catheters, is inserted in theatre. This allows one inlet for inflating the catheter balloon and another for the entry of irrigating solution, and an outlet for drainage of the bladder contents. Sodium chloride solution (0.9% w/v) is introduced into the bladder from a 3 litre bag suspended from an infusion stand, via an administration set connected to the catheter. In the immediate post-operative period the control clamp is left open fully to allow for continuous flushing of the bladder and of the eyes of the catheter. After several hours, depending on the degree of haematuria, the rate may be decreased. Volumes of irrigating solution ranging from 15–45 l may be required to treat the patient during the first 24 hours. The flow of such large volumes of fluid demands frequent attention by the nurse in maintaining input, discarding output and keeping records of both. In urological wards, anticipating needs and finding adequate storage space for large volumes of irrigation solutions can present problems. These may, to some extent, be alleviated by active involvement of the ward pharmacist who can, amongst other things, help to ensure that supply keeps pace with demand.

It should be remembered that hypertension (resulting from absorption of sodium) and perforation of the bladder may each result from this form of irrigation. Trained nurses in urology wards have particular responsibility therefore to ensure that close monitoring of the blood pressure and pulse (every $\frac{1}{2}$ hour at first), fluid balance, and pain is carried out. If the patient complains of pain, no matter how mild, irrigation should not proceed without seeking further advice. Whilst it is important not to alarm junior nursing staff, and hence patients, at this time, the possibility of perforation especially following transurethral resection of the bladder must never be forgotten.

General principles

When using any form of bladder washout the broad principles of medicine administration apply. The details of the solution are checked against the prescription, and the fluid should be visually examined before use, to make sure that it is free from any particulate matter. Any container whose contents are not clear should be rejected. In view of the high risk to the patient of microbial contamination, all procedures are carried out with full aseptic techniques. Ideally, solutions should be warmed to body temperature before use in a solution-warming cabinet. Improvised methods of warming solutions are not recommended since control of the solution temperature is impossible to achieve. In the absence of a solution-warming cabinet it is probably best to use the solution at room temperature.

Patients with an indwelling catheter who have been on continuous drainage for weeks or months, may have difficulty in tolerating the instillation of volumes of solutions in excess of 50 ml because of reduced bladder capacity or bladder irritability. When the patient indicates that the bladder feels uncomfortable and as though it cannot take in more fluid, then this must be taken as the maximal amount that can be instilled. As soon as possible following manipulations of a catheter, the catheter should be attached to a sterile closed drainage system. The drainage tubing should be stiff enough to reduce the likelihood of kinking and the drainage bag should be adequately supported on a floor stand positioned for ease of observation of the colour, consistency and volume of urine drained. Bag holders can become distorted, for example when lowering the height of the patient's bed. This increases the risk of the tubing becoming kinked. Also the drainage tap may come in contact with the floor, with obvious risk of contamination.

Bladder irrigation using an irrigation device

Requirements
 Sterile solution in plastic bag with catheter connection (irrigation device e.g. 'Uro-Tainer')
 Sterile replacement drainage system
 Incontinence pad
 Prescription sheet if required.

Procedure
1. Check details on irrigation device and with prescription if appropriate. Read the instructions for use. Examine solution visually for clarity. Identify patient.
2. Explain to patient what is involved.
3. Assist patient into relaxed position and expose catheter only. Place incontinence pad for maximum protection.
4. Wash hands.
5. Remove irrigation device from sterile package (Fig. 8.3A).
6. Close clamp of irrigation tubing (Fig. 8.3B).
7. Hold each end of rubber cap of irrigation device with fingers of both hands and twist (Fig. 8.3C).
8. Slide rubber cap on to plastic connector (Fig. 8.3D).
9. Withdraw rubber protector without touching connector.

10. Holding irrigation device in hand, use same hand to disconnect drainage system and hold drainage tubing erect until empty. Apply rubber protector to drainage tubing and discard. At the same time pinch catheter with other hand.
11. Insert connector into catheter (Fig. 8.3E).
12. Release clamp and allow solution to flow into bladder (Fig. 8.3F). If necessary, squeeze bag very gently to instil solution.
13. Close off clamp (Fig. 8.3G).
14. After 30 minutes or so, release clamp and hold bag downwards to drain rinsing solution (Fig. 8.3H).
15. Clamp tube and remove connector from catheter by turning gently.
16. Connect new drainage system to catheter.
17. Leave patient comfortable.
18. Wash hands.
19. Record administration.

Bladder irrigation using suction

Requirements
   Bottle(s) of irrigating solution
   Sterile bladder lavage pack containing
      jug (2 litre)
      catheter-tipped syringe (50 ml capacity)
      receiver
      gauze swab
      impermeable sheet
   Sterile replacement drainage system
   Pair of surgeon's gloves
   Large unsterile jug
   Incontinence pad
   Prescription sheet.

Procedure
1. Check bottle label with prescription and examine solution visually for clarity. Identify patient.
2. Prepare trolley as for aseptic procedure.
3. Explain procedure to patient.
4. Assist patient into comfortable position and expose catheter only. Place incontinence pad beneath catheter.
5. Open packs. Position jug using outside of wrapping paper. Pour anticipated volume or irrigating solution into jug.
6. Wash hands using antiseptic (e.g. detergent chlorhexidine solution). Apply gloves.

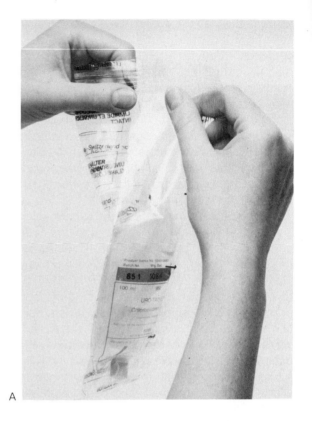

A

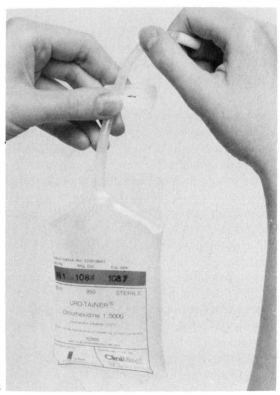

B

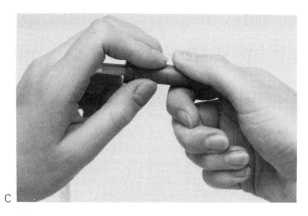

C

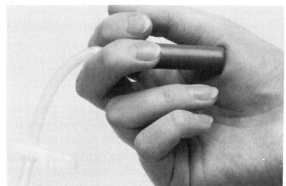

D

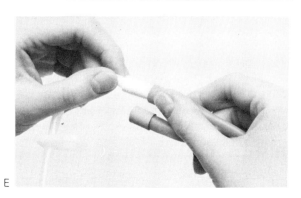

E

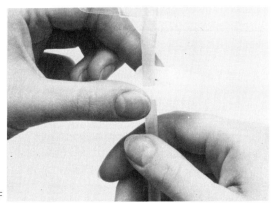

F

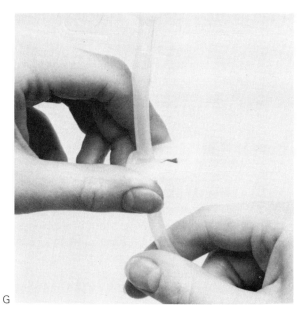

G

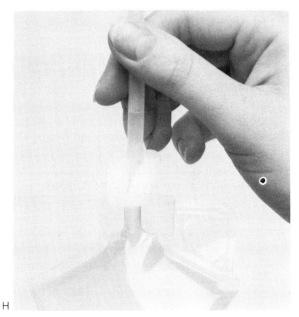

H

Fig. 8.3 A–H Uro-tainer

7. Place towel and receiver under catheter. Disconnect catheter from drainage tubing using 2 swabs.
8. Draw up approximately 50 ml solution into syringe, expel air and attach to catheter.
9. Inject solution at a steady rate and then pinch catheter.

10. Draw up a further 50 ml solution, release pinch on catheter and inject solution.
11. Pull back plunger and
    — if returned fluid is clear reinject same fluid a few times (3 or 4 times is as often as patients can tolerate each 50 ml).
    — if clots appear discard all fluid. Draw up further 100 ml solution for injecting. Repeat procedure always using fresh solution if clots are obtained, until returned fluid is clear.
12. Allow catheter to drain completely.
13. Attach new drainage system and place in stand.
14. Measure and record urine drained.
15. Clear away equipment.
16. Wash hands.
17. Record administration.

N.B. When the bladder is irritated by infection or is reduced in capacity by tumour, much smaller volumes of fluid may be tolerated. On occasion as small a volume as 10 ml is as much as the patient can hold. Infected fluid is never re-injected.)

Table 8.6 gives details of sterile solutions used in bladder irrigation and in Table 8.7 some drugs used in bladder instillations are indicated.

VULVAL AND VAGINAL MEDICATIONS

Procedural aspects

Gynaecological conditions are judged by many women to be a source of extreme embarrassment and fear. Patients express these feelings in different ways. Some are hesitant to ask for further explanation of their condition or treatment, showing a natural reservation about intimate matters. Others fear being thought of as unclean, embarrassed by odour, itching and perhaps staining of underclothes from vaginal discharge. Patients may fear discovery of a malignant condition or that they have developed an infection which has been sexually transmitted. Knowledge of anatomy and physiology of the female genital tract in some instances may be scant and attitudes to bodily functions may have been influenced by folklore.

Nurses working in gynaecological wards and clinics become accustomed to carrying out intimate procedures and discussing very personal issues with their patients. They may need to remind themselves of the importance of maintaining sensitivity to the feelings of each new patient. General ward nurses and district nurses are required to care for patients with gynaecological disorders from time to time, and so they should be ready to turn their attention to the special needs of these patients.

In all cases, embarrassment or attitude on the part of the nurse should never be allowed to interfere with establishing and dealing with the full nature of the problem. Tact, patience and gentleness are essential at all times.

Practical aspects

Hormones and anti-infectives are the main drugs used in treating vulval and vaginal conditions. To improve the quality of the vaginal epithelium and to increase natural resistance to infection, post-menopausal conditions such as atrophic vaginitis and kraurosis vulvae, may be treated with topical oestrogens in the form of a pessary or vaginal cream. They may also be used prior to vaginal surgery for prolapse when there is epithelial atrophy. So as to minimise the absorption of oestrogen, the dose and duration of treatment should be adhered to strictly. Some vaginal preparations contain lactic acid which lowers the pH of vaginal secretions and is used in the treatment of non-specific vaginal infections.

Identification of the causative organism is essential before treating infections such as vulval and vaginal thrush, genital herpes, trichomonal vaginitis and the bacterial invasion of gonorrhoea and syphilis. If treatment is to be successful and recurrence prevented, completion of the course, regardless of intervening menstruation, is important even when the signs and symptoms seem to have disappeared.

In sexually-transmitted infections, tracing and treating partners is vital. In previously undiagnosed diabetes mellitus, thrush may be the presenting feature and the nurse must be able to recognise this. In addition to diabetics,

Table 8.6 Sterile solutions used in bladder irrigation.

Active ingredient	Strength (all % w/v)	Pack or Presentation	Uses, indications and precautions
Chlorhexidine Chlorhexidine	1 in 5000 (0.02 %) 1 in 5000	100 ml 'Uro-Tainer' 500 ml bottle	Used for its mechanical effect. Also has a bacteriostatic action on organisms commonly found in the urinary tract.
Glycine	1.5%	3 l plastic bag	Used in transurethral resection of the prostate gland. Non-haemolytic, weakly ionised. Any glycine absorbed is metabolised, ammonia may be produced which has toxic effects. Cases of hyponatraemia have been reported, but these are rare.
Mandelic acid	1%	100 ml 'Uro-Tainer'	Used if resistance is encountered to chlorhexidine. Effective against pseudomonas and proteus.
Mannitol	3%	3 l plastic bag	Used as an alternative to glycine, but instruments may become caked with dried mannitol.
Noxythiolin	1% or 2.5%	2.5 g in rubber capped vial	Used for antibacterial and antifungal properties. It is made up into the required strength with sterile water, taking aseptic precautions. The solution has a limited shelf life (7 days).
Sodium chloride	0.9%	a variety of presentations e.g. 500 ml bottle or 3 l plastic bag.	Used for its mechanical effect. It is also used as a vehicle for certain drugs instilled into the bladder.
Sodium citrate	3%	500 ml bottle	Used primarily for the dissolution of blood clots
Solution R	6% citric acid 0.6% gluconolactone 2.8% magnesium carbonate 0.1% disodium edetate	100 ml 'Uro-Tainer'	Used to dissolve existing encrustations. Use between twice and four times a week for 2 weeks, before reverting to Solution G. Should not be used for a period of 10–14 days following prostatic surgery due to absorption of salts leading to electrolyte imbalance.
Solution G (Suby G)	3.23% citric acid 0.38% light magnesium oxide 0.7% sodium bicarbonate 0.01% sodium edetate	100 ml 'Uro-Tainer'	Used between twice daily and twice weekly to prevent the formation of encrustations. Should not be used for a period of 10–14 days following prostatic surgery due to absorption of salts leading to electrolyte imbalance

Table 8.7 Some drugs used in other bladder instillations

Drugs	Indications	Notes
Amphotericin Miconazole	Fungal infection of the bladder	The instillation is made up from the intravenous injection, diluted with sterile sodium chloride · 0.9% solution.

Cytotoxic drugs
  Doxorubicin
  Ethoglucid
  Thiotepa
	Superficial bladder tumours
	Rapidly recurring non-invasive bladder tumours
	Bladder tumours of low to medium grade malignancy
		A solution of appropriate strength is made up and a suitable volume instilled. The solution should be retained in the bladder for 1–2 hours depending on the drug used and condition being treated.

patients who are pregnant or patients receiving steroids or antibiotics are susceptible to candidal infection. Infections are usually treated with medicated pessaries, supplemented by cream to soothe vulvitis. Medicated tampons are sometimes used in place of pessaries. Antiseptic vaginal jelly may be used to lubricate dilators inserted to prevent stricture which can result from radiation fibrosis following treatment with vaginal radium or caesium.

Vulval and vaginal preparations which contain a drug should be prescribed, administered and recorded according to local policy. The genital area should be clean and traces of previously applied cream should be removed. Whenever possible, the patient should apply the preparation herself. The nurse must guarantee privacy for the patient whether she is explaining self-administration or actually carrying out the treatment. It is important to explain to which particular area the treatment is to be directed, the recommended times of administration and the need to complete the course. Disposable gloves should be worn by the nurse when administering vulval and vaginal preparations both to protect the patient and nurse from acquiring infection or the nurse from absorbing any of the medication. Whether nurse or patient carries out the procedure, the hands should washed before and after. Applicators should be washed in warm soapy water, rinsed and dried. A separate treatment kit should be assigned to the individual patient.

Insertion of vaginal pessaries

Requirements
    Pessary
    Applicator (if supplied)
    Disposable gloves
    Disposable wipes
    Disposal bag
    Prescription sheet.

Procedure
1. Compare details on pessary wrapper with prescription. Identify patient.
2. Explain procedure to patient.
3. Ensure privacy.
4. Encourage patient to empty bladder.
5. Assist patient into appropriate position, i.e. either supine with knees flexed and thighs abducted, or left lateral.
6. With clean hands and wearing gloves, lubricate pessary if directed or place pessary in applicator if supplied.
7. Insert pessary along posterior vaginal wall in an upwards and backwards direction for the full length of the vagina.
8. Wipe vulval area and leave patient comfortable. (The patient will feel more secure wearing a pair of pants or a sanitary pad.)
9. Wash applicator in warm, soapy water, rinse and dry.
10. Wash hands.
11. Record administration.

EYE PREPARATIONS

Procedural aspects

The eye is a delicate and vital structure which protects itself in several ways. The immediacy of the blink reflex is evidence of the protective response made to the slightest threat to the eye. Any ophthalmic procedure, be it the application of eye drops or ointment, is approached against this background. Despite the fact that many patients may tolerate more painful procedures with equanimity, procedures involving the eye may cause particular anxiety. Ophthalmic treatment calls for a manner which conveys confidence to the patient, helping to ensure he is relaxed before, during and after the procedure. As with all procedures a clear explanation is given to the patient to gain his co-operation.

Infection risks must be guarded against by washing the hands with a suitable antiseptic cleansing solution before and after each procedure. When applying eye medication the standard procedures for administering and recording medicines are followed. A damaged eye is particularly susceptible to infection, so that whenever possible a single-use presentation of the eye drop is used. This is especially important when a suspected corneal abrasion is being examined using fluorescein. Where single-dose units are not available, or when larger volumes are required, a separate multi-dose container should be used for each patient. Care must be taken not to contaminate the dropper or nozzle of eye preparations.

All containers should be labelled with the patient's name and the date of opening. The label on the eye preparation should be compared with the prescription. The special points to note are the name of the medication, the strength (usually expressed as a percentage), the amount, which eye is to be treated if not both, the time and frequency of administration and that the preparation is in date. As with other forms of medication, eye drops may be administered once only, (including pre-operatively) or on a regular basis. Intensive treatment may also be indicated, e.g. in the case of an infection. In order to convey all the necessary information it may be necessary to use a prescription sheet specially designed for the purpose (Fig. 8.4A and B).

In order that the medication is safely and effectively administered, it is important to position the patient suitably. The head requires to be tilted back and maintained in a steady position so that the risk of the patient damaging the eye by contact with the equipment in use is minimised. To achieve this, the patient should be lying or else sitting , in which case the head should be supported by a pillow or the back of the chair. If possible the nurse should work from behind the patient so that she is close to the working area and in greater control of the procedure. When the patient is confined to bed this may not be possible and so the approach should be made from the patient's side.

As always, safety aspects should be considered. Good lighting is essential for carrying out procedures on delicate structures such as the eye. Light should be from above and behind the nurse. With photophobic patients, consideration must be given to light reaching the patient, otherwise he may be unable to open his eyes. Movements of the hand should be gentle and controlled. Gloves are not worn, as the disposable type are seldom close fitting and therefore there is a

danger of their causing damage if allowed to touch the sensitive corneal surface of the eye. In all cases, the nurse must be alert for any sign of adverse reaction to a drug used locally in the eye. This may take the form of a worsening of inflammation or spread of inflammation to surrounding skin.

In the event of the wrong preparation being administered or the wrong eye being treated, the doctor must be notified *at once* so that any corrective action can be taken without delay.

Teaching patients to administer eye medications

When teaching a patient to administer an eye medication the special points to emphasise are

1. the need for scrupulously clean hands.
2. the need to avoid contamination
3. the importance of using only the prescribed medications.

Because of the systemic toxicity of many ophthalmic drugs it is especially important that all eye preparations are kept out of the reach of children. Similarly, safe disposal of any remainder when treatment is discontinued, or the container is changed, is essential.

Patients may be helped to select for themselves a suitable position in which to administer the medication. To instil eye drops, some patients find that lying flat and feeling for the lower eyelid is a succcessful method with gravity assisting. This may be inconvenient or impossible for others and they may prefer to work in front of an upstanding mirror although co-ordination of the hand and eye may take time to master by this method. Self-application of an eye ointment and removal or insertion of a contact lens or artificial eye are best performed in front of a mirror.

Eye drops

Eye drops are sterile aqueous solutions or suspensions, presented in multiple application dropper bottles which may be of glass fitted with a removable glass dropper and teat. An alternative presentation is a flexible plastic container with orifice through which drops are expelled with pressure of the fingers. Both types of container are suitable for use by individual patients in the community. Although eye

1. ONCE ONLY EYE MEDICATION

DATE PRESCRIBED	DRUG and FORM	STRENGTH	EYE	DOSE	DIRECTIONS FOR ADMINISTRATION	PRESCRIBER'S SIGNATURE	DATE GIVEN	TIME GIVEN	GIVEN BY	CHECKED BY

2. PRE-OPERATIVE INTENSIVE DILATATION

DRUG		STRENGTH	EYE	DOSE		TIMING FROM START	TIME GIVEN	GIVEN BY	CHECKED BY
Phenylephrine	EYE DROPS	10%		1 drop	TOPICAL	0 min.			
Cyclopentolate		1%		1 drop		+ 5 mins.			
Cyclopentolate		1%		1 drop		+ 10 mins.			
Cyclopentolate		1%		1 drop		+ 15 mins.			
Phenylephrine		10%		1 drop		+ 20 mins.			

Date prescribed _____ Prescriber's signature _____ Date to be given _____

3. POST-OPERATIVE INTENSIVE DILATATION

DRUG		STRENGTH	EYE	DOSE		TIMING FROM START	TIME GIVEN	GIVEN BY	CHECKED BY
Phenylephrine	EYE DROPS	10%		1 drop	TOPICAL	0 min.			
Cyclopentolate		1%		1 drop		+ 5 mins.			
Cyclopentolate		1%		1 drop		+ 10 mins.			
Cyclopentolate		1%		1 drop		+ 15 mins.			
Phenylephrine		10%		1 drop		+ 20 mins.			

Date prescribed _____ Prescriber's signature _____ Date to be given _____

Intensive dilatation: the time of administration commences when the first dose of Phenylephrine 10% is instilled. The times of the subsequent doses follow from this, i.e. the first dose of Cyclopentolate 1% is given 5 minutes after the Phenylephrine 10%, the second dose of Cyclopentolate is given 10 minutes after the Phenylephrine 10% and so on.

A

Fig. 8.4 A and B Ophthalmic prescription form containing six sections

4. REGULAR PRESCRIPTIONS

	Date	Time / Tick	6	7	8	9	10	11	12	13	14	15	16	17	18	19	20	21	22
Drug																			
Form																			
Strength																			
Eye																			
Directions																			
Started																			
Date																			
Doctor's Signature																			
Discontinued																			
Date																			
Doctor's Signature																			

5. OTHER PRE-OPERATIVE MEDICATION

DATE TO BE GIVEN	DRUG AND FORM	STRENGTH	EYE	DOSE	DIRECTIONS FOR ADMINISTRATION	PRESCRIBER'S SIGNATURE	GIVEN BY	TIME	CHECKED BY

6. INTENSIVE EYE MEDICATION

DATE TO BE GIVEN	EYE DROPS	STRENGTH	EYE	DOSE	DIRECTIONS FOR ADMINISTRATION	PRESCRIBER'S SIGNATURE	GIVEN BY	TIME	CHECKED BY

GENERAL INSTRUCTIONS

1 No eye medication must be given unless prescribed on this sheet.
2 Each prescription and cancellation should be signed by a doctor.
3 Prescription details must be written in block capitals.
4 When the same drug is being prescribed for both eyes, indicate clearly L+R.
5 Administration times on Chart 4 (Regular prescriptions) should be indicated by the prescriber with a tick ( ) in the appropriate column.
6 On Charts 4, 5, and 6, the nurse records administration of the medication by signing initials in the appropriate box.
7 On Charts 4, 5, and 6, the nurse records checking of the medication by signing initials in the box to the right.

B

Table 8.7 Outline of topical ophthalmic preparations

Therapeutic classification	Example	Eye drops Usual strengths % w/v	Eye ointment % Usual strengths w/w	Notes
Antimicrobial Anti-bacterial	Chloramphenicol	0.5%	1%	Systemic absorption has been reported.
	Framycetin sulphate	0.5%	0.5%	
Anti-viral	Acyclovir	—	3%	Apply 5 times a day
	Idoxuridine	0.1%	0.5%	Apply eye drops every hour during day. Eye ointment 2 hourly at night.
	Vidarabine	—	3%	Apply 5 times daily until corneal re-epithelialisation has occurred then apply twice daily for 7 days.
Anti-fungal	Flucytosine	1.5%	—	
Anti-inflammatory	Betamethasone Sodium Phosphate	0.1%	0.1%	May be combined with an antibiotic e.g. neomycin. May produce a steroid glaucoma.
	Clobetasone 17 — butyrate	0.1% 0.1% with 0.5% Neomycin	—	
	Dexamethasone	0.1%		As with other topically applied corticosteroids checks should be made on intraocular pressure.
	Hydrocortisone	0.5% with Framycetin	0.5% with Chloramphenicol	
Mydriatic and cycloplegic	Atropine sulphate	0.25% 0.5% 1%	0.5% and 1%	May be absorbed causing toxic systemic reactions.
	Cyclopentolate	0.5% and 1%	—	May precipitate an acute attack of glaucoma in patients with narrow angle.
	Phenylephrine	10%	—	As cyclopentolate
	Tropicamide	0.5% and 1%	—	Should not be used in patients with a narrow angle between the iris and cornea.
Reduction of Intraocular Pressure	Guanethidine with adrenaline	Guanethidine Adrenaline 1% with 0.2% 3% with 0.5% 5% with 0.5% 5% with 1%		Systemic effects due to adrenaline absorption have been reported including tachycardia and elevated blood pressure.
	Pilocarpine hydrochloride	0.5, 1. 2. 3. 4%	—	A miotic with a duration of action of 3–4 hours.
	Timolol maleate	0.25, 0.5%	—	A beta-adrenoceptor blocking agent

Table 8.7 Outline of topical ophthalmic preparations (con't)

Therapeutic classification	Example	Eye drops Usual strengths % w/v	Eye ointment % Usual strengths w/w	Notes
Local anaesthetics	Amethocaine hydrochloride	0.5, 1%	—	May cause stinging on application
	Benoxinate (oxybuprocaine)	0.4%	—	Prolonged applicaton of local anaesthetics may damage the cornea
	Cocaine hydrochloride	4%	—	
Tear deficiency	Hypromellose	0.3%	—	
	Liquid paraffin	available as liquid and Eye ointment		
Diagnostic agents	Fluorescein	1%	—	Used to locate
	Rose Bengal	1%	—	damaged corneal tissue.

In special units ophthalmic preparations are aseptically dispensed to meet the needs of individual patients.

drops in multiple application units contain preservatives there is always risk of contamination in use. A multiple application container should be used for not more than one month, after which the original container should be rejected and a new container should be started.

Single-application containers (e.g. 'Minims' or 'Opulets') should always be used in surgical procedures. Solutions presented in this way do not contain preservatives. A new single-use unit should be used for each application.

The question of the number of drops which can be instilled into the eye requires clarification. One drop from the normal eye dropper is 50 microlitres (μl) and will overload the average conjunctival sac, which has a capacity of 25 μl (Lessar & Fiscella 1985). To overcome this, where more than one drop of the same preparation is to be instilled (or another preparation used) an interval of 5–10 minutes should elapse before instilling the second drop. This may present difficulties in ophthalmology units where a considerable number of patients may be receiving several different forms of drops in succession. If there is a high rate of tear secretion, aqueous solutions will be quickly diluted or eliminated from the eye into the nasolacrimal duct, thus becoming unavailable for ophthalmic absorption but available for systemic absorption. This may result in systemic side-effects (e.g. dry mouth with atropine). Some practitioners recommend pressure over the punctum after administration

as a means of restricting tear flow into the duct. The frequency of instillation of drops varies and will depend on, for example, the degree of infection or inflammation. In the treatment of acute glaucoma, a very intensive regime of instillation is followed initially which is then gradually reduced in frequency to hourly, continuing until the intraocular pressure is controlled and the pupil pinpoint.

Every effort is made to avoid causing irritation to the eye. Drops used straight from the refrigerator cause discomfort for the patient. If eye drops have been refrigerated, sufficient time should be allowed for the drops to gradually attain room temperature before use. A drop instilled from a height greater than 2.5 cm directly onto the cornea will cause stinging. Any irritation caused by faulty technique will result in increased tear secretion with consequent loss of therapeutic benefit due to a dilution effect. In addition, the patient will often react by squeezing the lids in an accentuated blink reflex, expelling the solution between the lids or down the nasolacrimal duct.

If, after the instillation of drops, the patient complains of irritation of the skin or a feeling of heat and tightness, an allergic reaction should be suspected and the doctor informed.

Instillation of eye drops (see Fig. 8.5)
Where the eyes are sticky this procedure is preceded by bathing of the eyes using sterile sodium chloride 0.9% solution.

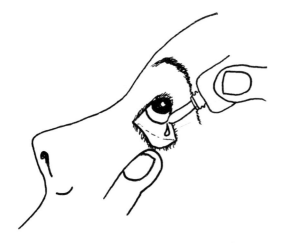

Fig. 8.5 Instillation of eye drops to left eye

Requirements
   Eye drops
   Cotton wool balls or absorbent tissues
   Prescription sheet.

Procedure
   1. Check details of eye drops against prescription and identify patient.
   2. Gain patient's co-operation through explanation.
   3. Assist patient into suitable position either lying flat or sitting with head tilted back and supported.
   4. Encourage patient to relax and ensure lighting is adequate.
   5. Wash hands using cleansing solution, e.g. a detergent/antiseptic handwash.
   6. Approach patient from behind or in front depending on ease of access and ask him to open eyes and to look upwards.
   7. Holding cotton wool ball in one hand, gently evert lower eyelid with pad of one finger of the same hand.
   8. Using other hand, approach eye from below, with bottle outside patient's field of vision. Warn patient that drop is coming, then instil drop into lower fornix allowing drop to fall no more than 2.5 cm before striking the eye but without allowing the dropper to touch any part of the eye. Replace cap if using multiple application bottle.
   9. Use cotton wool ball to mop excess, and

discourage patient from rubbing eye. Reassure patient that some blurring of vision is normal and will pass.
   10. Leave patient comfortable.
   11. Wash hands.
   12. Record administration.

There is some debate as to which aspect of the eye, drops should be instilled. Since the tears pass from the lacrimal glands situated on the lateral aspect of each eye across the eyeball before draining into the nasolacrimal duct, it would seem logical to instil drops into the outer aspect of the lower fornix so that they are washed across with the tears allowing time to take effect before draining away. Some authorities do however advocate using the middle or the inner aspect. The method which can be achieved by nurse and/or patient may be the deciding factor.

Eye ointments
In addition to the more commonly used eye drops (see Table 8.7.) many ophthalmic drugs are available as eye ointments. Eye ointments are essentially dispersions of the active ingredient in a sterile bland base, such as soft paraffin or polyethylene glycol. Useful properties of eye ointments include longer duration of action than eye drops, an emollient soothing action, ease of application and long shelf-life. Eye ointments soften crusts thus preventing adherence of eyelids and eyelashes when the patient is asleep. However, there may be some interference with vision due to the smearing of the cornea with the ointment base.

Application of eye ointment (see Fig. 8.6)

Requirements
   Tube of eye ointment
   Prescription sheet.

Procedure
   1. Check details of eye ointment against prescription and identify patient.
   2. Gain patient's co-operation through explanation.
   3. Assist patient into comfortable position either lying or sitting with head supported.

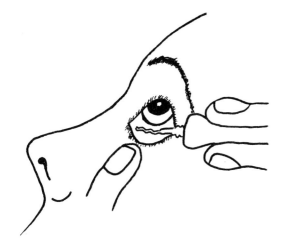

Fig. 8.6 Application of eye ointment to left eye

4. Encourage patient to relax and ensure lighting is adequate.
5. Wash hands using a detergent/antiseptic handwash.
6. Approach patient from front and ask him to open eyes and to look upwards.
7. Using pad of finger of one hand, gently evert lower eyelid. Warn patient that he will feel the ointment being applied.
8. Using other hand, squeeze ointment out of tube along lower lid from inner canthus outwards without allowing the nozzle to touch any part of the eye. Ask patient to close eyes for a minute or so after replacing cap on tube to prevent contamination of the nozzle.
9. Leave patient comfortable and reassure him that some blurring of vision is normal and will pass. Discourage patient from rubbing eye.
10. Wash hands.
11. Record administration.

Rodding

This procedure is done to prevent formation of adhesions between the eyelid and the eyeball which can arise as the result of chemical burns of the conjunctiva. In the first few days after injury the procedure is likely to be uncomfortable and a local anaesthetic such as amethocaine 0.5% eye drops is instilled in advance. Sterile petroleum jelly is used to lubricate the rod in most cases although sometimes an anti-biotic ointment may be used instead, if prescribed. Any adhesions which are forming are broken down and a film of grease is left between the two surfaces.

Requirements
Local anaesthetic eye drops
Sterile smooth, slim glass rod
Sterile petroleum jelly or antibiotic eye ointment if ordered
Sterile wool mops
Gallipot, sterile.
Sachet of sterile sodium chloride 0.9% solution
Disposal bag.
Prescription sheet.

Procedure
1. Prepare patient as for instilling eye drops.
2. Stand behind patient.
3. With thoroughly washed hands, grease rod by coating with petroleum jelly or antibiotic ointment
4. Pass rod under the upper eyelid and move from side to side exerting slight pressure outwards.
5. Wipe any excess jelly from eyelids with moist wool mop.
6. Leave patient comfortable.
7. Clear equipment. Wash and dry rod and pack carefully for re-autoclaving.
8. Wash hands.
9. Record administration.

Eye bathing

Requirements
Sterile pack containing: impermeable sheet
two gallipots
cotton wool balls
Sachet of sterile 0.9% sodium chloride solution
Alcohol swab
Disposal bag.

Procedure
1. Wash hands using e.g. a detergent/antiseptic handwash.
2. Clean tray or trolley as for surgical dressing.

3. Explain to patient what is involved.
4. Open pack and lay gallipots ready.
5. Swab sachet of saline with alcohol swab. Open and pour half of contents into each gallipot.
6. Assist patient into comfortable position lying flat or sitting with head supported. Protect pillow and clothing with impermeable sheet.
7. Wash hands again.
8. Approach patient from the front. Start with the uninflamed, uninfected or operated eye. Ask patient to look down to allow bathing of upper lid and to look up to allow bathing of lower lid. Reserving one hand for picking up each cotton wool ball and the other for treating the patient, bathe eye with each cotton wool ball which should be immersed first in the solution and then wrung out. Swab gently from the inner canthus out to prevent infection of the punctum, the lacrimal apparatus and the other eye. Use each swab once and discard. Ensure neither swabs nor fingers touch the cornea. Always use moist swabs (dry wool may leave wisps attached to the eyelashes).
9. Leave patient comfortable.
10. Dispose of and clean equipment in the usual way.
11. Wash hands.
12. Adjust nursing care plan as necessary.

Irrigation of the eye

This procedure is carried our mostly in accident and emergency departments and occupational health centres for the emergency removal of caustic substances such as lime.

Requirements
    Undine or syringe (sterile)
    Sterile sodium chloride 0.9% solution
or a sterile prefilled disposable undine.
    Bowl of warm water, to warm solution.
    Sterile gauze swabs
    Kidney dish (medium size)
    Lotion thermometer
    Protective cape
    Disposal bag.

Procedure
1. Wash hands using detergent/antiseptic handwash.
2. Clean tray or trolley as for surgical dressing.
3. Explain to patient what is involved and apply cape.
4. Assist patient into position lying flat or sitting with head supported.
5. Wash hands again.
6. Fill undine with lotion at body temperature.
7. Ask patient to hold kidney dish firmly against appropriate cheek and to tilt head slightly towards dish.
8. Stand behind patient and warn him that you are about to begin.
9. Allow patient to become accustomed to the temperature of the lotion by pouring a little over the cheek first.
10. Hold eyelids apart using thumb and first finger and direct fluid in a steady stream over eyeball from inner canthus outwards.
11. Ask patient to move eyeball up, down and from side to side so that entire eye is cleansed.
12. When eye is thoroughly clean, gently dry eyelids and cheek.
13. Leave patient comfortable and apply eyepad if instructed.
14. Clear away equipment.
15. Wash hands.
16. Adjust nursing care plan as necessary.

Cutting eyelashes

This procedure is carried out pre-operatively so that the ophthalmic surgeon has a clear area in which to operate. (Although this procedure does not involve the use of any medicaments, it is included for the sake of completeness).

Requirements
    Sharp, blunt-ended scissors
    Petroleum jelly
    Gauze swabs
    Disposal bag
    Good lighting.

Procedure
1. Prepare the patient as for instilling eye drops.

2. Wash the hands and stand behind the patient.
3. Apply petroleum jelly to scissor blades with a swab.
4. Starting with the upper lid lashes first, ask the patient to look down. Warn the patient that you are about to start. Gently holding the upper lid with the index finger, cut the lashes very close to the lid margin.
5. Remove lashes and petroleum jelly frequently from the scissors with a swab and apply more jelly to the blades.
6. Cut the lower lashes in a similar way but with the patient looking up.
7. If necessary, irrigate the eye with sterile normal saline to remove any lashes which may have fallen into the conjunctival sac.

Care of an artificial eye

Patients who have had enucleation of an eye performed and have been fitted with a temporary shell or prosthesis, should have the prosthesis removed twice a day, or according to the surgeon's preference, to allow it and the socket to be cleaned with sterile normal saline. The prospect of this activity calls for some degree of fortitude on the part of the nurse but quickly her mind will be concentrated on the technique involved and on the great need to provide the patient with encouragement.

At first the patient is likely to be understandably tense and frightened that the procedure will be painful. He should be warned that he will feel the presence of something in the socket but that there will be no pain.

After a few days, when it is felt that the patient is ready to look at himself in a mirror and when he feels he wants to become involved in the care of his eye, the nurse must be prepared to spend time with the patient. About 3–4 days following the operation, the prosthesis is replaced with an artificial eye. He should be allowed to handle the artificial eye and become familiar with its shape. The notch on the nasal side of the eye which accommodates the trochlea serves as a guide for positioning.

To remove the artificial eye, the patient should be seated. He is asked to look up and using the little finger, the lower edge of the artificial eye is eased up whilst the lower margin is drawn down. Gentle pressure exerted on the upper lid will allow it to slip out.

To insert an artificial eye, the upper lid is raised and the upper edge of the artificial eye is slipped under. It is then held in place whilst the lower lid is drawn down and the lower edge of the eye is slipped into the lower fornix.

The patient may be taught to carry out eye toilet in front of a bathroom mirror. Until he becomes fully confident, a towel may be placed in the washhand basin to protect the artificial eye from damage should it slip through his fingers. By the time the patient is discharged, he should be quite confident with the procedure. When the socket is completely healed, the patient will be able to rinse his artificial eye under running water and come to no harm.

Contact lenses

Because of the increased use of contact lenses and the very discreet nature of many of them, nurses must make a conscious effort to ask patients if they wear contact lenses or to observe if they are in use. This should be done on the patient's admission to hospital. Lenses should be removed before any general anaesthetic for safekeeping. They should also be removed prior to any eye procedure to prevent irritation and so as not to be spoiled, unless medical advice has been given to the contrary. Great care must be taken in storing them since they are easily damaged, and are both costly and inconvenient to replace. They are normally kept in a specially supplied contact lens case although in an emergency a suitable alternative may have to be found. The container should be labelled with the patient's name, ward and unit number and stored in a safe place. Handling of lenses should be kept to a minimum and they should not be allowed to dry out because of the danger of cracking. Lens solution is normally brought into hospital by the patient but if this is not available sterile normal saline serves just as well, provided that the case with lens and solution are regularly subjected to heat treatment (e.g. 80°C for 40 minutes) to reduce microbial contamination.

To remove a lens, the hands should be washed, rinsed and dried leaving no trace of soap which could be conveyed to the lens and irritate the eye. The patient is asked to tilt his head back as recommended for any eye procedure and to look up. The lens is gently slid downwards using the index finger on to the bulbar conjunctiva and then lifted off the conjunctiva with the thumb and index finger. The utmost care is required not to drop a lens as it may then be very difficult to find.

Drugs and contact lenses

Consideration needs to be given to contact lenses and the concurrent administration of medicines. Some patients find that inserting contact lenses is painful and so they may be prescribed local anaesthetic eye drops to instil in advance. It is now well recognised that plastic materials, notably PVC, can absorb certain preparations instilled into the eye. Coloured eye drops such as Rose Bengal will stain soft contact lenses permanently. Adverse effects from drugs taken systemically have been reported. For example, anticholinergic drugs may cause a reduction in tear secretion and blurred vision while oral contraceptives may also cause ocular complications. Rifampicin used in the treatment of tuberculosis colours body secretions, including the tears, an orange-red leading to pigmentation of the contact lens. In certain conditions, however, the water absorption property of the lens can be used to advantage; a soft hydrophilic lens may be inserted to avoid repeated instillation of drugs such as pilocarpine in the treatment of glaucoma.

EAR AND NOSE PREPARATIONS

Procedural aspects

Procedures relating to disorders of the ear and nose involving the use of drugs follow somewhat similar lines. As always, the standard procedure for prescribing and recording medications must be followed. To prevent cross-infection, the hands should be washed before and after each procedure and each patient should have a separate medicine container. When checking ear and nose preparations against the prescription, special note should be made of the strength of the medication and for example the number of drops to be instilled and whether both ears/nostrils are to be treated. Explanation of the procedure is important in order to gain the patient's co-operation so that the medication is allowed to take maximum effect and minimal discomfort is caused for the patient. Correct positioning of the patient helps to minimise discomfort and ensure penetration of the medication to the part where it is intended to take effect. Ear and nose procedures are usually carried out with the nurse working at the side being treated. Before instilling ear or nose drops, instructions may be given by the doctor to mop the ear canal or nasal passage using a cotton-tipped applicator for better penetration of the medication. Care should be taken when patients have a history of epistaxis. Because of the delicate membranous structures involved it is important to administer such preparations at a suitable temperature. Ear drops should be used in the temperature range between room and body temperature. If ear drops are instilled from a bottle recently stored in a refrigerator they may cause a mild vertigo. Patients at home may prefer to warm the drops by holding the bottle in the hand or standing them in a bowl of hot water for a few minutes. Nasal drops do not have to be warmed as this will happen as the drops pass over the nasal mucosa although they should be allowed to reach room temperature prior to instillation if previously stored in the refrigerator.

The patient may be helped to feel more secure throughout the procedure if he is given an absorbent tissue to hold. If, for any reason, he has to rise quickly, the tissue may be used to mop excess medication which would otherwise run out of the ear or nose. For patients receiving ear drops who are unable to maintain the required position, a wisp of cotton wool may be *gently* placed in the ear canal to ensure that the drops remain in contact with the epithelium. The prescribed volume of ear drops may range from 2–5 ml. On every occasion it is important to check that the top of the glass dropper used is not chipped or cracked. Patients using any of these preparations at home should be reminded to use only a preparation intended for themselves, to keep it away from children, and to safely discard the container and any remaining medication at the end of the course of treatment.

Locally applied ear preparations

Ear drops are solutions or suspensions of active ingredient(s) in water, propylene glycol or other suitable vehicle. Some of the more commonly used ear drops are described in Table 8.8

Ear ointments have similar properties to ointments in general (see p. 99). An ear ointment commonly used for its antibacterial and anti-inflammatory actions contains neomycin 0.5% and hydrocortisone 1.5%. This ointment has similar nursing implications as framycetin ear drops (see Table 8.8). Another ear ointment used frequently contains tetracycline 1% and should be applied with the same precautions as clioquinol ear drops (see Table 8.8).

Some eye ointments may also be used for ear conditions.

Instillation of ear drops

Requirements
    Ear drops
    Paper towel
    Cotton wool balls
    Cotton-tipped applicators
    Absorbent tissue
    Disposal bag
    Prescription sheet.

Procedure
1. Check details on bottle with prescription. Identify patient.
2. Explain to patient what you are going to do.
3. Assist patient into position either sitting with head tilted to one side or lying on side with ear to be treated uppermost.
4. If instructed, gently mop external auditory meatus with cotton-tipped applicator.
5. Wash hands.
6. Having shaken bottle (if it contains a suspension), draw required amount into dropper.
7. Gently pull cartilaginous part of pinna up

Table 8.8 Characteristics of some commonly used ear drops

Active ingredient(s) % w/v	Indications/properties	Nursing implications
Aluminium acetate 8% or 13%	inflammation in otitis externa/astringent	
Betamethasone sodium phosphate	eczematous inflammation in otitis externa/anti-inflammatory	
Chloramphenicol 5% or 10%	bacterial infection in otitis externa/antibacterial	vehicle is propylene glycol which may cause local sensitisation
Clioquinol 1% with flumethasone pivalate (corticosteroid)	infection associated with inflammation, mild antibacterial antifungal, anti-inflammatory action.	stains skin and clothing and may cause local sensitisation
Framycetin 0.5% (also available with hydrocortisone)	bacterial infections/anti-bacterial	may cause sensitisation, prolonged local use to be avoided, possible ototoxicity; fungal overgrowth may also occur.
*A bland oil, almond or olive oil normally used	when warm helps to soften accumulations of ear wax	
*Sodium bicarbonate	used in conjunction with ear syringing to remove ear wax	
*Proprietary preparations containing 'wetting agents' or organic solvents to assist in the removal of ear wax.		local irritation may be caused by organic solvents

*Eardrops used prior to syringing the ear

and back. (For a child, pull the pinna down and back)

8. Instil drops in external canal without allowing dropper to come into contact with ear.
9. Massage gently over tragus to help work in drops.
10. Encourage patient to maintain position for several minutes to allow drops to reach eardrum. If necessary, *gently* insert wisp of cotton wool into external auditory canal.
11. Wipe excess medication.
12. Wash hands.
13. Record administration.

(A wick soaked in ear drop solution is sometimes inserted for 24 hours and topped up with the same solution three times during this period.)

Ear ointments

The customary way of introducing an ointment into the ear is to insert ribbon gauze which has been impregnated with the ointment. The wick is left in for 24 hours. Oral analgesics may be required prior to removal of the wick each day.

Syringing the ear

This procedure is carried out to remove plugs of wax which block the ear causing discomfort and deafness or when closer inspection of the eardrum is required. It is often preceded for several days by a course of wax-softening drops such as a bland oil or sodium bicarbonate solution. Because of the potential danger of perforating the tympanic membrane, either the ear is examined by a doctor using an auriscope before syringing takes place or enquiries from the patient are made to ensure that there is no history of perforation.

Requirements
Auriscope
Ear syringe
Jug containing warm (36.9°C) tap water. A 1% solution of sodium bicarbonate in warm water may be used.
Large kidney dish
Protective cape
Cotton wool balls

Cotton-tipped applicators
Disposal bag.

Procedure
1. Wash hands.
2. Prepare equipment.
3. Explain to patient what is involved.
4. Seat patient comfortably in upright chair and apply protective cape.
5. Ask patient to hold kidney dish against neck just below ear to be treated.
6. Fill syringe with water and expel air.
7. Gently pull pinna up and back.
8. Without undue force but at a steady rate, direct fluid along roof of auditory canal.
9. Observe content of fluid returned.
10. Repeat until all wax has been removed. Check using auriscope.
11. Gently but thoroughly mop external auditory meatus dry.
12. Leave patient comfortable.
13. Wash equipment in hot, soapy water, rise and dry. Send for autoclaving
14. Wash hands.
15. Record result.

Nasal preparations
In Table 8.9 nasal preparations are classified according to their therapeutic use and examples given of each type.

Instillation of nasal drops

Requirements
Nasal drops
Paper towel
Absorbent tissues
Small bowl
Cotton-tipped applicators
Disposal bag
Prescription sheet.

Procedure
1. Check details on bottle with prescription. Identify patient.
2. Explain to the patient what is involved.
3. Unless contraindicated for example postoperatively ask patient to blow nose or if necessary, clean nasal passages gently with a cotton-tipped applicator.

Table 8.9 Classification of nasal preparations

Therapeutic classification	Example	Usual strength	Notes
Drugs used to treat allergic conditions	betamethasone (corticosteroid)	0.1% drops	Prolonged use should be avoided in children and patients receiving oral corticosteroids.
Nasal decongestants	ephedrine oxymetazoline	1% drops	As with most nasal preparations, avoid excessive use.
Anti-infective preparations	chlorhexidine/neomycin	available as a cream containing 0.1% chlorhexidine and 0.5% neomycin.	The value of applying anti-infective preparations to the nasal mucosa has not been established.

4. Wash hands.
5. Assist patient into supine position with head hyperextended e.g. with head over edge of bed or with pillow under shoulders.
6. Assist patient if necessary to close off one nostril at a time and insert drop(s) in the other. Avoid touching any part of the nose with the dropper.
7. Ask patient to sniff liquid into back of nose or, if unable, to maintain position for about one minute. Ask patient not to blow nose. Offer patient bowl into which excess drops collected in the throat can be spat out.
8. Wipe excess drops from anterior nares with paper tissue.
9. Leave patient comfortable.
10. Wash hands.
11. Record administration.

Instead of instilling nasal drops, they may be sprayed into the patient's nose in powder form using a nasal insufflator. A nasal spray is also available which is inserted into the anterior nares. The container is squeezed two or three times to instil the medication.

Packing the nose
Nasal packs may be used to control severe epistaxis and as a rule are inserted by the doctor. The patient is understandably often very alarmed by the blood loss and requires a nurse to stay with, and reassure, him. Diazepam may be given orally and may be continued until the acute episode is over and the pack is removed. The insertion of a nasal pack is done with the patient sitting up with clothing suitably protected. Using a suitable size of nasal speculum, the doctor inserts sterile ½″ (1 cm) ribbon gauze which has been soaked in vaseline with the aid of forceps.

Alternatively, a Brighton catheter or a Foley catheter may be inserted into the nose and inflated to stop the bleeding. Patients appreciate a mouthwash after a nose bleed and may get rid of clots from the back of the throat by gargling. It is often advisable to administer an oral analgesic prior to removal of a nasal pack, which with drying becomes painful to remove. To begin with, only half of the packing should be gently pulled out to see what happens. If there is no bleeding the remainder can be removed, but if the first stage has caused bleeding, the remainder of the pack should be left in place and a further attempt made later.

Preparation for nasal surgery
Although nasal operations are mostly done under general anaesthetic, the nurse has an important part to play in applying local anaesthetic to the nose pre-operatively.

Requirements
    5 ml syringe
    Needle (to draw up solution)
    Intravenous cannula
    Solutions, e.g. lignocaine 4%
                        adrenaline 1 in 1000
    Gallipot
    Cotton wool balls
    Disposable towel
    Absorbent tissues

Bowl (to spit into)
Disposal bag
Prescription sheet.

Procedure

1. Check details on bottle(s) with prescription and identify patient
2. Wash hands. Make up solution of 3 ml lignocaine 4% and 3 ml adrenaline 1 in 1000.
3. Explain to patient what is involved.
4. Assist patient into recumbent position with two pillows under shoulders so that neck is hyperextended.
5. Give patient absorbent tissue to hold in each hand. Explain to the patient not to swallow solution as it will numb the throat.
6. Gently instil approximately 1.5 ml solution into each nostril using cannula attached to syringe making sure entire nasal mucosa and back of nose are treated.
7. Soak two pieces of cotton wool with solution, squeeze and use to plug each nostril.
8. Instil remainder of solution into each nostril.
9. Allow patient to spit out excess solution.
10. Ask patient to maintain position for about 10 minutes.
11. Observe for side effects of the solution (e.g. swelling of throat, tachycardia, collapse) and report *at once* to doctor if occasion arises.
12. Leave patient in comfortable position in readiness for theatre.
13. Wash hands.
14. Record administration

ORAL HYGIENE

The need to carry out oral hygiene in one form or another to rid the mouth of debris is part of everyday living. When illness presents, the need for oral hygiene is much greater. For example, in anorexia, vomiting, constipation, fever and dehydration, the tongue (and the teeth especially) becomes dry and coated and if left uncared for results in a foul taste, bad smell and the development of oral sepsis.

Where fluid intake has to be restricted the mouth quickly becomes dry, as it does when a patient is mouth-breathing or receiving continuous oxygen therapy. Patients who are immunosuppressed, as the result of a disease such as leukaemia or treatment such as radiation or cytotoxic drugs, are prone to mouth infections. The large number of situations which could be regarded as high risk for developing some form of discomfort of the mouth is evidence of how important this procedure is for nurses.

Some patients can be left to attend to this aspect of their care, some simply need to be prompted or given encouragement. Other patients are capable of carrying out the procedure for themselves but may need assistance in gathering together the necessary equipment. Many other patients are wholly dependent on the nurse to meet every need. The purpose is to remove, and prevent the build up, of sordes, to stimulate the flow of saliva and reduce the risk of complications such as candidal infection and parotitis. The three direct methods employed are brushing the teeth with toothpaste and water, rinsing the mouth with mouthwash solution and swabbing the mouth with a gloved finger. Wherever possible patients should be encouraged to brush their teeth in the usual way. Some authorities claim that a soft toothbrush could and should be used more often not only for cleaning the teeth but to deal with the problem of a heavily coated tongue and in edentulous patients for cleaning the gums and cheeks also. The act of cleaning one's teeth is an important and beneficial part of any programme of rehabilitation for disabled patients. Stroke patients, for example, can be helped to regain independence and to overcome a lack of awareness which many of them have of one side of the face.

Mouthwashes are easier for the patient to manage when he feels weak and is rather unwell. They should always be used in preference to a toothbrush by patients with a reduced platelet count whose gums are very liable to bleed. Swabbing with the finger, though not a pleasant procedure for the patient, is essential for those who are acutely ill, unconscious, or in the terminal stages of their illness.

This approach needs to be gentle yet effective. The airway of the unconscious or semiconscious patient must be protected at all times. Because of the danger of inhalation, any excess of the solution used for cleaning the mouth should be wrung out of the swab before use. Man-made woven swabs are less inclined to fray and are therefore safer. Care must be taken to ensure that the sponge of an applicator is not retained in the mouth by accident. With conscious patients, the tongue and roof of the mouth should be touched carefully not to make the patient 'gag'. Although oral hygiene is not a sterile procedure, a disposable pack is used for each patient to prevent cross-infection. Gloves are worn by the nurse for her own protection and care should be taken to dispose of soiled materials safely. Ideally, food debris should be removed from the teeth after each meal. Patients appreciate being given the opportunity to rinse dentures after meals. Very ill patients will require to have the mouth cleaned at least every 2 hours.

There are additional ways of helping to keep the mouth of conscious patients clean and moist. Apart from encouraging and facilitating nasal breathing, imaginative ideas of suitable food and drinks, if permitted, may be put into practice. Flavoured ice lollies or cubes, boiled sweets and chewing gum may help. Fruit juices, especially those containing lemon, stimulate the flow of saliva and are cleansing and refreshing but may cause the mouth or lips to sting if the mucosa is irritated or broken.

In summary, the role of the nurse in oral hygiene is:

— to assess the state of the patient's mouth
— to select the appropriate method of oral hygiene for the patient
— to estimate the amount of assistance the patient requires with the procedure
— to assist the patient with oral hygiene as required
— to observe, report and record details of the condition of the patient's mouth
— to teach aspects of oral hygiene to patients and relatives.

As with other fundamental nursing procedures, most patients are highly appreciative of the care given to make the mouth feel more comfortable. The contribution mouth care can make to improving the appetite and boosting morale cannot be overemphasised. It is a nursing responsibility to ensure that oral hygiene is accorded the high priority it so often warrants.

Requirements
  Gauze swabs
  2 gallipots
  Sponge applicators   oral hygiene pack
  Wooden spatula
  Sodium bicarbonate solution 1 : 160
  Mouthwash solution or solution tablets
  Vaseline
  Disposable gloves
  Disposal bag
  Torch
  Denture carton
  Toothpaste and toothbrush
  Patient's towel.

Procedure
  1. Wash hands.
  2. Explain to patient, if appropriate, what is involved.
  3. Where possible, assist patient into position which allows for ease of access.
  4. Open pack, pour solutions and put on gloves.
  5. Remove patient's dentures if appropriate.
  6. Examine mouth using spatula and torch and identify area requiring greatest attention, e.g. tongue.
  7. Wrap each swab round forefinger, dip into solution, squeeze excess solution from swab and gently wipe each area of mouth from inside out. Using one swab at a time, work systematically round oral cavity using sodium bicarbonate solution and then repeat the process with mouthwash solution.

  For example: right cheek along upper gum to centre, right cheek along lower gum to centre. Repeat on left side, hard palate and tongue.

  Carefully discard each swab into disposal bag.

8. Re-inspect mouth.
9. Apply Vaseline sparingly to lips.
10. Brush dentures and replace.
11. Discard gloves and pack into disposal bag and tie.
12. Leave patient comfortable.
13. Wash hands.
14. Adjust nursing care plan as necessary.

Preparations used in general care of the mouth

The preparation selected for use will depend on local guidelines as contained in a nursing formulary (see p. 94) or laid down in some other way. The properties of four commonly used preparations are described below.

Mouthwash solution tablets

One tablet dissolved in 60 ml of water yields an aromatic, pleasant-tasting alkaline solution containing thymol which has mild antimicrobial and deodorant properties.

Compound glycerin of thymol

This product, when diluted with three times its volume of water, yields a solution with similar properties to that produced by dissolving a mouthwash solution tablet. Both solutions are used to freshen the mouth and for mechanical cleansing. Most patients with a sore mouth will appreciate the soothing properties of warm mouthwashes. Some patients, especially if they are pyrexial, may welcome the refreshing effect of a cold mouthwash.

Care must be taken to avoid microbial contamination of thymol mouthwashes by rejecting any unused solution on completion of the procedure. Thymol, in the concentrations normally present in mouthwash solutions, is only a very weak antimicrobial agent. If solutions become contaminated, bacterial growth can occur with consequent risk of infection especially in immunosuppressed patients (Stephenson et al 1985).

Sodium bicarbonate aqueous solution 1 in 160 (0.625% w/v)

The action of sodium bicarbonate would seem to be to render mucus less viscous, thus facilitating mechanical cleansing. Unfortunately this solution does not have a particularly pleasant taste but is very economical in use.

Hexetidine solution 0.1% w/v

This solution has antibacterial and antiprotozoal activity. It is used in the treatment of gingivitis, pharyngitis and for oral hygiene generally. The solution should normally be used undiluted, although some patients may find the taste rather unpleasant.

Hydrogen peroxide solution 6% w/v

Hydrogen peroxide is an oxidising agent which, when in contact with organic matter effervesces, releasing oxygen. This has some mechanical cleansing action. This solution is particularly useful in dealing with anaerobic organisms that cause acute gingivitis, or where the tongue is so heavily furred that other solutions are rendered ineffective. To minimise the likelihood of local irritation the mouth should be well rinsed with water or normal saline when the procedure has been completed.

Preparations used in the care of the mouth in special situations

Mouthwashes are administered after tonsillectomy to remove blood clots from the throat. Using the mouthwash as a gargle may help to clear the throat by mechaniccal action. The solutions used in this situation are intended to:

- cleanse and refresh (thymol mouthwash solution)
- detach blood clots and debris (hydrogen peroxide solution)
- ease pain using local anaesthetic (benzydamine hydrochloride solution)
- treat or prevent infection (povidone-iodine solution).

Patients who have had an epistaxis appreciate rinsing the mouth with a thymol preparation to rid the mouth of any foul taste and of blood which may have run down the back of the nose. In the special situations described below the appropriate preparation would be prescribed in the normal way.

Post-radiation inflammation of the throat may be soothed without aggravating the existing reaction by using sodium bicarbonate solution or povidone-iodine solution as a mouthwash or gargle.

Fungal infections of the mouth, principally candidiasis, are especially likely to arise in patients who are debilitated or immunosuppressed. The commonest groups affected are the very young, the elderly and those receiving a course of broad-spectrum antibiotic or cytotoxic medication.

Nystatin, which is available as a suspension or pastilles is commonly used, although amphotericin may be substituted in cases resistant to nystatin. It has to be remembered that oral suspensions have a local action and that patients require to be counselled in their use. Before administering nystatin, dentures should be removed. The patient is encouraged to retain the medication in the mouth for as long as possible. Preferably, the suspension is swallowed as the oesophagus may also be infected. For maximal local benefit, food and fluids are withheld for a short time after treatment. It is essential to ensure that the care of dentures takes into account the fact that they may be a source of reinfection.

Herpes infections of the mouth, if severe, may respond to tetracycline mouthwash. Idoxuridine 0.1% paint may be used to treat herpetic lesions.

Salivary substitutes are obtainable in the form of a spray or drops and contain small quantities of sodium, potassium, calcium and magnesium salts, sorbitol and carboxymethylcellulose. These are indicated when salivary flow is reduced such as occurs with:

- certain drugs, e.g. anticholinergics or drugs having anticholinergic side-effects
- radiotherapy near the mouth or throat
- infection of a salivary gland
- inflammation of the mouth or throat
- dental or oral surgery.

An alternative approach may be to use a pastille specially formulated to increase salivary flow.

Measures taken to keep a patient's mouth clean and comfortable are generally only required for as long as the patient is acutely ill. As the patient's general state of health improves there is usually concurrent improvement in the condition of the mouth.

Aphthous ulcers

These very painful lesions (non-specific mouth ulcerations) may be treated with one of the following products:

Benzydamine solution to relieve pain and inflammation.

Hydrocortisone lozenges to relieve inflammation.

Triamcinolone oral paste to protect and relieve inflammation.

This condition is difficult to treat, since it is difficult to maintain an adequate concentration of drug in contact with the lesions.

PEDICULOSIS

Contrary to popular belief, head lice are not confined to dirty long hair. In fact they flourish in a clean environment and are passed from person to person when one head touches another. The head louse would appear to have a preference for the blood of children. The reason for this is not understood. As boys get older they are much less susceptible to infestation than girls. The 'at risk' group includes schoolchildren and some women. Mixing at home, at school or while playing increases the risk to all children. There is never a single case of head lice.

Lice are born, live and die on the host leaving the head only to transfer to a similar environment. They spend their time feeding off the scalp and reproducing. The eggs laid are glued to the base of a strand of hair and are well camouflaged as they change in colour to match the skin. Once the eggs incubate, each hatches to produce a louse which left untreated will eventually sap the person's strength and leave them generally unwell. The empty shells remain firmly glued as the hair continues to grow and they change to a pure white colour distracting attention from any new live eggs which are always laid at the base of a hair. It is the white shell which is left behind that is called a nit.

Nurses in the community, at school and in

hospital should exercise diplomacy when dealing with affected patients or explaining the condition to a child's mother. While not wanting to create offence or embarrassment, the nurse in her role as a health educator, must ensure that this particular problem is not allowed to go unchecked.

Treatment of head lice

Modern lotions for the treatment of head lice are now regarded as safe, effective and unlikely to cause resistance. (Lotions are preferred to medicated shampoos which do not achieve sufficient contact time of the active ingredient.) When applying a lotion to the head it should be remembered that it is the scalp that has to be treated rather than the hair. The hair should be parted while it is still dry and the lotion, (e.g. malathion), sprinkled into the partings until the whole scalp has been moistened taking care to avoid contact with the eyes. The scalp is massaged gently, paying particular attention to the back of the head and to the areas behind the ears. The hair may then be combed and should be allowed to dry naturally. The application is removed 12 hours later using ordinary shampoo. A fine-tooth comb may be used to remove the nits. If necessary, the treatment is repeated a week later.

If one member of a family is affected, the whole family must be treated to make certain that they are all free of infestation. Classmates should be treated similarly. Mothers should be advised to make a regular check on their chil-dren's heads and to encourage combing of the hair especially at bedtime. In summary, good grooming prompt detection and effective treatment can help to keep this condition under control.

REFERENCES

Lessar T S, Fiscella R G 1985 Antimicrobial drug delivery to the eye. Drug Intelligence and Clinical Pharmacy 19: 642–654
Norton D 1973 Treating pressure sores (Letter to the Editor). Nursing Mirror 136: 35–36
Norton D, McLaren R, Exton-Smith A N 1975 An investigation of geriatric nursing problems in hospital. Churchill Livingstone, Edinburgh
Stephenson J R, Heard S R, Richards M A, Tabaqchalis 1985 Outbreak of septicaemia due to contaminated mouth wash. British Medical Journal 289:1584

FURTHER READING

Greenhow M M 1983 Topical treatments — a simple guide. Nursing Add-on Journal of Clinical Nursing 2 (10): 281–284
Lascelles I 1982 Wound dressing techniques. Nursing Add-on Journal of Clinical Nursing D 2(8): 217–219
Stoma care nurses and Smith J C 1983 Prescribers' Journal vol 23(1): 21–28
Doering K J, La Mountain P 1984 Flowcharts to facilitate caring for ostomy patients. 4 part series. September — December
Nursing Mirror Clinical forum 1983 Stoma care. September 14.
Roughneen M J 1983 Ear syringing. Nursing Add-on Journal of Clinical Nursing 2(18): 530–531
The Royal Marsden Hospital 1984 Manual of clinical nursing policies and procedures. Harper and Row, London
Scholes M E, Wilson J L, Macrae S 1982 Handbook of nursing procedures. Blackwell, Oxford

9 ENTERAL AND PARENTERAL NUTRITION

Over the past 10 to 15 years there has been an increasing awareness of the requirement for nutritional support. It has been suggested that 5–15% of all acute hospital admissions might require nutritional support and up to 2–4% of these require intravenous support (Lee, 1980). A patient unable to tolerate a normal diet does not necessarily require parenteral nutrition. It is often possible to provide all nutritional requirements via the enteral route in these patients with the aid of specialised tube feeds and fine-bore enteral tubes. There is no doubt that enteral nutrition is superior but it is not always possible to use this technique. Parenteral nutrition can be life-saving or considerably reduce the morbidity of many conditions. If a patient loses more than 30% of his body weight, his chances of survival in an acute illness are remote since immunocompetence is impaired resulting in increased susceptibility to infection.

ENTERAL NUTRITION

Advances in the management of severe illness and trauma have meant that more patients survive the initial phase of their illness and require continuing supportive treatment. There has been growing awareness of the importance of full nutritional support during this time and great care must be taken in the provision of appropriate fluids, electrolyte and nutritional requirements. When gastrointestinal function is adequate, enteral nutrition should always be used in preference to parenteral nutrition. Enteral nutrition is a safer and much less costly procedure than total parenteral nutrition (TPN). In particular, it avoids the risk of sepsis and other complications associated with the invasive aspects of TPN. Although knowledge of techniques and formulae of products used is required, the time and expertise are generally less than that required for TPN. Complications do occur during enteral nutrition but these usually present as less severe clinical problems than with TPN.

Administration of enteral nutrition

Administration of enteral nutrition via a fine bore tube is a technique which is now used frequently in many hospitals in the nutritional management of critically ill or debilitated patients. Tube feeding may be carried out using the nasogastric, nasoduodenal, gastrostomy or jejunostomy routes.

Nasogastric feeding

This is the simplest and most widely used approach. In the past it was standard practice to pass a rubber Ryles tube into the stomach. This tube was poorly tolerated and the incidence of side-effects was high. There was increased danger of regurgitation and aspiration due to the presence of a large tube in the lumen of the cardia, and the incidence of oesophageal ulceration and stricture was relatively high.

The introduction of the fine-bore tube has alleviated these problems and as a result revolutionised the whole concept of nasogastric feeding. A wide range of proprietary products and delivery systems is now available making the advice of the dietician invaluable. In certain clinical conditions, according to the British National Formulary, some foods have characteristics of drugs and the Advisory Committee on Borderline Substances advises as to the circumstances in which such substances may be regarded as drugs. To produce the desired formula for individual patients, dietitians may make additions to a proprietary product.

To reduce risk of bacterial contamination, correct preparation and storage of feeds are necessary. All individually prepared feeds should be refrigerated at 4°C until required for use. The feeds must be clearly labelled to indicate the date and time by which they must be used. Reservoirs and giving sets should be thoroughly cleaned between each volume of feed and renewed once every 24 hours. In warm environments, it is advisable to use only 500 ml volumes at a time thus exposing the feed to a high ambient temperature for only a short period. To minimise the risk of growth of micro-organisms no feed should be used that has been exposed to room temperature for more than 5 hours. Regular bacteriological testing of the feeds should also be carried out, i.e. quality control procedures should be introduced both in the diet kitchen and at ward level. Feeds prepared on the ward include those which require reconstitution with water and also proprietary products which are ready to use.

The importance of ensuring correct positioning of a nasogastric tube becomes even more essential when it is of a fine calibre. Following all manipulations of fine-bore feeding tubes it is recommended that in all cases the position is checked by X-ray to increase safety. In addition, regular checks are made either by aspiration of stomach contents and testing with pH-indicating paper or by syringing a small volume of air down the tube and at the same time listening over the epigastrium with a stethoscope. This precaution is taken for as long as the patient is on the feed and is especially important in comatosed or drowsy patients and in those with respiratory problems. In the event of the tube becoming partially withdrawn, no attempt should be made to re-insert the tube as there is danger of the tube becoming kinked or entering the lungs.

The availability of nutritional preparations, diverse in composition and nutrient ratios, permits the selection of a feed to meet the specific requirements of the patient. Nutritional support must be designed to suit the particular metabolic needs of each individual. Careful assessment of the patient's nutritional state is required before the decision to use a particular product is made. This is normally carried out by the dietitian who obtains information from a variety of sources including the patient, relatives, doctor and nursing staff. Close liaison between dietetic, medical and nursing staff is of great importance. An ideal arrangement, not currently operating in any UK hospital, is to have a clinician with a specific responsibility for dietetic staff. Whatever the local policy, doctors and nurses require access to details of the daily regimen, which has been worked out for each patient being fed by tube, including:

- a breakdown of energy, protein and electrolyte values
- the total volume
- whatever vitamins or minerals have been added
- instructions regarding the volume of feed to be given per hour, how many hours in a 24 hour period the 'drip' is to span, or overnight administration only.

In acutely ill patients it is important to establish that the stomach is emptying properly before full nasogastric feeding is established. A satisfactory method is to give 25 ml water via the nasogastric tube initially, aspirating 4 hourly, and increasing to 50 ml then 75 ml hourly as tolerated. This is an important precaution to take and can prevent potential hazards such as vomiting, with aspiration pneumonia. If after 24 hours or sooner it is clear that the stomach is emptying, a dilute feed may be given for the next 24 hours, followed by a more concentrated feed, then a full-strength feed thereafter if tolerated. It is important that the volume and strength of feed given is increased gradually, particularly in patients who have received nothing via their gut for several days, in order to prevent gastrointestinal side-effects. Occasional nausea and abdominal distension may be induced if the feed is administered too quickly. Continuous administration can alleviate this problem using either gravity drip or pump-assisted feeding. Continuous drip administration can also alleviate the problems of diarrhoea which is often induced by administering bolus feeds, particularly if these are hyperosmolar. Pump-assisted feeding will help in patients who have some impairment in gastrointestinal function as the flow rate can be controlled to meet their absorptive capacity. Patients whose condition is stable (e.g. after stroke), who require tube feeding will usually tolerate full-strength feeds straight away if given by continuous 'drip'.

Whatever method of feeding is used, accurate entries should be made on the patient's fluid balance chart and a record kept of the patient's tolerance of the feed. 'Today's feed tolerance will influence tomorrow's feeding regimen.'

In summary, the nurse has a considerable contribution to make in the care of the patient fed by tube. She is involved in:

- assisting in the assessment of the patient's nutritional state
- storing feeds carefully
- initiating and supervising the feed
- observing the patient's colour and tolerance of the feed
- providing the patient with encouragement
- keeping accurate records
- communicating with dietetic and medical staff

Administration of medicines via enteral feeding tube

Enteral tubes provide a useful alternative route for the administration of medicines. When prescribed by this route medicines are administered in the form of a solution, suspension, or emulsion. If the drug is not normally available in a liquid form the pharmacist can advise and assist with this problem. It may be possible for a liquid form of the drug to be prepared in the pharmacy using a suitable formulation that takes account of the properties of the drug such as stability in an aqueous vehicle. Crushing of tablets into the necessary fine powder cannot be satisfactorily achieved on the ward. If tablets are insufficiently powdered, there is a risk of the tube being blocked with consequent risk of under-dosage. It should also be borne in mind that some solid dose forms cannot be crushed, even to give a coarse powder. In some cases the crushing of a tablet may destroy the essential properties of the product. Apart from using an oral liquid it may be acceptable to administer the injectable form of the drug via the enteral tube. If this procedure is adopted, clear instructions must be given by the prescriber on the patient's prescription sheet. Before the procedure is adopted the pharmacist should be consulted to ensure that the procedure is satisfactory and that there is no suitable alternative approach.

Adding a medicine to a feed is not recommended as chemical or physical interactions may adversely affect the drug or the feed, or both. There is also the problem of loss of an unknown quantity of drug if the feed is altered or some is lost due to spillage or leakage from the delivery system.

The standard procedure for checking the position of the tube must be followed before administering medicines via the tube. Following their administration a volume of water (e.g. 20–30 ml) should be run in to ensure that the medicine has passed through the tube and into the stomach. There is greater certainty then that the patient has received the medicine and that the tube will not be blocked. The total volume of fluid given, i.e. the medicine and the additional water, should be recorded.

Continuous nasogastric feeding using a fine-bore tube

Correct positioning of the tube should be confirmed by X-ray before the feeding regimen is commenced.

Requirements
   Reservoir
   Giving set
   Feed — stored in refrigerator at 4°C
   Stethoscope
   2 ml syringe
   Small container of 30 ml tap water
   Fluid prescription sheet.

Procedure
1. Compare details of feed with prescription. Identify patient.
2. Explain your intentions to patient and ensure he is comfortable.
3. Wash hands
4. Fill reservoir with feed (not more than 500 ml). Attach giving set and run feed through to expel air
5. Check nasogastric tube is in position by auscultation
6. Connect giving set to nasogastric tube
7. Regulate flow and volume of feed according to instructions
8. Make necessary documentation of feed
9. Ensure patient is comfortable and reas-

sure him that continual observation will be made to ensure all is in order.
10. Wash hands

Continuing care
1. Check flow rate hourly or more frequently as instructed.
   If rate of flow becomes sluggish, check that nasogastric tube and giving set are functioning properly.
   If the fault is in the tube, it should be flushed through with water.
   If the fault is in the giving set, it should be disconnected and cleaned or the set should be replaced.
2. Check that the tube is in position at least 2 hourly by auscultation
3. Check the tube by aspiration 4 hourly using a 2 ml syringe. (The tube will collapse if a larger syringe is used.)
4. Run 20–30 ml water through the tube 4 hourly or as necessary.
5. Stop feed, as directed, within the 24 hour period to rest the liver.
6. If feed is stopped for any reason (e.g. X-ray visit), flush tube through with 20–30 ml water before connecting a fresh feed to ensure complete patency.
7. Change reservoir and giving set at least every 24 hours.
8. If tube starts to protrude, even as little as 1 centimetre, remove tube completely and prepare for fresh tube to be passed. *Never* push back down a tube which has been partially removed.
9. Record administration of feeds.

PARENTERAL NUTRITION

Because of the complexity and expense of parenteral nutrition, this method of nutrition is only used to correct or prevent malnutrition when no other route is suitable.

Indications
1. Pre-operative. To correct existing nutritional deficiency (e.g. recent weight loss greater than 10%). Patients with carcinoma of the stomach or oesophagus are often malnour-

ished and pre-operative nutrition may be beneficial. However to be of significant benefit, at least 2 weeks of parenteral feeding is necessary prior to surgery.

2. Acute illness. Intensive care patients are frequently acutely hypercatabolic due to trauma, septicaemia, multi-organ failure, or burns. Intravenous nutritional support has proved successful in reducing complications as well as lowering the mortality rate in injuries such as burns. Many of the serious metabolic consequences of extensive burns are attributed to the increased energy requirement, part of which depends on water evaporation from the burned surface. The evaporation of one litre of water requires 2.4 MJ (580 kcal).

3. Post-operative. When complications such as prolonged post-operative ileus, sepsis or fistulae prevent a return to normal eating.

4. Chronic therapy. For some cases of chronic gastrointestinal tract disease or short bowel syndrome.

5. Premature infants. When they are very small and have difficulty in receiving nutrition by other means.

Nutritional assessment

In addition to the visual appearance of the patient it is essential to have a reliable method of assessing nutritional status. Useful measurements for building up a profile of the nutritional status of a patient include the following:

1. Body weight — recent weight loss greater than 10%
2. Triceps skin fold thickness
3. Mid-arm muscle circumference
*4. Serum albumin
*5. Serum transferrin
6. Creatinine excretion index
7. Total lymphocyte count

*These are prognostic signs not directly related to nutrition. They are affected by infection or as a response to trauma.

Nursing responsibility will encompass the measurement of weight and collection of urine samples. The nurse should make specific enquiry about previous weight loss and current diet. In some cases where a nutritional team operates, a specially trained nurse may under-

take other anthropometric measurements and collection of blood samples.

Nutritional therapy

Once the nutritional status of the patient has been assessed, it is necessary to decide what nutritional therapy, if any, should be given. The body has only limited reserves of immediately available energy and nitrogen sources. In the absence of adequate food ingestion, energy is derived from stores of glycogen in the liver, muscle protein, and from fat in adipose tissue. The glycogen stores are limited and are exhausted within the first 24 hours of starvation. Over the next few days muscle protein is broken down to provide glucose. In more prolonged starvation, fat is used to provide the energy source and the brain adapts to utilise ketone bodies. When the fat stores have been utilised, accelerated protein breakdown resumes and leads eventually to death. The aim of intravenous nutrition is to arrest catabolism due to these losses and restore the patient to positive nitrogen balance. This can be accomplished by administering calories, nitrogen, fluid, electrolytes, vitamins and trace elements.

Protein

If nutrition is deficient, not only does the patient lose weight by the loss of skeletal muscle, but also tissue repair and immune mechanisms are significantly inhibited as these processes require active cell turnover and therefore new protein formation. Amino acids are the building blocks of protein. They can be considered in two groups. Essential amino acids i.e. those such as leucine, threonine and valine which can not be synthesised by the body and the non-essential amino acids which include arginine, glycine and tyrosine. Although non-essential amino acids can be synthesised in the body (e.g. by transamination), these reactions require adequate enzyme function which may be deficient in ill patients. Thus it is important that nutrition solutions should contain not only a balanced content of essential amino acids but also a broad spectrum of non-essential amino acids.

Infants and children have a strikingly greater need for nutrients in relation to body weight. During periods of rapid growth and tissue repair, demands for certain non-essential amino acids such as histidine, proline, alanine and cysteine may exceed endogenous synthesis so that they become essential or 'semi-essential'.

The ability of amino acid solutions to increase tissue protein anabolism or to decrease tissue protein catabolism is assessed by studies of nitrogen balance. One gram of nitrogen is equivalent to 6.25 g protein. The protein requirements of a normal adult are approximately 0.2 g nitrogen/kg body weight daily. Nitrogen losses can be estimated and nitrogen requirements adjusted accordingly. Protein is supplied by solutions of crystalline amino acids.

Energy

Energy is provided as carbohydrate or fat. The caloric needs of a resting adult are 6.3 MJ (1500 kcal) per day but in burns patients these requirements may increase to 8.4–16.8 MJ or more per day (2000–4000 kcal or more daily). To effect complete amino acid anabolism up to 840 kJ (200 kcal) per gram of nitrogen must be supplied. In sepsis and major traumas the ratio of nitrogen: calories increases.

Glucose which provides 16.8 kJ (4 kcal) per g is the best carbohydrate for intravenous use but, unfortunately, glucose solutions of high calorific value are hypertonic and must be infused by a central vein to provide rapid dilution. This avoids venous thrombosis which would occur if these hypertonic solutions were infused peripherally. Fat emulsion in the form of Intralipid is also used as an energy source providing 37.8 kJ (9 kcal)/g. In addition to its use as an energy source, Intralipid is also used to treat or prevent essential fatty acid deficiency which would occur if no fat emulsion were administered. The fat emulsion is hypotonic and can be infused by peripheral vein. Indeed, in neonates the nutrients can be continuously infused along with fat emulsion via a peripheral vein often in the scalp. Peripheral feeding can be carried out in adults where fat emulsions are incorporated using the 3 litre pack commonly called the 'Big Bag' system. A maximum of 1.5 g/kg body weight is recommended daily as in excess of 2 g/kg daily, fat

has been shown to accumulate in the reticulo-endothelial system impairing antibody production. In gram negative septicaemia administration of fat should be discontinued as endotoxin inhibits the utilisation of fat. Lipid cannot be used as the sole caloric source; 40–50% of carbohydrate is required otherwise increased gluconeogenesis from amino acids will ensue. Where glucose intolerance occurs insulin may be required and blood glucose levels should be carefully monitored.

Electrolyte and trace elements

Electrolyte levels in intravenous solutions vary according to the individual requirements of the patient. Sodium is the predominant cation in the extracellular fluid and maintains the integrity of the cell membrane along with potassium. Sufficient quantities must be given not only for maintenance (1–1.4 mmol/kg body weight daily) but also to replace any significant losses. The major intracellular cation is potassium which is required for the transport of glucose across the cell membrane and normally 0.7–0.9 mmol potassium/kg body weight is required daily for adults.

A continuous calcium supply is necessary to form and maintain the skeleton and to maintain homeostasis in nerve and muscle tissue. In parenteral nutrition a daily calcium supply of 0.1 mmol/kg body weight is recommended. Magnesium is an important factor in many enzyme reactions and 0.04 mmol/kg body weight may be required daily (Wretlind, 1972). Although some phosphate is available in Intralipid, additional amounts are necessary and are added as potassium phosphate. Sodium acetate, a bicarbonate precursor, is incorporated to regulate the acid–base balance.

It is necessary to incorporate trace elements into the intravenous admixture. Iron is required for haemoglobin synthesis, and copper is involved in the release of iron from the liver. Many enzyme functions rely on zinc. Cobalt is an essential constituent of vitamin B_{12}. Manganese is involved in calcium and phosphorus metabolism, iodine is required in the synthesis of thyroid hormones, fluoride in the maintenance of the skeleton and a chromium deficiency leads to glucose intolerance.

Vitamins

All vitamins can be supplied parenterally. The fat-soluble vitamins, namely vitamins A, D, E and K, are available in commercial preparations. One of the major functions of vitamin E is to prevent the destructive oxidation of polyunsaturated fats. When polyunsaturated fat intake is high, increased amounts of vitamin E may be required. Commercial water-soluble vitamin preparations for addition to parenteral nutrition solutions contain some or all of the following — ascorbic acid, thiamine, riboflavine, niacin, pyridoxine pantothenic acid, vitamin B_{12}, folic acid and biotin.

Preparation of intravenous solutions

Standardised total parenteral nutrition formulations may be acceptable for many patients because of the kidney's extraordinary ability to maintain homeostasis. However, no single parenteral regimen would be ideal for all patients with a wide variety of pathological processes, or for all age groups, or for the same patient during all aspects of a particular disorder. This has led to tailoring specific parenteral nutrient regimens. The composition of the solution is determined from day-to-day by constant monitoring of a number of variables, both clinical and chemical. Figure 9.1 shows an example of an intravenous nutrition prescription sheet to simplify the ordering of parenteral nutrition solutions. The patient's name, age, weight, etc. are filled in by the prescriber and also the date, day of prescription, duration of prescription, volume of amino acids and glucose solutions, quantities of both electrolytes and other additives. The pharmacist, in calculating electrolytes to be added to the infusion, must take into consideration the quantities already present in the commercial amino acid preparation. Additional sodium is in the form of chloride or acetate, the acetate being a bicarbonate precursor. Potassium can be added either as the chloride or as the phosphate, depending on the patient's requirements. Calcium is added as gluconate and magnesium as sulphate; zinc is added as zinc sulphate. Special additives such as vitamins, trace elements, insulin and heparin are also catered for.

Initially the solutions were prepared and supplied in 500 ml and 1000 ml bottles. This system had, perhaps, the advantage that by using several bottles, potential incompatibilities could be avoided by separating the possible incompatible ingredients into different bottles. However, the system of supplying all nutrients in a 3 litre bag has distinct advantages, namely:

1. Errors made in putting up the wrong bottle if the sequence is not closely followed are avoided.
2. The increased risk of contamination by frequent bottle changes and the use of airways and connectors is avoided.
3. The 3 litre bag system has advantages as far as staff time and training are concerned since it requires changing only once in 24 hours.
4. It can be used for peripheral feeding where fat emulsion is incorporated.

The preparation of parenteral solutions presents problems of pharmaceutical calculations, drug stability, incompatibilities, solubility and sterility. These are all pharmaceutical in nature and, as such, the intravenous admixtures are best prepared in the pharmacy. This is underlined by the fact that clinicians and nurses are largely unaware of physical and chemical incompatibilities which can occur. Furthermore, the ward preparation room is an unsuitable location for aseptic procedures, which should be carried out in the aseptic suite in the pharmacy. Regular checks of airborne contamination both by particle counts and settle plates must be carried out. The operators undertake a set procedure for scrubbing up and donning clean-room clothing. All solutions and equipment are assembled on a tray in a preparation room and then passed through a hatch into the aseptic suite. Double doors on the hatch maintain the integrity of the aseptic suite. The manipulations are carried out under a laminar flow hood in which a constant supply of filtered air passes over and around the assembled items.

Admixtures are carried out in the centre of the screen well inside the outer edge of the work surface, and interruptions to air flow

CONSULTANT	PATIENT'S SURNAME SMITH	UNIT NUMBER 789101
HOSPITAL ARI	FIRST NAME(S) JOHN	
WARD 23	AGE 45	WEIGHT 62 Kg

Date........14/6/85.......... Day..........1.......... of Intravenous Nutrition

Duration of prescription: for 24 hours from .....14/6/85........... to .....15/6/85...........

Infusion Rate........................130.................... ml. per hour.

Solution Requested		Volume Requested	Solution Supplied	Volume Supplied	Batch No.
Amino Acids VAMIN GLUCOSE		1000 ml.	Amino Acids	ml.	
Glucose	20 %w/v	500 ml.	Glucose %w/v	ml.	
Intralipid	20 %w/v	500 ml.	Intralipid %w/v	ml.	
Basic Volume before Additives =		ml.	Basic Volume before Additives =	ml.	

	Ionic Requirement		FOR PHARMACY USE ONLY				
Ion	m.mol./ 24 hrs.	In form of	Volume Added	Prep. Added	Calc. By	Checked By	Batch No.
Acetate	70	Sodium Acetate					
Sodium	120	Sodium Chloride					
Phosphate	20	Potassium Acid Phosphate					
Potassium	80	Potassium Chloride					
Calcium	10	Calcium Gluconate					
Magnesium	4	Magnesium Sulphate					
Zinc	0·06	Zinc Sulphate					
Special Additives/24 hrs.							
......1...... vial Solivito							
......10...... ml. Addamel							
.... units Soluble Insulin							
......6000...... units Heparin							
......10...... ml Vitlipid Adult							

Total Volume Supplied .... ml.

INTRALIPID %.............. ml. plus.............. ml. VITLIPID ADULT

Fig. 9.1 Intravenous nutrition prescription for adults

should be guarded against. The amino acids and glucose solutions are run into a 3 litre ethyl vinyl acetate pack. Additions of vitamins, electrolytes, and other small volume components are made by injecting through an additive port.

Incompatibilities

It is essential to consider the potential incompatibilities or the degradation rates of certain ingredients in the presence of others. In most cases the incompatibilities can be avoided or corrected. Insulin is unstable in the presence of bicarbonate. Furthermore, insoluble carbonates may form if bicarbonate is added to calcium or magnesium. It is simpler therefore to use a bicarbonate precursor such as sodium acetate.

Some vitamins are unstable in hypertonic intravenous solutions especially in the presence of light. By using a freshly prepared solution and protecting it from bright light, the reaction can be slowed. On *no* account should total parenteral infusion be used as a means of administering drugs. In addition to the danger of contamination, many chemical changes can occur e.g. penicillins are rapidly degraded in amino acid solutions and tetracyclines form insoluble complexes with calcium and magnesium.

Care must be taken when fat emulsion is added since high levels of electrolytes, particularly calcium and magnesium, may crack the fat emulsion. If calcium and phosphate are present above a certain level, a precipitate of calcium phosphate may form particularly if the solution is stored in a refrigerator. Thus it is essential that solutions are examined prior to setting up, and again during infusion, since precipitates may only appear after a few hours or even days.

Administration of parenteral nutrition

Insertion of a central line

TPN is normally administered via a central vein, preferably the superior vena cava. This may be approached via the subclavian vein, the jugular vein, the upper cephalic vein or the antecubital fossa-basilic vein. A central line should be inserted by the doctor with full aseptic surgical technique, where possible in theatre under local or general anaesthetic. Responsibility for the care of the line is a combined one between medical and nursing staff, the overall aim being to ensure no harm comes to the patient. The nurse must provide explanations and reassurance for the patient and therefore she should be fully aware of what is entailed. Assistance will be required to position the patient optimally, that is, lying flat with a rolled-up towel placed between the scapulae and the head

turned away. The skin site may be prepared first by using acetone to degrease the skin and then by cleansing with chlorhexidine 0.5% in spirit or povidone-iodine. The administration set is assembled using additional filters and an extension set, and is primed using, for example, injection of sodium chloride 0.9% w/v to test the patency of the catheter. An intravenous pump/controller is made available.

The catheter should be inserted through a subcutaneous tunnel, about 10–12 cm (4–5 inches) across the chest wall. In this way the skin entry site is separated from the venepuncture site and the incidence of sepsis is reduced. Once the catheter is sited and the administration set connected up, a suitable occlusive dressing is applied and the clear infusion solution run in slowly. The position of the catheter is always confirmed by chest X-ray which should be examined for a pneumothorax.

Care of the patient receiving intravenous nutrition

Patients receiving parenteral feeding should be closely observed for the early detection of complications. Urinalysis should be performed every 4–6 hours to note the presence of glucose or ketone bodies. A 24 hour urine collection for measurement of urea level is used to estimate the nitrogen balance. The patient should be weighed regularly (e.g. twice weekly). Four hourly recordings of temperature, pulse and blood pressure are made and the character of the respirations observed. Very strict recordings of the intake and output of fluid must be kept. Care must be taken to maintain accuracy of fluid recordings especially on completion of one chart and the commencement of the next (e.g. at midnight). As with any infusion, regular checks should be made that the prescribed rate of flow is being maintained and that sufficient volume of feed remains in the infusion pack.

Transparent dressings allow for easy visualisation of the catheter insertion site; any evidence of swelling, discolouration or pain should be reported at once. No medications should be added to any part of the system nor should it be used for blood sampling or central venous pressure monitoring. A special cover can be obtained for placing over a 3 litre bag to protect the feed from strong sunlight and in addition an administration set made of ultra-violet absorbent material may be used. As well as minimising the entry of micro-organisms, the nurse has a vital role in vigilant monitoring of the rate of the infusion. Three litre bags must be used in conjunction with some form of infusion pump but this is not a substitute for frequent checking and if necessary making minor adjustments to the infusion rate. No attempt should be made to 'catch up' if the infusion is behind time.

By virtue of the fact that he is receiving nutritional therapy, the patient is malnourished and therefore debilitated to some degree. He requires every encouragement at this time. General physical care increases in importance including skin care, mouth care and exercise within the limitations of the infusion. Bowel activity, which may be reduced, should be carefully noted.

Changing the infusion pack

When changing the infusion pack, the usual precautions are required. Accurate identification of the patient is essential. Details on the pack must be compared carefully with the prescription. The infusion solution should be checked to ensure that it is not out of date, that the solution is free from precipitate and that there is no evidence of the bag having been damaged, rendering it unsterile. Care is needed to connect up the new infusion bag aseptically. This can be achieved by thorough handwashing and careful introduction of the giving set needle into the infusion pack. The utmost care should be taken to avoid perforating the bag. Before setting the rate controller and restarting the infusion, the giving set must be free of air bubbles. A record of the new pack, its batch number, and starting time is made and initialled by the nurses involved. The volume of solution which has been administered is recorded on the patient's fluid balance chart.

Changing the administration set

To reduce chances of allowing the culture of

micro-organisms, the intravenous infusion tubing should be changed to the level of the catheter hub every 24 hours. This aseptic procedure is performed by a doctor assisted by a nurse or, in some centres, by a specially trained nurse. For all tubing changes, the patient must be lying flat and all connections of the intravenous system should be made secure to prevent air embolism.

Checking the dressing

Transparent dressings need only be removed if there is local redness or swelling, or if the dressing starts to detach itself from the skin. These dressings are normally changed weekly and are used in conjunction with a catheter extension piece which ensures that all daily tubing changes are carried out well away from the catheter entry site.

Traditional dressings should be changed approximately every second day and this may be carried out at the same time as the tubing is changed. A normal surgical dressing technique is used but extra precautions are required in respect of skin care. Acetone or ether used to prepare the skin should not be allowed to come into contact with the catheter. The skin area is cleansed for example using povidone-iodine for two minutes. Tincture of benzoin compound spray may be applied over the skin area but again should not be in contact with the catheter. Povidone-iodine ointment may then be applied over the catheter entry point. The site is covered with fitted swabs leaving the hub of the catheter exposed. A firm airtight dressing is applied with the patient's head turned away and his arm abducted to allow movement to be unrestricted. It is secured with broad adhesive tape e.g. 10 cm (4 inches) to cover the area and zinc oxide tape to secure the sides although still leaving the hub exposed.

Removal of the catheter

Intravenous catheter removal carries with it the risk of air embolism. The procedure is done by a doctor assisted by a nurse. Again, the patient must be in the supine position. About an hour prior to removal of the catheter, the rate of the infusion should be slowed. The catheter is shut off by means of the control clip and the intravenous system always left connected. The site is cleaned with isopropyl alcohol or chlorhexidine in spirit. The suture securing the catheter is cut and while the patient performs the Valsalva manoeuvre, the catheter is removed slowly. (The Valsalva manoeuvre is used to increase thoracic pressure so that venous return to the heart is momentarily reduced and is achieved by a forced expiration with the mouth and nose closed.) Great care should be taken to ensure that the entire length of the catheter has been removed. The puncture site should be covered immediately with an airtight dressing and firm pressure applied. The area should be kept covered for 24 hours. The tip of the catheter is cut off using sterile scissors and sent to the bacteriology department for culture studies.

Parenteral nutrition at home

Training is given prior to discharge from hospital. Nutritional requirements are supplied by the pharmacy in pre-assembled packs which the patient stores in a refrigerator and changes under clean conditions at home. The patient reports to hospital on a regular basis in order that checks can be carried out and, where necessary, the nutritional components altered accordingly.

Summary

Safe intravenous nutrition has been developed by doctors, pharmacists, biochemists, bacteriologists and nutrition experts. The role of the nurse in this form of therapy (whether undertaken in a specialist centre or in the patient's own home) is increasing. Ideally, a senior nurse with specific responsibility for nutrition patients is appointed. In any event, a high standard of nursing care including assessment of the patient, meticulous levels of hygiene, close observation, accurate recording and prompt reporting, is of fundamental importance. Where care at this level is assured, the maximum benefit to the patient of this technique, which may be life-saving, is within reach.

REFERENCES

Lee H A 1980 Parenteral nutrition; its indications and limitations. British Journal of Intravenous Therapy 1: 26–32
Wretlind A 1972 Complete intravenous nutrition. Nutrition and Metabolism Supplement 14: 1–57

FURTHER READING

Allison S P 1984 Enteral and parenteral nutrition. Prescribers' Journal 24 (1): 2–11
Metheny N M 1985 20 ways to prevent tube-feeding complications. Nursing 85 January: 47–50
The Royal Marsden Hospital 1984 Manual of clinical nursing policies and procedures. Harper and Row, London
Wilhelm L 1985 Helping your patient to 'settle in' with TPN. Nursing 85 April: 60–64

10 THE ADMINISTRATION OF MEDICINES

GUIDELINES FOR MEDICINE ADMINISTRATION

1. The hands should be clean prior to any procedure involving medicines.
2. Health authority policy established from legal requirements, DHSS/SHHD guidance and recommendations made by the UKCC and the RCN regarding storage and checking of medicines must be adhered to.
3. Six items of information must be present on a written prescription before administration can take place. These are:

   a. the date of prescribing of each individual medicine which should be co-incidental with the date of commencement. As far as possible, medicines should not be prescribed prospectively although it is recognised that pre-operative medicines and diagnostic agents may be prescribed prospectively.
   b. the name of the medicine prescribed printed in full in block letters using the approved name or if the product has more than one active component, (compound formulation), the proprietary name.
   c. the dosage of the medicine prescribed using the metric system. Substitutes for actual dosage, e.g. tabs., caps., vials, etc. must be avoided except in the case of compound formulations. Decimal fractions should be avoided, e.g. 250 micrograms and not 0.25 mg, 500 micrograms and not 0.5 mg. When writing prescriptions micrograms should

be written in full and not abbreviated to avoid confusion with mg.

d. the route of administration should be indicated and abbreviated as follows:

IV—Intravenous
SL—Sublingual
PR—Per Rectum
SC—Subcutaneous
IM—Intramuscular
TOP—Topical
INHAL—Inhalation
ID—Intradermal

'Oral' and other forms of administration should be written in full. Further requirements for giving the medicine may have to be stated specifically, e.g.

- 'Oral after food'
- TOP to both eyes.
- INHAL via 'Lifecare' mask 24% at 2 litres per minute

e. the time(s) or time interval.

For 'as required' prescriptions, the prescribing instructions must include the symptoms to be relieved and must be written in English stating the maximum frequency (e.g. 'As required for Headache — every 4 hours.').

f. the full signature of a registered (or provisionally registered) practitioner for each individual prescription.

If any part of the prescription is unclear or absent, the nurse must seek clarification before proceeding.

4. Pharmaceutical products are only used if they are in date and their colour, appearance/consistency and smell are unaltered. Unsuitable medicines should be returned to the pharmacy. The help and guidance of the ward pharmacist are invaluable here.

5. The nurse must be alert to those occasions when it would be unsafe to proceed in giving a medicine exactly as prescribed. For example, digoxin is only administered if the pulse rate is 60 beats per minute or more. Narcotic analgesics should not be given in the early post-operative period unless the systolic blood pressure is greater than, say, 100 mmHg. Depending on the patient's baseline blood pressure and the severity of pain, permission may be granted to give a reduced dose. Permission to use an alternative route of administration should be sought following, for example, an upper endoscopy when the throat has been anaesthetised or when a patient is being fasted. When a dose has had to be omitted or reduced (or the medicine is refused by the patient or not immediately obtainable) a record of the fact must be made giving the reason and initialled by the member(s) of staff involved.

6. The label or packaging nearest to the product must be checked before administration. It is not sufficient to check the outer box or packet in which a bottle or blister pack is contained.

7. The patient must be identified correctly. Address the patient by name or ask him to state his name and check the name on a bed label or chart kept at the bedside. Factors contributing to ease of identification include knowing the patients in your care, checking medicines with a second nurse and making proper use of identification bracelets. However, shift work, staff shortages, movement of staff from ward to ward or from team to team and a high turnover of patients can create difficulties in knowing patients well. Not all staff like patients to be 'labelled' (i.e. using identification bracelets) or to ask the patient to state his name. Encouragement of patients to be more mobile and to socialise away from the bedside, e.g. in day rooms, can add to the problems while deafness and confusion can compound them.

Not uncommonly, patients with the same name appear in a ward. It is of paramount importance that the nurse in charge draws the attention of the patients concerned and all staff to this occurrence. The hospital unit number, unique to the patient, is the only safe means of distinguishing patients in this situation.

8. For safety and comfort, patients should be suitably positioned in advance of being given a medicine, e.g. an upright posture will assist the swallowing of a solid dose form.
9. Small quantites of unwanted medicines should be disposed of by flushing. Larger quantities should be returned to the pharmacy. The pharmacist will advise on any special disposal problems. The disposal of cytotoxic drugs is carried out according to local policy (see p. 168).

Summary of the guidelines for medicine administration

- The hands should be clean.
- Regulations for storage and checking must be adhered to.
- The prescription must be clear and complete.
- The medicines must be in good condition and suitable for use.
- The medicine may be contraindicated.
- The innermost label must be checked.
- The patient must be identified accurately.
- The patient should be positioned appropriately.
- Unwanted medicines should be disposed of safely

In spite of the gradual disappearance of task organisation in nursing, the majority of medicines are still issued to patients consecutively on medicine rounds. The outline of a medicine round using documents (see Figs. 10.1 & 10.2) of the Grampian Health Board for prescribing and recording of medicines is given. Specially designed prescription forms are required in certain situations, e.g. for total parenteral nutrition for topical therapy and for diabetics.

Medicine round

The hands should be socially clean.

1. Obtain keys from nurse in charge
2. Detach trolley from wall and unlock
3. Ensure sufficient spoons/medicine glasses
4. Proceed systematically, e.g. clockwise round ward or in order of 'Kardex'.
5. For each patient read:

a. Prescription sheet — full name
   — any known medicine sensitivity
b. Recording sheet — full name
   — check medicines not already given
c. Prescription sheet — date
   — medicine
   — dose
   — route
   — time
   — doctor's signature.

6. Select medicine.
7. Compare name and strength of medicine with name and dose prescribed. Check expiry date.
8. Make any calculation necessary.
9. Place tablet or capsule in spoon or glass (by transferring it first into the bottle cap or by pushing it through the foil side of a blister pack). For a liquid medicine, first shake the bottle and holding the measure at eye level measure the required volume without defacing the label.
10. Recheck details on label with prescription before replacing in trolley.
11. Enter appropriate code letter on recording sheet.
12. Repeat 5 c–11 with each medicine due.
13. Take medicines on tray to patient.
14. Identify patient.
15. Administer the medicine(s).
    Tell him of any special instructions regarding use of tablets by the sublingual route (e.g. buprenorphine tabs), suspensions which are held in the mouth before being swallowed (e.g. nystatin), or pastilles for sucking.
16. Witness the medicine(s) being taken.
17. Initial recording sheet.
18. On completion of round wash spoons/glasses, wipe sticky bottles and replenish stock.
19. Attach trolley to wall and lock.
20. Return keys to nurse in charge and pass on any relevant comments.

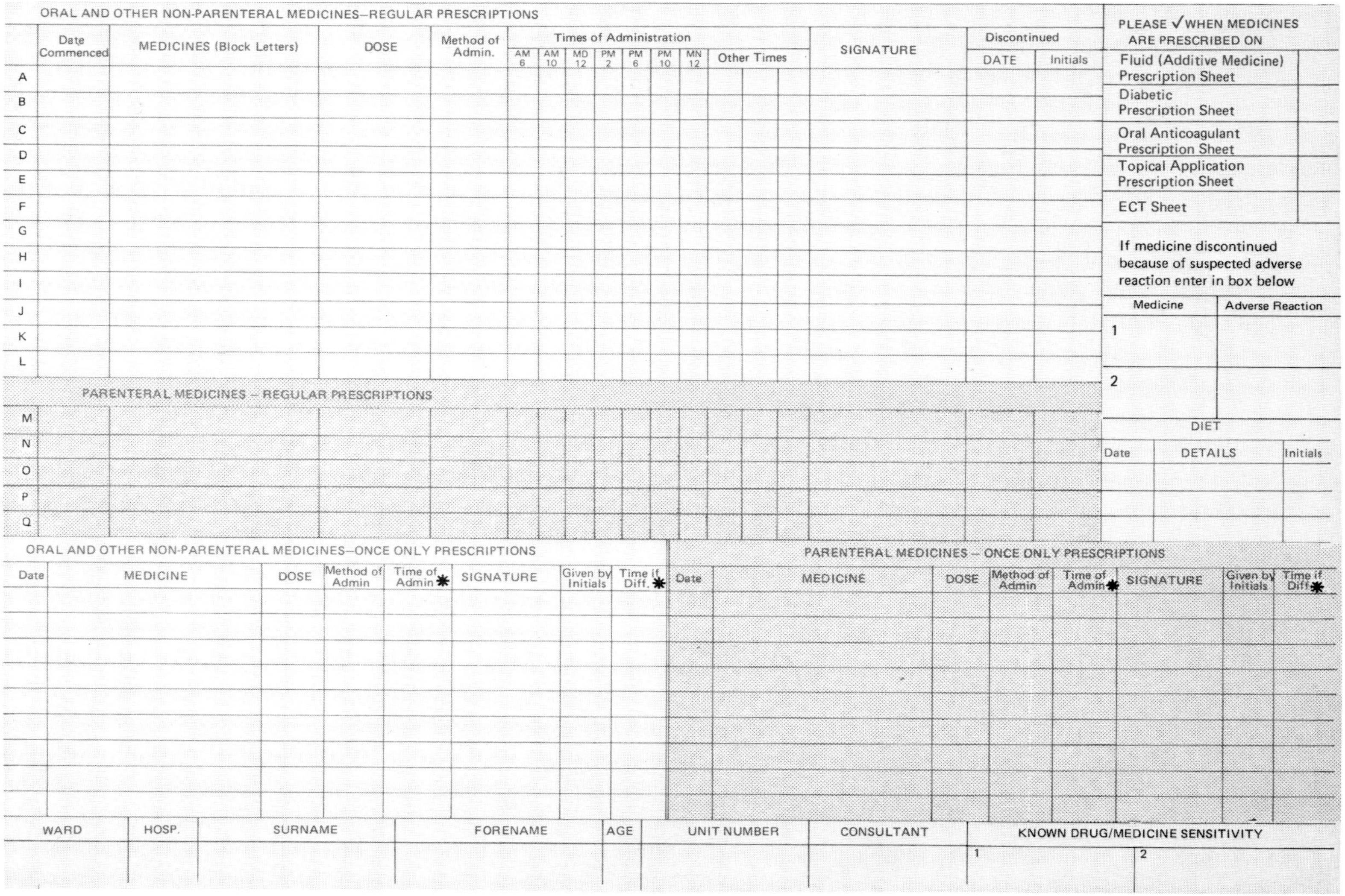

ORAL AND OTHER NON-PARENTERAL MEDICINES–REGULAR PRESCRIPTIONS

	Date Commenced	MEDICINES (Block Letters)	DOSE	Method of Admin.	AM 6	AM 10	MD 12	PM 2	PM 6	PM 10	MN 12	Other Times			SIGNATURE	Discontinued DATE	Discontinued Initials
A																	
B																	
C																	
D																	
E																	
F																	
G																	
H																	
I																	
J																	
K																	
L																	
PARENTERAL MEDICINES – REGULAR PRESCRIPTIONS																	
M																	
N																	
O																	
P																	
Q																	

PLEASE √ WHEN MEDICINES ARE PRESCRIBED ON

Fluid (Additive Medicine) Prescription Sheet	
Diabetic Prescription Sheet	
Oral Anticoagulant Prescription Sheet	
Topical Application Prescription Sheet	
ECT Sheet	

If medicine discontinued because of suspected adverse reaction enter in box below

	Medicine	Adverse Reaction
1		
2		

DIET

Date	DETAILS	Initials

ORAL AND OTHER NON-PARENTERAL MEDICINES–ONCE ONLY PRESCRIPTIONS

Date	MEDICINE	DOSE	Method of Admin	Time of Admin *	SIGNATURE	Given by Initials	Time if Diff. *

PARENTERAL MEDICINES – ONCE ONLY PRESCRIPTIONS

Date	MEDICINE	DOSE	Method of Admin	Time of Admin *	SIGNATURE	Given by Initials	Time if Diff *

WARD	HOSP.	SURNAME	FORENAME	AGE	UNIT NUMBER	CONSULTANT	KNOWN DRUG/MEDICINE SENSITIVITY	
							1	2

Fig. 10.1 Main prescription sheet

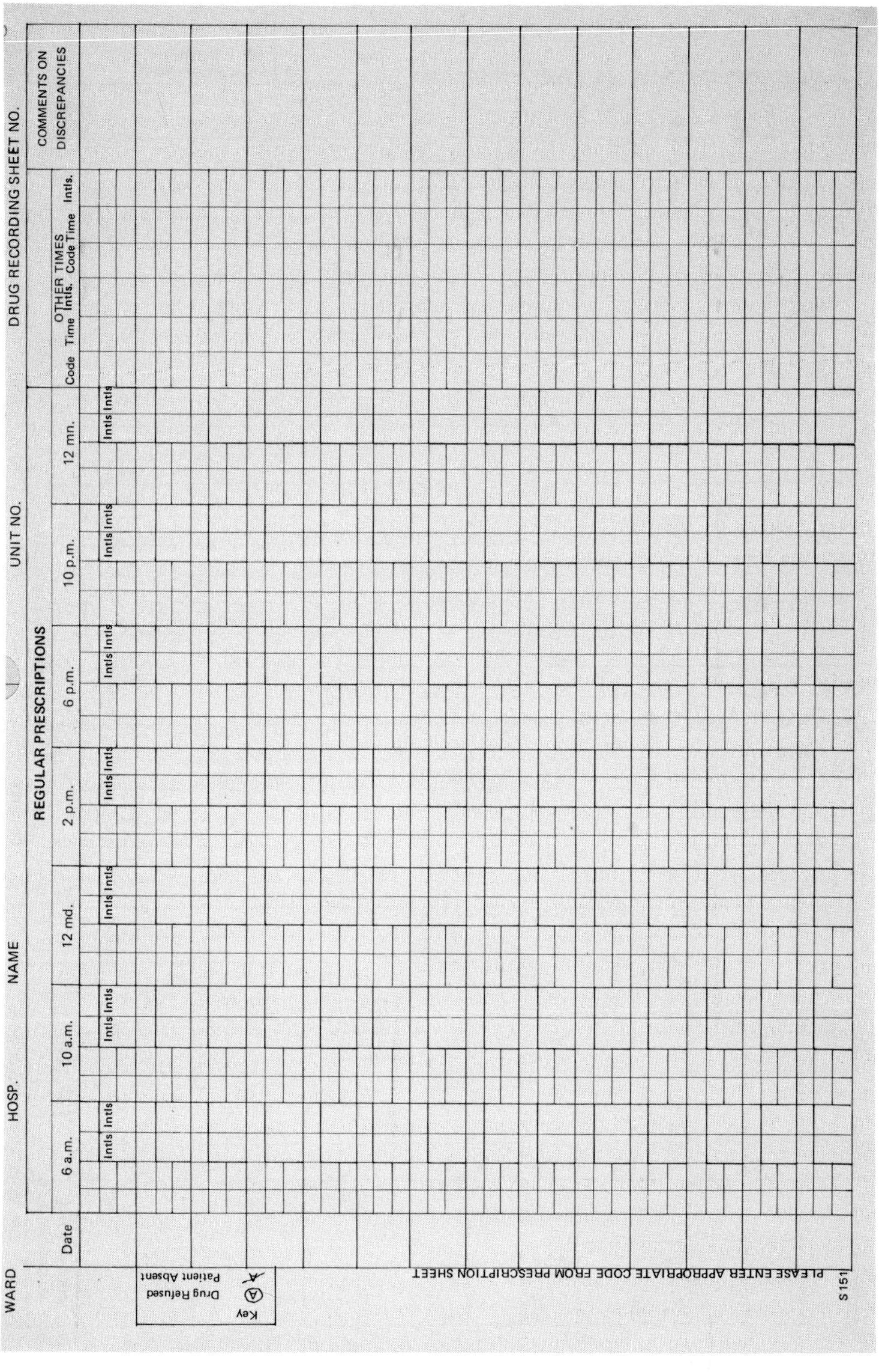
WARD
HOSP.
NAME
UNIT NO.
DRUG RECORDING SHEET NO.
Date
REGULAR PRESCRIPTIONS
6 a.m. Intls Intls
10 a.m. Intls Intls
12 md. Intls Intls
2 p.m. Intls Intls
6 p.m. Intls Intls
10 p.m. Intls Intls
12 mn. Intls Intls
OTHER TIMES
Code Time Intls. Code Time Intls.
COMMENTS ON DISCREPANCIES
Key
Ⓐ Drug Refused
Patient Absent
PLEASE ENTER APPROPRIATE CODE FROM PRESCRIPTION SHEET
S151

Fig. 10.2 Medicine recording sheet

Special prescription forms — diabetes

The management of diabetes mellitus involves the keeping of records which will reflect clearly a patient's diabetic state and also allow for the prescribing and recording of hypoglycaemic drugs. Special documentation is required to accommodate this. Examples of documents which combine this information are illustrated in Figures 10.3–10.6

Diabetic prescription sheet for adults

The boxes in the top, left-hand corner of the prescription sheet (Fig. 10.3) are completed on the doctor's instructions giving details as follows:

Diet — completed by medical staff or dietitian.
— e.g. 150 g CHO

Urinalysis — frequency requested and, in special cases, ratio of drops of urine to drops of water when other than 5:10

Blood Glucose — frequency requested.

Insulin Dose Test — instructions entered as appropriate depending on the calculation used, e.g. fixed, direct, reverse.

Basis — if direct or reverse, it should be stated whether the calculation is based on blood glucose or urine test results.

Fixed — means the dose of insulin is ordered irrespective of urine/blood testing results.

Direct — means the dose of insulin to be given is selected according to the result of urine or blood testing *at that time.*

Reverse — means the dose of insulin to be given is selected as follows:
Breakfast insulin according to previous day's tea-time urine or blood result.
Tea-time insulin according to same day's breakfast urine or blood result.

Specific instructions. Occasionally when a patient is only having a once daily insulin dose before breakfast, the instructions may have to be written out in full, e.g. on pre-lunch test. (Direct and reverse calculations may be described as types of sliding scale.)

Recording ward blood glucose and urinalysis results

Results of blood glucose testing at ward level are entered as number of mmol/litre corresponding to the date and time of their estimation.

The amounts of glycosuria and ketonuria are recorded in graph form by entering a dot in the space which corresponds to the date and time of their estimation.

Where the ferric chloride test is used, the result is entered in the appropriate column as positive or negative.

Prescribing of hypoglycaemic agents

1. All hypoglycaemic agents, except those added to infusions, are prescribed on this sheet.
2. Insulin may be prescribed on a sliding scale, i.e. the number of units corresponding to the amount of glycosuria or to the result of a ward tested blood glucose specimen, is entered in the 'no. of units of insulin' column, or, as with other hypoglycaemic agents, as regular and/or once only prescriptions.
3. The actual time of administration may be replaced by the abbreviation, BB, BL, BT (Before Breakfast, etc.) and when these abbreviations are used, the meaning is indicated in the appropriate section at the foot of the chart.

Recording administration of hypoglycaemic agents

1. Once only prescriptions are recorded as illustrated on page 157.

2. Regular prescriptions are recorded by entering the code letter(s) in the appropriate box(es) when the medicine is selected.
3. Where the dose of insulin is on a sliding scale, the code letter and the number of units of insulin selected are entered in the appropriate boxes.

In 2 and 3, the actual time of administration and nurses' initials are entered when the dose has been administered.

Diabetic coma/insulin infusion sheet

This special adult diabetic chart is used for patients who are receiving intravenous insulin therapy or when frequent recordings of a patient's diabetic state require to be made. For diabetic patients undergoing surgery, the diabetic prescription sheet is replaced temporarily by the diabetic coma/insulin infusion sheet (see Fig. 10.4). This sheet differs slightly from the diabetic prescription sheet.

1. The date and times columns are completed at any time an entry requires to be made on the chart.
2. Results of blood and urine tests are entered as follows:

   blood glucose as mmol per litre, e.g. 10
   glycosuria as %, e.g. $\frac{1}{2}$
   ketonuria as number of pluses, e.g. ++
   blood chemistry — figures entered for each as per laboratory report.

3. Records may be kept of central venous pressure, cm of water, e.g. 5.
4. Insulin is prescribed in the following ways:
   Intravenous infusion
   — *regular*
   — *sliding scale*, i.e. number of units per hour corresponding to the result of a ward tested blood glucose specimen.
   Intramuscular or subcutaneous injection — *once only*
5. The column headed 'Solution' is completed to show the number of units of insulin in a given volume of a given fluid.

Example 1: 50 units in 50 ml normal saline
Example 2: 12 units in 500 ml 10% glucose.

6. At the start or on completion of a prescription of insulin by infusion, the doctor enters the time along with his/her initials in the appropriate column. In this way, the chart serves both as a prescribing and recording sheet.

Paediatric diabetic prescription sheets

The management of diabetes in children requires slightly different records to be kept although a similar type of chart may be used as for adults (see Figs. 10.5 & 10.6). It is important to record the child's age and weight to allow for calculation of insulin dosages. Allowance should also be made for the much wider range of results of urinalysis. Oral hypoglycaemic agents are not used in paediatric practice and for most children a 'sliding scale' of insulin is not used. Because of the need for extreme accuracy in the management of diabetic coma and/or when the child is receiving an insulin infusion, more detailed prescribing of insulin is recommended than is necessary with adults. As well as the name of the insulin and the strength of the solution to be used, the exact rate of the solution including the number of ml per hour, units per hour, and units per kg per hour should be stated.

CALCULATIONS

With the development of ward and clinical pharmacy services and the introduction of ready-to-use unit packs, the need for nurses to undertake calculations in connection with the administration of medicines and other pharmaceutical products has declined over recent years. Situations will, however, still arise when nurses need to perform basic calculations accurately and with confidence. Apart from the need to calculate how to obtain a particular dose for an individual patient a sound understanding of SI (Systéme International) units of

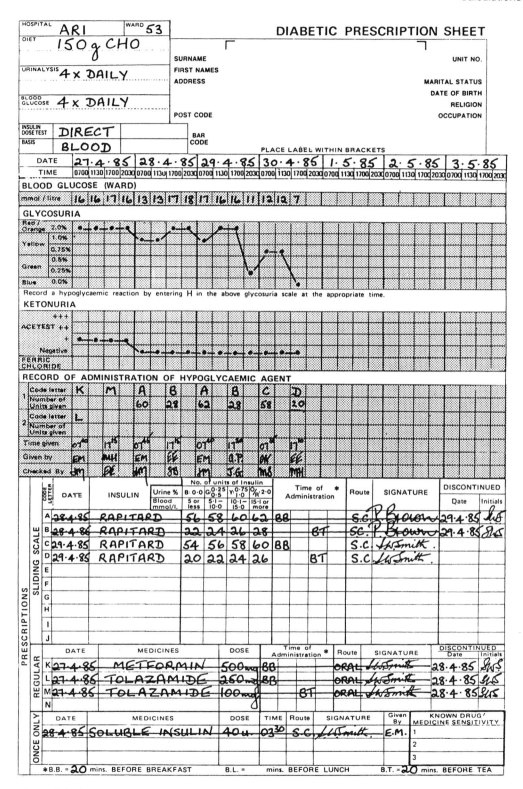

Fig. 10.3 Adult diabetic prescription sheet

HOSPITAL	W.G.H.	WARD 8M	DIABETIC COMA / INSULIN INFUSION SHEET		

CONSULTANT	Dr. Forsyth	SURNAME		UNIT NO.
BLOOD GLUCOSE	Hourly	FIRST NAMES		
		ADDRESS		MARITAL STATUS
URIN-ALYSIS	4 hourly		12·3·21	DATE OF BIRTH
				RELIGION
		POST CODE		OCCUPATION
INSULIN TEST DOSE		BAR CODE	PLACE LABEL WITHIN BRACKETS	

DATE	27·10·85																	
TIME	7am	8	9	10	11	12	1pm	2	3	4	5	6	7	8	9	10	11	12
BLOOD GLUCOSE mmol. per litre																		
LABORATORY	23·3			17·2												9		
WARD	22	22	22	22	13·3	13·3	13	13·3	13·3	13	10	22	22	13	13·3	10	10	10
GLYCOSURIA																		
%	2						-ve		-ve									
KETONURIA																		
INDICATE '+' SIGNS	++++						-ve		-ve									
BLOOD CHEMISTRY																		
Na	136			142												134		
K	4·1			3·9												3·5		
HCO₃	16			-												24		
UREA	5·5			5·8												6·8		
CREATININE																		
pH																		
pO₂																		
CENTRAL VENOUS PRESSURE																		
Cm. of Water																		

PRESCRIPTIONS – I.V. INSULIN INFUSION

	START			INSULIN	SOLUTION	UNITS PER HOUR	SIGNATURE	STOP		
	DATE	TIME	INITIALS					DATE	TIME	INITIALS
REGULAR	27·10·85	7am	aW	ACTRAPID	50u in 50ml N. SALINE	3	a Walker	27·10·85	3pm	IG
	27·10·85	3pm	IG	ACTRAPID	50u in 50ml N. SALINE	2	Gordon	27·10·85	11pm	G
	27·10·85	11pm	IG	ACTRAPID	15u in 45ml N. SALINE	1	Gordon			

	START			INSULIN	SOLUTION	UNITS PER HOUR				SIGNATURE	STOP		
	DATE	TIME	INITIALS			4 or LESS	4.1–7.0	7.1–13.0	13.1 or MORE		DATE	TIME	INITIALS
SLIDING SCALE													

PRESCRIPTIONS – I.M. OR S.C. ONCE ONLY

DATE	INSULIN	DOSE	TIME	ROUTE	SIGNATURE	GIVEN BY	CHECKED BY

Fig. 10.4 Diabetic coma/insulin infusion sheet — adult.

PAEDIATRIC DIABETIC PRESCRIPTION SHEET

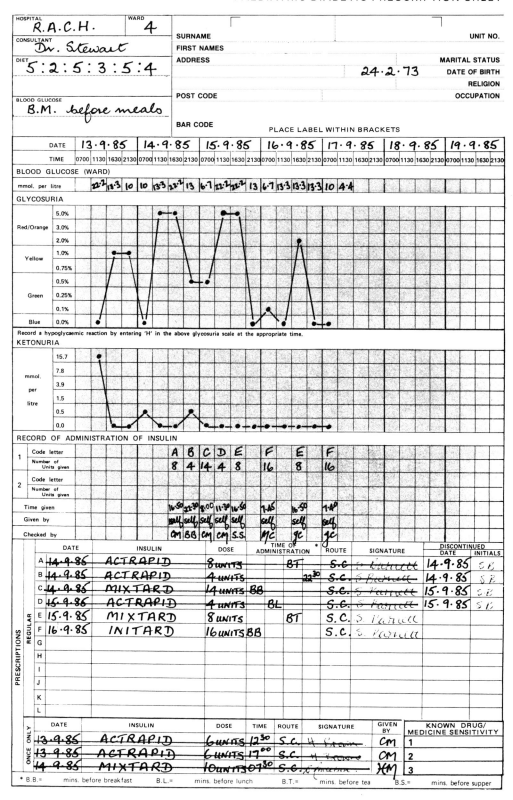

HOSPITAL R.A.C.H.	WARD 4

CONSULTANT Dr. Stewart

DIET 5:2:5:3:5:4

BLOOD GLUCOSE B.M. before meals

SURNAME

FIRST NAMES

ADDRESS

POST CODE

BAR CODE

UNIT NO.

MARITAL STATUS

DATE OF BIRTH 24.2.73

RELIGION

OCCUPATION

PLACE LABEL WITHIN BRACKETS

DATE	13.9.85	14.9.85	15.9.85	16.9.85	17.9.85	18.9.85	19.9.85

TIME: 0700 1130 1630 2130 (repeated for each date)

BLOOD GLUCOSE (WARD)

mmol. per litre: 22.2 18.3 10 10 13.3 22.2 13 6.7 22.2 22.2 13 6.7 13.3 13.3 13.3 10 4.4

GLYCOSURIA

Red/Orange 5.0% 3.0% 2.0%
Yellow 1.0% 0.75%
Green 0.5% 0.25% 0.1%
Blue 0.0%

Record a hypoglycaemic reaction by entering 'H' in the above glycosuria scale at the appropriate time.

KETONURIA

mmol. per litre: 15.7 7.8 3.9 1.5 0.5 0.0

RECORD OF ADMINISTRATION OF INSULIN

1	Code letter				A	B	C	D	E		F		E		F			
	Number of Units given				8	4	14	4	8		16		8		16			
2	Code letter																	
	Number of Units given																	

Time given: 16.50 | 22.30 | 8.00 | 11.30 | 16.50 | 7.45 | 16.50 | 7.45

Given by: self | self | self | self | self | self | self | self

Checked by: CM | BB | CM | CM | S.S. | MC | JC | JC

		DATE	INSULIN	DOSE	TIME OF ADMINISTRATION *	ROUTE	SIGNATURE	DISCONTINUED DATE	INITIALS
	A	14.9.86	ACTRAPID	8 UNITS	BT	S.C.	S. Parnell	14.9.85	SB
	B	14.9.85	ACTRAPID	4 UNITS	22.30	S.C.	S. Parnell	14.9.85	SB
	C	14.9.86	MIXTARD	14 UNITS BB		S.C.	S. Parnell	15.9.85	SB
	D	15.9.86	ACTRAPID	4 UNITS	BL	S.C.	S. Parnell	15.9.85	SB
	E	15.9.85	MIXTARD	8 UNITS	BT	S.C.	S. Parnell		
	F	16.9.85	INITARD	16 UNITS BB		S.C.	S. Parnell		
	G								
	H								
	I								
	J								
	K								
	L								

PRESCRIPTIONS REGULAR

	DATE	INSULIN	DOSE	TIME	ROUTE	SIGNATURE	GIVEN BY	KNOWN DRUG/ MEDICINE SENSITIVITY
ONCE ONLY	13.9.86	ACTRAPID	6 UNITS 12.30	S.C.	H. Brown	CM	1
	13.9.86	ACTRAPID	6 UNITS 17.00	S.C.	H. Brown	CM	2
	14.9.86	MIXTARD	10 UNITS 07.30	S.C.	H. Brown	HM	3

* B.B.= mins. before breakfast   B.L.= mins. before lunch   B.T.= mins. before tea   B.S.= mins. before supper

Fig.10.5 Paediatric diabetic prescription sheet

PAEDIATRIC DIABETIC COMA/ INSULIN INFUSION SHEET		SURNAME			UNIT NO.	
		FIRST NAMES				
HOSPITAL R.A.C.H.	WARD 4	ADDRESS		14·1·73	MARITAL STATUS DATE OF BIRTH RELIGION	
CONSULTANT Dr. Stewart		POST CODE			OCCUPATION	
CHILD'S WEIGHT 32·1 kg	AGE 12	BAR CODE	PLACE LABEL WITHIN BRACKETS			

DATE	12·9·85				13·9·85														
TIME	19⁰⁰	22⁰⁰	23⁰⁰	24⁰⁰	01⁰⁰	02⁰⁰	03⁰⁰	04⁰⁰	05⁰⁰	06⁰⁰									

BLOOD GLUCOSE mmol. per litre

LABORATORY	32	11·8						8·1							
WARD	22·2	13·3	13·3	13·3	4·4	10	10	13	10	10					

GLYCOSURIA

%	5							5							

KETONURIA

mmol. per litre	7·8							0·5							

BLOOD CHEMISTRY

Na	134	140						140							
K	5·2	3·5						4·5							
HCO_3	16	18						23							
UREA	8·2	5·8						5·1							
CREATININE															
pH	7·3														
pO_2															

CENTRAL VENOUS PRESSURE

Cm. of Water															

PRESCRIPTIONS – I.V. INSULIN INFUSION

START DATE	TIME	INTL⁵	INSULIN	STRENGTH OF SOLUTION	ML. PER HOUR	UNITS PER HOUR	UNITS PER KG. PER HR.	SIGNATURE	STOP DATE	TIME	INTL⁵
12·9·85	19⁰⁰	PH	ACTRAPID	60u in 60ml SALINE	3	3	0·1	P. Hill	13·9·85	12³⁰	PH
13·9·85	12³⁰	RW	ACTRAPID	60u in 60ml SALINE	1·5	1·5	0·05	R. Whyte	13·9·85	20⁰⁰	RW
13·9·85	20⁰⁰	LS	ACTRAPID	60u in 60ml SALINE	3	3	0·1	L. Scott	13·9·85	21⁰⁰	LS

PRESCRIPTIONS – I.M. OR S.C. ONCE ONLY

DATE	INSULIN	DOSE	TIME	ROUTE	SIGNATURE	GIVEN BY	CHECKED BY

Fig. 10.6 Paediatric diabetic coma/insulin infusion sheet

mass and volume as well as percentages is essential if medicines, disinfectants etc. are to be used safely and effectively. It may be that the need to perform calculations can be avoided by appropriate use of the pharmaceutical service, not because the nurse is lacking in the necessary skills, but so as to improve accuracy of dosage. In paediatric practice for example, it is much better to use a paediatric dosage specially dispensed for the purpose, than to attempt to obtain the required dose from a product intended primarily for adult use, although, on occasions, there may be no practical alternative to this approach. It is against this background that the following paragraphs should be studied.

SI units

The international system of units for mass and volume are:

Mass
  1 kilogram (kg) = 1000 grams
  1 gram   (g) = 1000 milligrams
  1 milligram (mg)= 1000 micrograms
  1 microgram (μg)* = 1000 nanograms
                           (ng)*

Volume
  1 litre   = 1000 millilitres (ml)
  1 millilitre = 1000 microlitres (μl)

*It must be noted that this abbreviation is not to be used in prescription writing because of the possibility of confusion with the abbreviation for milligram.

The mole and millimole (mmol)

The strength of a pharmaceutical preparation used in electrolyte replacement therapy is normally expressed in millimoles per tablet or millimoles per given volume of solution. (In addition the strength will be expressed as a percentage).

    A millimole is one thousandth of a mole, which is the molecular weight of a substance expressed in grams. Nurses will not normally be expected to calculate millimoles from molecular weights, but may have to determine how much of a given solution to measure to obtain a particular dose prescribed in millimoles. Not only is the term millimole used to express the strength of electrolytes, the

concentration of other substances can also be expressed similarly, providing their molecular weights are known. Millimoles are widely used in hospital laboratories, and clinical chemistry and haematology laboratory reports will use these units.

Percentages

The strength of a pharmaceutical product may be expressed as a percentage, meaning parts per 100 parts.

Percentage weight in volume (% w/v)
The expression 5% w/v indicates that 5 g of active ingredient is present in 100 ml of product.

Percentage weight in weight (% w/w)
The expression 5% w/w indicates that 5 g of the active ingredient is present in 100 g of product.

Percentage volume in volume (v/v)
The expression 5% v/v indicates that 5 ml of an active ingredient is present in 100 ml of product.

Percentage volume in weight (% v/w)
The expression 5% v/w indicates that 5 ml of an active ingredient is contained in 100 g of product.

Example 1
A solution contains 17.5 g of a substance in 2 litres of liquid. What is its strength in percentage terms?
$$\% \text{ w/v} = \frac{17.5}{2000} \times 100 = 0.875\%$$

Example 2
A solution has a strength of 0.875% w/v. How many grams of active ingredient are contained in 2 litres?
$$\frac{0.875}{100} \times 2000 = 17.5 \text{ g}$$

Methods of expressing the strength of active ingredient(s) in medicines and other pharmaceutical products

Solid dose forms
In most cases the strength of the active ingredient(s) present in each tablet or capsule will be expressed on the label of the product in grams, milligrams or micrograms. Quantities of

less than 1 gram should always be expressed in milligrams, thus the expression 500 mg is used and not 0.5 g. Similarly, quantities of less than 1 milligram should always be expressed in micrograms. This approach should always be followed when prescribing, recording the administration, ordering or dispensing medicines. This approach reduces the need to use the decimal point, which if incorrectly placed can lead to massive errors in drug administration. The need for the decimal point to be used remains when doses such as 37.5 mg are required.

Strengths of some solid dosage forms are expressed in units of activity, vitamin D, enzymes such as chymotrypsin being examples.

Products used for electrolyte replacement therapy, in addition to a strength of active ingredient being given in grams or milligrams will also have the strength quoted in millimoles (mmol). A slow release potassium chloride tablet, for example, contains 600 mg of potassium chloride or 8 mmol of K^+ and Cl^-.

Liquid ora dosage forms

The amount of active ingredient per given volume is usually given for the strength of preparations such as antibiotic syrups. An ampicillin syrup will bear a label stating that the product contains 250 mg in 5 ml, or a paediatric digoxin elixir contains 50 micrograms in lml. It is in connection with the administration of liquid medicines (oral and parenteral) that calculations are often required.

Liquid parenteral dosage forms

Small volume injections. Two main approaches will be encountered depending on the volume of the product. Small volume injections will normally bear a label expressing the strength of the product in a similar manner to that used for oral liquids. An injection will be shown to contain 25 mg per 1 ml but care should be taken to note the volume in each ampoule, since if the ampoule contains 2 ml the amount of active ingredient in the ampoule is 50 mg. The strength of some small volume injections of local anaesthetics such as lignocaine. are commonly expressed as a percentage w/v.

In parenteral products for electrolyte replace-ment therapy (large or small volume) the strength is frequently expressed as a percentage, mass per given volume, and mmol per given volume. Examples are as follows:

A strong, sterile solution of potassium chloride contains:

potassium chloride 15% w/v
potassium chloride 150 mg per ml (= 1.5 g in 10 ml)
approx. 2 mmol each of K^+ and Cl per ml.

Sodium chloride intravenous infusion contains:

sodium chloride 0.9% w/v
sodium chloride 9 g per litre
150 mmol each of Na^+ and Cl^- per litre.

The strength of adrenaline injections is still frequently expressed as 1 in 1000. This indicates that 1 gram of active ingredient is contained in 1000 ml of product. Of more value to the nurse is the fact that 1 ml of the injection contains 1 mg of adrenaline.

When a product is supplied in an ampoule as a dry powder for reconstitution before use, the label will give the amount of dry powder contained in the ampoule or rubber-capped vial. When reconstituting such products prior to injection the total volume produced by adding the diluent to the powder must be known if only a part of the dose in the ampoule or vial is to be administered. (see p. 165 for calculation).

The strength of certain biological materials such as insulin and heparin is expressed in units of activity per given volume e.g. 100 units per 1 ml (insulin) or 5000 units per 1 ml (heparin).

Large volume parenteral products. Labels on containers of large volume infusion solutions will generally give information on the strength of the product in percentage terms. Solutions of sodium chloride may contain 0.9% w/v or a glucose (dextrose) infusion may contain 5% w/v. Solutions for electrolyte replacement therapy will also contain information on the number of millimoles per given volume (see p. 161).

Other pharmaceutical products

The strengths of such products as lotions, sterile topical solutions, irrigations, antiseptic solutions etc, will generally be expressed as a percentage i.e. liquid preparations as a percentage w/v, solid or semi-solid preparations as a percentage w/w. When very dilute antiseptic solutions are in use the strength may be expressed as the number of parts of active ingredient in a given volume of fluid, e.g. 1 in 5000, 1 in 2000. In the first example 1 gram of the active ingredient is contained in 5000 ml of product, in the second case 1 gram is contained in 2000 ml of product.

General approach to calculations

For many calculations two different approaches are possible: a method based on 'first principles' or a method involving the use of a simple formula. In practice the nurse may use one method in preference to the other. As an additional check it is worthwhile wherever possible to use both methods for a particular calculation.

Method 1 (First principles)
A dose of 50 mg of a drug is required. The product available on the ward contains 200 mg in 5 ml.
Firstly calculate the amount of drug in 1 ml of product
i.e. $\frac{200}{5} = 40$ mg.

The product available contains 40 mg in 1 ml.

So for a dose of 50 mg, $\frac{50}{40} \times 1$ ml $= 1.25$ ml must be measured.

Method 2 (Formula)
This is based on simple proportion and uses the following formula:

$$\frac{\text{Dose required (mg)}}{\text{Strength available (mg)}} \times \frac{\text{dose volume (ml) of}}{\text{available product}}$$
$= $ volume (ml) containing the required dose

$$\frac{50}{200} \times 5 = \frac{50}{40}$$
$$= \frac{5}{4}$$
$$= 1.25 \text{ ml}$$

To obtain a dose of 50 mg, 1.25 ml would be measured.

As a simple memory aid it may be helpful to think of the formula as $\frac{\text{'want'}}{\text{'got'}}$. This is of course no substitute for a clear understanding of this method of calculating.

Solid dose forms

Calculations involving solid dose forms will generally cause few problems, but as with all calculations the need for accuracy can hardly be overstated. Sometimes it will be necessary

to subdivide a tablet or to give a number of tablets to obtain the prescribed dose.

Example 1

The dose required is 50 micrograms but the product available contains 100 micrograms
It is obvious that the tablet must be divided to obtain the required dose since the product available is twice the strength of the dose required. A general formula can be used in situations of this kind.
It is essential that the strengths are expressed in the same units, in this case micrograms.

$$\frac{\text{Dose required}}{\text{Strength available}} \times 1 = \begin{array}{l}\text{proportion of original}\\ \text{dosage form to give re-}\\ \text{quired dose.}\end{array}$$

$$\frac{50}{100} \times 1 = \tfrac{1}{2} \text{ tablet required.}$$

Example 2

The dose required is 100 micrograms but the product available contains 25 micrograms.

$$\frac{\text{Dose required}}{\text{Strength available}} \times 1 = \begin{array}{l}\text{number of tablets}\\ \text{required}\end{array}$$

i.e. $\frac{100}{25} \times 1 = 4$ tablets required

Example 3

Regrettably on some occasions it may be necessary to convert fractions of a milligram into micrograms. This should rarely be required, since for quantities less than 1 milligram the prescriber should use micrograms and the label on the container should bear the strength expressed in micrograms. However, situations might arise where the dose is expressed in micrograms and the product available is labelled in milligrams or vice versa.

A dose of 50 micrograms of a drug is required, and the tablets available are labelled 0.1 mg.
The formula $\frac{\text{Dose required}}{\text{Strength available}} \times 1$ can again be used

but the dose required and strength available must be expressed in the *same terms*, in this case micrograms.
1 milligram = 1000 micrograms
0.1 milligram = 100 micrograms (the decimal point is moved one place to the left)

Using the formula
$$\frac{\text{Dose required}}{\text{Strength available}} \quad \frac{50}{100} \times 1 = \tfrac{1}{2} \text{ tablet required.}$$

Example 4

If the strength on the prescription is written as 0.05 mg and the strength of the product is expressed as 100 micrograms it is obviously necessary to convert 0.05 mg into micrograms.

1 milligram = 1000 micrograms
0.1 milligram = 100 micrograms (decimal point moved one place to the left)·
0.05 milligram = 50 micrograms ($\div$ 2)

Complete the calculation as above.

Oral liquids

Calculations involving liquid dosage forms are essentially similar to those for solid dosage forms, being based on the first principles method (see p. 163) or the formula (see p. 163).

Example 1
The dose required is 200 mg but the product available contains 250 mg in 5 ml
or (divide by 5) 50 mg in 1 ml

So for a dose of 200 mg, $\frac{200}{50} \times 1$ ml = 4 ml required

Using the formula
$\frac{\text{Dose required (mg)}}{\text{Strength available (mg)}} \times$ dose volume (ml) of available product
= volume (ml) containing the required dose

i.e. $\frac{200}{250} \times 5$
= 4 ml

The required dose is contained in 4 ml of the available product. It is important to note that the dose required and the strength available must be expressed in the same units, in this case milligrams.

Example 2
It is required to give a dose of 45 mg but the product available contains 30 mg in 5 ml.
From first principles: If there are 30 mg in 5 ml, then 1 ml contains 6 mg.

For a dose of 45 mg, $\frac{45}{6} \times 1$ ml = 7.5 ml

Using the formula
$\frac{\text{Dose required (mg)}}{\text{Strength available (mg)}} \times$ dose volume (ml)
= volume (ml) to be measured to give required dose

i.e. $\frac{45}{30} \times 5 = 7.5$ ml must be measured to give the required dose

Parenteral products
A similar approach to calculations can be adopted.

Example 1
The dose required is 50 micrograms but the strength available is 500 micrograms in 2 ml.
$\frac{\text{Dose required (in micrograms)}}{\text{Strength available (in micrograms)}} \times$ dose volume (ml) of available product
= volume (ml) containing the required dose

i.e. $\frac{50}{500} \times 2$ = 0.2 ml of the available product required.

The figures obtained by this means can (and should) always be checked by a second nurse, preferably using first principles.

The strength available   is 500 micrograms in 2 ml,
or ÷ 2, i.e. 250 micrograms in 1 ml
then ÷ 5, i.e. 50 micrograms in 0.2 ml
It will be obvious that a sound knowledge of SI units and decimals is essential if these simple calculations are to be accurately performed. As with solid dose forms it may be that the dose required is contained in a multiple of the standard dosage form.

Example 2
The dose required is 7.5 mg but the strength available is 5 mg in 5 ml.

$\frac{\text{Dose required (mg)}}{\text{Strength available (mg)}} \times$ dose volume (ml) of available product
= volume (ml) containing the required dose

i.e. $\frac{7.5}{5} \times 5 = 7.5$ ml contains required dose.

Checking from first principles,
product available contains   5 mg in 5 ml
or ÷ 5, i.e. 1 mg in 1 ml
So for a dose of 7.5 mg, 7.5 ml of the available product is required.

Example 3
In some situations it may be necessary to administer a given mass of an active ingredient using a product where the strength of the available product is expressed as a percentage.
The dose required is 17.5 g but the strength available is 5% w/v i.e. it contains 5 g in 100 ml. To calculate how to obtain the 17.5 g dose required the general formula can again be used.

$\frac{\text{Dose required}}{\text{Strength available}} \times$ dose volume (ml)
= volume (ml) needed to obtain the required dose

In this situation the formula is expressed as follows:

$\frac{\text{Amount of active ingredient required (dose) g}}{\text{Amount of active ingredient in grams per 100 ml of solution available}}$
× 100 ml = volume (ml) to give dose required

i.e. $\frac{17.5}{5} \times 100 = 350$ ml

Again the calculation can be checked from first principles,
a 5% w/v solution contains 5 g in 100 ml
or × 3   15 g in 300 ml
or ÷ 2   2.5 g in 50 ml
So   17.5 g is contained in 350 ml

Example 4
Strong solution of potassium chloride contains 2 mmol each of K^+ and Cl in each ml. Calculate the volume required to obtain a dose of 10 mmol of K^+.
$\frac{\text{Dose required}}{\text{Strength available}} \times$ dose volume (ml)
= volume (ml) to give required dose

i.e $\frac{10}{2} \times 1 = 5$ ml required to give a dose of 10 mmol K^+

Example 5.
Heparin injection contains 5000 units per ml. Calculate the volume required to obtain a dose of 3000 units.
$\frac{\text{Dose required}}{\text{Strength available}} \times$ dose volume
= volume (ml) to give required dose

i.e. $\frac{3000}{5000} \times 1 = 0.6$ ml required to give 3000 units.

Topical antiseptics
Although antiseptic solutions are commonly

produced in a ready-to-use form, calculations may still be required in connection with the dilution of antiseptics.

Example 1
Chlorhexidine is available as a 5% concentrate and 1 litre of a 0.05% w/v solution is required for use as an irrigation.
   Again the general formula can be used, on this occasion using the percentages.

$$\frac{\% \text{ required}}{\% \text{ available}} \times \text{ volume required (ml)}$$

= volume of concentrate required to be diluted to 1 litre

i.e. $\frac{0.05}{5} \times 1000 = 10 \text{ ml}$

   So 10 ml of a 5% w/v solution must be diluted to 1000 ml to give a 0.05% w/v solution.

Calculations involving reconstitution of injections

When an injection has to be reconstituted from a powder before use, it should be noted that the resulting volume is in excess of the volume of diluent added, due to the displacement effect of the powder. This must be taken into account if a dose less than that contained in the vial is required.

Example
A vial contains 500 mg of a drug but the dose required is 200 mg. The addition of 5 ml of diluent yields a volume of 5.25 ml when drawn into the syringe. In this case it is useful to use the general formula.

$$\frac{\text{Dose required (mg)}}{\text{Strength available (mg)}} \times \text{ dose volume (ml)}$$

= volume (ml) to be measured

i.e. $\frac{200}{500} \times 5.25 = $ 2.1 ml required to obtain a dose of 200 mg.

Dosage calculations involving body surface area (see p. 192).

PROMOTING THE EFFECTIVENESS OF MEDICINES

In addition to administering medicines correctly, the nurse has a responsibility to do her utmost to promote their effectiveness. A knowledge of how groups of medicines (e.g. antacids, anticoagulants) act or fail to act, along with helpful prescribing, allows the nurse to play a considerable part in improving efficacy of the drugs the patient is receiving. For example:

1. The absorption of some antibiotics (e.g. ampicillin) taken by mouth is decreased by the presence of food in the gut and so it is advisable to give the medicine before a main meal.
2. By restricting salt in the diet of those patients receiving diuretic therapy, there is less sodium to be reabsorbed by the renal tubules. Less water will be absorbed, therefore more urine is manufactured.
3. In the terminal stages of a painful illness where comfort has become the primary concern, strict timing of the giving of analgesics is often essential to obtain complete pain relief. By so doing, the medicine can relieve pain just as it is due to break through, the only drawback being that this may mean wakening the patient.

MONITORING THE EFFECT OF MEDICINES

A further aspect of the nurse's role is her participation in monitoring the effect of medicines. The following indices regularly recorded by nurses reflect the effect of commonly used groups of medicines.

Temperature
Body temperature will be reduced using an appropriate antibiotic for bacterial infection, by using an antipyretic, such as aspirin, where there is disturbance of the heat-regulating centre or by administering antithyroid drug (e.g. carbimazole) to the thyrotoxic patient.

Pulse
Cardiac glycosides (e.g. digoxin) slow, steady and strengthen the heart rate while anticholinergic drugs and thyroxine increase the pulse. The radial and apical rates may require to be measured by two nurses simultaneously.

Respirations
The rate and pattern of breathing are likely to be improved by diuretics, bronchodilators and antibiotics. Analgesics, by relieving pain may make breathing more comfortable, but in high doses may depress respiration to a dangerous

level. The forced expiratory volume (FEV_1) may be ascertained using a peak flow meter before and after inhaling bronchodilators.

Blood pressure

Corticosteroids (e.g. hydrocortisone) have the effect of raising the blood pressure and are used in the treatment of collapse.

Antihypertensives (e.g. atenolol, hydralazine, methyl dopa) are used to treat high blood pressure but may cause the blood pressure to fall sharply when the patient stands up. Close monitoring, including records of lying and standing blood pressure, is essential.

Strong analgesia lowers the blood pressure and extreme caution is needed in states of shock and following anaesthetic.

Urinary output

Diuretics (e.g. frusemide) increase urine formation while corticosteroids may cause retention of fluid with subsequent oliguria. A record of both intake and output of fluid helps to monitor fluid balance.

Weight

A record of the patient's weight taken at the same time each day in the same clothing is probably the most accurate method of measuring diuretic effect or fluid retention.

Urinalysis and capillary blood glucose testing

The urine of diabetic patients is tested for glucose, although testing a sample of capillary blood taken from the thumb or ear lobe is a more accurate reflection of diabetic control. Dosages of insulin and sulphonylureas (e.g. glipizide, tolbutamide) are often estimated from these results.

Corticosteroids and thiazide diuretics (e.g. bendrofluazide) can precipitate diabetes mellitus and therefore urine testing for glucose at regular intervals may be ordered.

Laboratory blood tests

These are not carried out by nurses but results are often received by nurses. Prothrombin times (PT) are used to calculate daily dosages of anticoagulant drugs, such as warfarin. While maximum anticoagulation is the aim in the prevention of thrombus formation, extreme caution is required to prevent over anticoagulation and subsequent bleeding.

The white blood count (WBC) of patients receiving immunosuppressant or cytotoxic therapy is checked at frequent intervals as these drugs can reduce the count to a dangerously low level and hence lower the patients resistance to infection.

Medicines should not replace nursing care

Simple nursing measures alone may fail to achieve for example, pain relief, regular evacuation of the bowel or sleep. Nevertheless, they must be attempted initially and if medicines have to be prescribed, the appropriate nursing care should be continued. For example:

1. The use of analgesics does not replace the need for good communication and reassurance of the patient, careful positioning and adequate rest, as well as the possible use of local heat or massage.
2. A generous intake of fluid and high fibre foods, increased mobility, maximum use of the gastrocolic reflex, especially after breakfast, and provision of privacy for toilet purposes are all still necessary in spite of a temporary need for laxatives.
3. Peace of mind, a comfortable bed and a quiet, uninterrupted environment are especially necessary for the patient who suffers insomnia whether or not he is being treated with hypnotics.

Alleviation of unavoidable side-effects

In many patients unavoidable side-effects result from taking some medicines and so precautions may have to be taken. Many of the strong analgesics (e.g. diamorphine) make patients feel sick and this can be especially distressing post-operatively or, for example, following myocardial infarction when stress should be kept to a minimum. It is therefore common practice to give an antiemetic (e.g. prochlorperazine) at the same time. Sedatives can make patients disorientated as well as drowsy. The erecting of bed sides may be necessary and it may be advisable to position the patient's bed within view of the nursing staff especially at night.

Diuretics are given early in the morning so that urinary frequency has worn off by the middle of the day allowing freedom of activity for the remainder of the day. Incontinence of urine can be precipitated (as can falling) in an attempt to reach the toilet in time. In geriatric wards with large numbers of dependent patients, arrangements are sometimes made to administer diuretics slightly later to fit in with the number of staff available to provide the necessary assistance with toileting. Where applicable, the patient should be told what to expect, be shown some means of summoning assistance and should have his bed positioned close to the toilet or have a commode placed at the bedside. Oral iron preparations colour the stools black and the patient should be warned accordingly. This can be especially alarming to him if he has a history of passing blood in the stools and he mistakes the discolouration for a recurrence of bleeding.

Of course, not all patients receiving medicines require active nursing. Despite having serious conditions, some feel fairly well, are ambulant and are independent. Their appearance may be deceptive however and the nurse must not omit a routine scrutiny for possible adverse effects.

SAFETY IN DRUG ADMINISTRATION — CYTOTOXIC DRUGS

The hazards associated with the handling of cancer chemotherapeutic agents have received increasing publicity in the last few years, partly because of the acceleration in their use but mainly as the result of several claims of actual and postulated adverse effects on personnel involved in their reconstitution and administration.

Evidence in support of this growing concern can be found by reviewing the literature. Mutagenic substances have been detected in the urine of nurses handling cytotoxic agents (Falck et al, 1979). Cyclophosphamide can be detected in the urine of nursing and pharmacy personnel who make it up, and a report from Finland documented liver damage in three head oncology nurses after years of handling cytotoxic drugs. (Sontaniemi et al, 1983). These are but a few examples. Some of the reports available are, however, inconclusive and continuing research is necessary if the precise risk associated with low-level occupational exposure to cytotoxic drugs is to be determined.

The dangers encountered in the handling of cytotoxic drugs fall into two categories. As the result of their extremely irritant effects, immediate damage to the skin and eyes can result. The long-term consequences of absorbing materials, which may be carcinogenic or teratogenic, through the skin, the lungs or the gastrointestinal tract, though still somewhat theoretical, are sufficient to warrant energetic implementation of policies by health authorities to reduce any risks to their staff to the minimum.

Location for reconstituting cytotoxic drugs
All manipulations involving cytotoxic drugs should be undertaken only in areas specifically designated by local policy for the purpose. Such areas should be placed centrally, such as in the pharmacy department or in a side room within an oncology ward or department. The only sure way of providing protection during reconstitution of such drugs is to use a laminar flow cabinet. Such a device creates constant recirculation of air and removes contaminants through its filters to produce clean conditions in a contained environment. It is however recognised that this facility is not always available.

Where a side room of a ward or similar designated area is used this should be away from normal ward traffic and food areas, and the windows and door should be kept closed. These areas should be equipped with a work bench having an impervious surface. A sink and running water should be available. Work should not be done at a position where draughts, mechanical ventilation or the air-conditioning system might convey aerosols or dusts to another occupied area. Drugs should be reconstituted over a disposable sterile tray which should contain any spillage.

Training and designation of personnel

Doctors, nurses or pharmacists involved in the handling of cytotoxic drugs should be instructed in the dangers, precautions and techniques of their preparation and administration. Training may be given by a suitably experienced senior member of the medical, nursing or pharmacy staff and *only* those so trained should be responsible for the handling of these drugs. All personnel involved in the handling of cytotoxic drugs should be familiar with the written guidelines on the handling of these drugs and be given a personal copy. During the first three months of pregnancy, staff should not be exposed to cytotoxic drugs.

Protection against occupational exposure

Protection against exposure to cytotoxic drugs or their metabolites is essential.

Clothing

All individuals should wear the following protective items during the preparation of all cytotoxic drugs to protect the skin and eyes, and to prevent inhalation of aerosolised drug particles.

Disposable gloves. PVC gloves will normally be suitable but rubber gloves may be required in some circumstances as indicated by the manufacturer of the drug.

Gown or disposable plastic apron

Disposable sleeves. These may be required for those staff not wearing a long-sleeved uniform or gown.

Goggles/protective glasses (complying with BS 2092C). All staff should wear regulation eye protection. Ordinary spectacles do not provide all-round protection.

Disposable face mask

Technique

Every effort should be made to reduce aerosolisation. Ampoules, including those containing diluents, should be opened with care using a file if necessary and plastic ampoule breaker to avoid cuts and scratches. The exact volume required should be drawn into a syringe and the remainder discarded (see below) or used immediately for another patient. Air from the syringe should be expelled into the empty ampoule over sterile cotton wool or a gauze swab. The sheath should then be placed over the needle.

Drugs in powder form must be reconstituted with care. The drugs may be released as a fine spray through the needle hole if excess pressure is produced in the vial. This may be avoided by removing an appropriate amount of air from the vial before injecting the diluting fluid or by the use of a special venting needle (Fig. 10.7).

Filled syringes should be labelled as appropriate and placed in a receiver ready for immediate use.

Disposal of surplus drugs and contaminated equipment

Solid waste. Surplus drugs and contaminated bottles and ampoules together with syringes, needles, vials, swabs and infusion equipment should be placed into designated containers. The use of disposable equipment is recommended whenever practicable. Swabs should be discarded in disposable plastic bags.

Liquid waste. Small volumes are best disposed of by placing the ampoule or vial containing the waste in a needleproof, leakproof disposal bin.

Parenteral administration of cytotoxic drugs

The peripheral blood count, weight and height of each patient should be measured and the results compared with previous findings. Any major discrepancy should be investigated.

The dose of chemotherapy should be

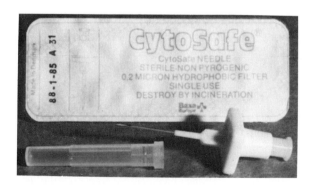

Fig. 10.7 Special venting needle

prescribed by the doctor only after consultation with a senior member of the medical staff. The calculation of the dose, volume and concentration should be checked and recorded.

Syringes should be clearly labelled with the name and the dose of the drug. Any solutions made up in this way and remaining unused must be disposed of safely as previously described. The used vial(s) or ampoule(s) should be placed with the loaded syringe(s) in a receiver bearing the patient's name and/or prescription to enable a final check to be made.

Prior to administration of the drug to the patient, the prescription should be checked together with the patient's name, the drugs and their doses in the syringes and the used ampoules/vials. Before the person preparing the drug proceeds to administer it, these items should first be checked by a second qualified person and recorded in accordance with agreed procedure.

Obviously, risks of contamination are present throughout the entire procedure from reconstitution of the drugs to their administration and disposal of equipment. Protective clothing as already described should therefore be worn throughout including the time of administration. Careful explanation of the purpose of the drugs and the precautions which are necessary, should be given to the patient at the onset of treatment. Most patients accept these needs, but in individual situations slight modifications may have to be made to the amount of protection used at the time of administration of the drugs if there is a likelihood of the patient being alarmed by the 'spaceman image' of the donor. For example, protective goggles and face mask may have to be removed after reconstituting the drugs.

The patient's clothing and arm should be protected by a disposable paper towel. A 'butterfly' needle is convenient when drugs, which require a dilution intravenous infusion, are used. For direct bolus administration, a fresh needle should be applied to the syringe. If there is any doubt about the siting of the needle the procedure should be abandoned and begun elsewhere.

Once the infusion is established, responsibility rests with the nurse to continue observing the patient and to provide him with physical and emotional support. The point of entry into a vein of the drug administration set should be observed for leakage. If extravasation should occur the manufacturer's recommended treatment — a medical responsibility — should be observed. A pack for the initial treatment of extravasation should be available always.

The following cytotoxic drugs are known to be particularly damaging and irritant on extravasation:

Dacarbazine	Mustine
Daunorubicin	Vinblastine
Doxorubicin	Vincristine
Mithramycin	Vindesine
Mitomycin C	

Vomitus, urine and faeces from treated patients may contain unchanged drug or active metabolites, therefore skin contact should be avoided by wearing gloves and a long-sleeved gown when disposing of excreta. Care should be taken to place disposable receptacles carefully in the waste-disposal unit to avoid splashing of the contents. The linen of incontinent patients receiving a course of cytotoxic drugs should be dealt with as infected linen. It is the responsibility of the nurse in charge of the ward to advise all members of the nursing staff of the patients for whom these precautions must be taken.

Procedure in the event of an accident

Spillage of a cytotoxic drug on to intact skin
1. If any cytotoxic drug, apart from dacarbazine (DTIC) and melphalan (Alkeran) comes into contact with the skin, flush the affected area with copious amounts of water.
2. If dacarbazine is spilled on to the skin, wash it off immediately with soap and water. In the case of melphalan, treat the contaminated skin with a solution of sodium carbonate 3% w/v. Note that a *fresh* solution of sodium carbonate should be available prior to handling melphalan injection.
3. After skin contamination with methotrexate, if transient stinging occurs

following washing with water, apply a bland cream (e.g. aqueous cream BP) to the affected area.

Spillage of a cytotoxic drug on to broken skin, into eyes or through needle penetration of the skin

1. If accidents involve cuts or needle-penetration of the skin, wash with copious amounts of water.
2. If any cytotoxic drug enters the eye(s), irrigate the eye(s) thoroughly with sterile normal saline.
3. Inform the doctor and person in charge of department, e.g. ward, clinic or pharmacy.

Spillage of a cytotoxic drug on to a hard surface

1. Isolate the contaminated area and inform person in charge of the department.
2. Wear protective clothing, i.e. gloves, goggles, face mask and plastic apron when cleaning up spillage.
3. Wipe up any spillage that remains with absorbent paper and place in polythene bag.
4. Wash contaminated surfaces with copious amounts of water. Dry off surface with absorbent paper and place also in polythene bag.
5. Seal polythene bag and place in designated receptacle.
6. Remove protective clothing and place any disposable materials in an incinerator bag. Tie off.
7. Send waste for disposal by incineration.

Cytotoxic drugs administered orally

Oral solid dose forms of cytotoxic drugs constitute no risk to the handler if a few simple precautions are taken. Coated tablets should not be broken, compressed tablets should not be crushed and capsules should not be opened. Tablets and capsules should be dispensed and administered using a non-touch technique. A stainless steel triangle, which should be washed after use, should be used when tablets require to be counted. In the event of contamination by free powder or the

contents of a capsule, the same principles for dealing with spillage of parenteral drugs apply. To prevent inhalation of powder, it is essential to use a well-fitting face mask. For mopping up spilled powder, the disposable towel used should first be made damp. Disposal is by incineration.

Conclusion

Without creating unnecessary alarm amongst staff or patients, a respect for cytotoxic drugs should be engendered in much the same way as exists for radioactive materials. Provided that staff make themselves fully conversant with the guidelines laid down on the safe handling of these drugs and are seen to incorporate the practical measures into their day-to-day work, protection for the user, the patient and all other personnel who may be working near treatment areas, should be guaranteed. The Health and Safety Executive in a Guidance Note (MS21, December 1983) recommended that a competent person should be appointed in writing to undertake responsibility for the safety arrangements connected with the use of cytotoxic drugs.

A multidisciplinary approach involving medical (clinical and occupational health), nursing and pharmaceutical personnel will be required together with an input from safety officers.

No completely reliable test is yet available for monitoring the degree to which individuals may be being exposed. Health authorities should however be prepared to offer health screening for regular handlers of parenteral cytotoxic drugs.

ERRORS IN THE ADMINISTRATION OF MEDICINES

With the present complexity of drug therapy and the need for many patients to receive multiple drug therapy, the potential for errors in the administration of medicines is great. To illustrate this, a medical ward with 30 beds may have as many as 60 products in use at any one time and could keep in stock a range of 200 medicinal products (excluding lotions, sterile fluids, etc.). Factors other than complexity of therapy contribute to errors in the administration of medicines and these will be discussed later.

An error in the administration of medicines can, at best, be inconvenient for the patient or, at worst, may be catastrophic. In order to gain a balanced perspective on such errors it is necessary to define them. This is best done by considering how, in practical terms, the overall objective of drug therapy (i.e. to achieve therapeutic benefit for the patient with minimal adverse effects) is most likely to be achieved. For the purposes of this discussion, the assumption is made that the prescriber has taken all relevant clinical factors into account when deciding to prescribe a particular drug, i.e. the choice of drug, dose, route, etc. is appropriate in all respects. To achieve therapeutic benefit for the patient it is obviously essential to ensure that the right dose of the right drug be administered at the right time by the correct route.

Adverse drug reactions and interactions must be avoided if at all possible. If adverse drug reactions are unavoidable, the effects on the patient should be minimised. It therefore follows that monitoring of the patient is required. All adverse reactions to drugs should be reported to the doctor. It is also important to ensure that the patient is sufficiently well informed about his medicines so that during his stay in hospital and subsequently, when discharged from hospital, compliance with the treatment can be expected with a reasonable degree of confidence. Adherence by all health care staff to hospital drug procedures is clearly a prerequisite at all times. Hazards to the nurse manipulating or administering any medicines must be avoided. Her colleagues working nearby must also be safeguarded.

On this basis, a drug error can be defined broadly as any act of commission or omission that militates against the achievement of the therapeutic objective i.e. benefit for the patient. Such acts may relate to one or more of the practical aspects discussed above. It is obvious that it is not possible to comply to the letter with *all* aspects of medicine administraiton throughout *all* courses of drug therapy for *all* patients. Clearly, it is essential that on every occasion the correct dose of the correct drug is administered by the correct route. However, it must be recognised that it is never possible to administer all medicines exactly at the time indicated on the prescription sheet for all patients in a given ward, simply due to the time required to complete the traditional medicine round. This is technically an error, but will seldom be of significance. On the other hand the timing of the administration of some medicines may be of vital importance to the patient (e.g. pre-operative medication). Furthermore, it is not always possible to carry out the many responsibilities indirectly associated with medicine administration for various reasons, the most common being lack of time. Nevertheless, the aim must be to eliminate errors by maintaining the highest possible standards of practice. Strategies for achieving this aim are discussed later in the chapter.

Sources of errors in the administration of medicines

Errors can arise for many reasons and are often compounded in a 'cascade-like' way. An error in dispensing may not be detected by the checking system in the pharmacy. Medical and/or nursing personnel may also fail to notice the error, which may finally result in a patient being given an incorrect dose or even the wrong drug.

The failure of professionals to adhere to the rules of good practice has been recognised by Ley (1981), in medical, nursing and pharmaceutical personnel. This failure is clearly a potential source of errors.

Having recognised that errors are often compounded, specific sources of errors that can be attributed to particular members of the health care team are now discussed.

The prescriber

Full responsibility rests with the prescriber to state clearly and without ambiguity the medicines the patient is to be given. The improved design of prescribing charts has undoubtedly contributed to more accurate and to safer drug administration. However, adherence to the prescribing policy is essential if errors are to be avoided, irrespective of the sophistication of the documents used. Bad handwriting is probably the commonest potential source of errors. Confusion between similar drug names is a well recognised cause of error e.g. Intal, Inderal; quinine, quinidine; chlorpromazine, chlorpropamide. When badly written these words have a similar shape. Those who prescribe, dispense, and administer medicines should not accept this all too common fault. Unofficial abbreviations for medicines are always open to misinterpretation and should not be used or accepted.

The omission of essential information (e.g. the strength of the drug), may tempt the nurse to administer what is readily available rather than that intended by the prescriber. Similarly the use of outdated abbreviations and symbols (e.g. PRN, ii) are misleading and dangerous and should never be used. Where cancellation of a prescription lacks precision, the medicine may continue to be given to the possible detriment of the patient.

The pharmacist

Errors in the administration of medicines may be due directly or indirectly to failures in the pharmaceutical service. As within clinical departments and wards, procedures in pharmaceutical departments are designed to ensure that, as far as possible, errors are eliminated. Nevertheless, errors can and do occur which may be due to failures to follow procedures and, on some occasions, to lack of effective communication with the prescriber or nurse in charge of a ward or department.

Errors or omissions in the labelling of medicines may cause difficulty, which may lead to an incorrect dose or even a wrong drug being administered. There is much debate about colour coding of labels/containers etc. but there can be no substitute for *reading* the label at all times.

On occasions medicines are required when a full pharmaceutical service is not available. This may result in delay in administering a medicine which may have serious consequences for the patient.

Regrettably, medicines are often supplied to wards with little or no background information as to the actions, uses or dosage of the product. Ward staff may then have to rely on their own limited information sources, especially if the pharmacy-based drug information service is not available. On fairly rare occasions a product or particular batch of a product may have to be withdrawn from use due to a fault or suspected fault. In such circumstances pharmaceutical staff must ensure the rapid flow of accurate information to wards and departments concerned.

When products are issued to wards for use in connection with a clinical trial it is very important that sufficient information is made available (without breaking the code) to the medical and nursing staff to enable the product to be used safely. Greater interest and co-operation of nurses would be shown if the background to, and reasons for a clinical trial were explained. It would also be helpful if the results of the work were made available to and discussed with those participating.

The role of the pharmacist in drug therapy has been described as that of 'safety net and overseer'. Any failure to discharge this role has serious implications for the safety and wellbeing of the patient.

The nurse

Nurses are responsible for the safe and accurate administration of medicines to most inpatients and some patients in the community. (Supervision of medicine taking may also be required in certain instances). In order to discharge these duties the nurse must interpret the prescription, select the correct medicine and make a record of the administration.

The administration of the medicine is the culmination of research, development, manufacture, prescribing and dispensing. All the skill and resources that have gone into making a particular medicine available can, at this stage, contribute nothing. The patient is now dependent on the nurse's skill and attention to detail. The responsibility to ensure safe and accurate administration of a medicine to a patient irrespective of his physical or mental condition should never be underestimated.

Identification of patient

An examination by the authors of drug errors

has shown that approximately 50% are due to the nurse's failure to identify the patient correctly. The bracelet is, as yet, the best method developed for identifying patients. However, it is only as safe as those who apply it and refer to it. While every precaution may be taken to insert accurately the information in the bracelet and to attach the bracelet carefully to the right patient, problems can still arise. Bracelets have, on occasions, to be removed, for example, when an intravenous infusion is being set up, and may not be replaced. The patient, unwittingly, may remove the bracelet or he may do so while on weekend leave. Writing on the bracelet may become indistinct with the passage of time. Even when the bracelet remains satisfactorily in position, reference must be made to it. Of course, it has never been intended that the bracelet should take the place of effective communication between nurse and patient, nor that it should obviate the need for regular updating of staff on the patients under their care.

There can be no doubt about the need for identification bracelets to be used in paediatric units, intensive care units, theatres and in all acute areas where a patient is unable to account for himself. Areas which pose particular difficulty are geriatric units and psychiatric wards. Patients in these wards may understandably have feelings of resentment at being 'labelled'. In addition, staff may feel that this procedure militates against their efforts to reduce any feelings patients may have of being institutionalised and that they know their patients anyway. However, as is discussed in the next chapter, there is special need for care in the use of medicines for the elderly and the mentally ill. Health authorities must devise workable policies which are in patients' best interests.

Errors in calculations are another significant source of error. A study made by MacPherson et al (1983) of 130 nurse learners demonstrated the considerable difficulty that some nurses have with basic calculations. Particular problems relate to the use of quantities less than one milligram. Efforts to convert, 0.125 mg into micrograms, have resulted in

gross overdosage of digoxin in paediatric practice. It has been suggested that there might be a place for calculators in assisting those who have such difficulty. If the individual's lack of numeracy is so severe as to call for this level of assistance, there must be grave doubts as to whether a calculator could be used safely. Indeed, the improper use of such equipment may be another source of error. Calculators have a place, but should probably only be used to check figures arrived at by other means.

Use of inadequate equipment may cause mistakes to be made. Pipettes with indistinct markings cannot safely be used to measure small volumes of liquid medicines. Potent liquid medicines are often used in paediatric practice where it is especially vital to ensure accuracy at all times.

Using medicines in an unorthodox way may lead to errors. Some tablets are designed to be broken if a fractional dose is required. Other tablets are not so designed. An attempt to break or divide such a product will almost certainly result in the administration of an incorrect dose. Similarly, the crushing of a slow-release tablet will destroy the essential properties of the formulation, any benefit to the patient being lost. Errors may arise due to the use of an unsuitable formulation such as a very large capsule or tablet which a patient may be unable to swallow.

The patient

The active co-operation of the patient is essential in order to achieve the therapeutic benefit of a course of drug treatment. Nurses and their medical colleagues should never take the patient's co-operation for granted or expect this to be given automatically. The patient's right to question or even reject any form of therapy must be respected. However, nurses must play their part in ensuring that, if a patient does decide to reject a particular treatment this decision is reached on the basis of a full understanding of the implications for the patient's health and well-being. It would obviously be unfair to attribute the patient's action or lack of action as a source of drug errors, but in some situations the patient will bear some responsibility if the treatment fails. The not uncommon occurrence of finding tablets in the patient's bed or under the cushions of a chair may or may not indicate failure on the part of the patient. This may be the first indication the nurse has that all is not well. Needless to say great tact and perception may be needed to establish the true cause of this rejection.

There are dangers in using medicines brought into hospital by patients on admission. Medicines dispensed for individual patients may have been inappropriately stored in the patient's home. Labels may have been altered or removed causing difficulty in identifying the contents of a container. In remote areas it may be that on a limited number of occasions it will be necessary to use the patient's own medicines when he is in hospital. Whilst those responsible for deciding to use the patient's own medicines when in hospital have a heavy responsibility, it is vitally important that the patient provides accurate information on his current drug therapy.

Error avoidance/reduction

Given that drug errors often arise as a result of a series of failures by the health professionals involved, it follows that programmes designed to improve matters must have the active support of prescriber, pharmacist and nurse. Against the background of the discussion of the role of nurse managers and practising nurses that follows, the assumption should not be made that actions by nurses alone, important as these are, will be all that is required to eliminate or reduce errors. A non-nursing aspect that is of particular concern to nurses, relates to the minimal amount of curriculum time that appears to be devoted to teaching medical students the procedural aspects of prescribing, administration and recording of medicines. As a result of the low priority given to this, medical and nursing staff time is often wasted when prescriptions have to be amended to comply with hospital policies and procedures. Not surprisingly relationships become strained and drug errors may occur.

The first line manager

Since one of the roles of a first line manager is to create an environment which is conducive

to safety and efficiency, guidance relating to drug administration for the nurse in charge of a ward is offered first.

Whenever possible, the nurse in charge should avoid delegating the administration of medicines to nurses who are unfamiliar with the identity of patients in the ward. Examples include nurses who have recently been appointed to the ward, have just returned from a period of absence or have been sent to assist on a temporary basis from another ward. It is important also to assign appropriate members of staff to the administration of medicines. It is irresponsible to ask nurses to participate in the administration of medicines unless they have been taught the theoretical aspects of it. The Royal College of Nursing publication *Drug Administration — A Nursing Responsibility* (1983) recommends that the role of the nursing auxiliary or assistant in relation to drug administration is

'to see that the patient has a drink with which to take the drug, to help the patient into a suitably comfortable position to take the drug, and to report to the person conducting the drug round if for any reason the patient fails to take the drug'.

The nurse in charge of a ward bears a heavy responsibility to ensure that her staff comply with the policies laid down. In addition the nurse in charge has many, less obvious, responsibilities. For instance, she must ensure that up-to-date relevant information on drugs is readily available at ward level. All wards and departments should have an up-to-date copy of the British National Formulary. Great emphasis is rightly placed on the need for the accurate administration of medicines, but it is also essential to ensure that medicines are discontinued when a course of treatment is complete. Where an instruction to discontinue therapy has not been given, and where it is clear that the medicine does not constitute replacement or other long-term therapy, the continuing need for the medicine should be questioned. Prime responsibility for discontinuation of treatment must of course rest with the prescriber.

Insisting on accurate prescribing practice is one of the most demanding aspects of the ward sister's role. It will be to her benefit and the benefit of her patients to make her standards known when there is a change of doctors on the ward.

Efforts should be made to discourage discussion with patients' visitors or visiting members of staff during procedures involving the administration of medicines. It may be useful to display a notice on the medicine trolley — DO NOT DISTURB — with the intention of minimising interruptions during medicine administration.

In the event of there being duplications in patients' names in a ward, staff and the patients concerned, must be alerted. The nurse in charge must also ensure that identification bracelets are renewed and replaced as necessary.

Staff should be encouraged, and if necessary instructed, to keep accurate and legible records of drug administration. Prescribers should be asked to rewrite prescription sheets when they become untidy or when the use of two prescription sheets concurrently could be obviated. 'Kardex' or similar holders for prescribing and recording documents should be kept in good repair and the order of sheets should be rearranged to correspond with the movement of patients within the ward. Nursing staff must adopt a safe and efficient system of storing medicines in the medicine trolley and withdraw medicines which are no longer required. Advice can be sought from pharmacy staff on appropriate levels of ordering, expiry dates, etc.

Complacency may creep in to long-stay units or during periods when wards are exceptionally quiet and so ward sisters must strive to maintain standards of safety with medicines and to stimulate staff interest. Using medicine rounds however, at any time, for teaching *about* medicines is to be avoided. It is safer when administering medicines to concentrate fully on the procedure and to leave the discussion of uses, actions, side-effects, etc. for a more appropriate time.

The administration of medicines should be kept high on the list of priorities in a ward. The nursing staff's awareness of medicines in use in their ward may be increased by referring to patients' prescription sheets in conjunction with the giving of a verbal report on the patients, for example, at the changeover of staff. If time permits, a separate reporting session specifically on the medicines in use and any related difficulties that the patient or nurse may have with them can be valuable to the nurse in charge as well as to more junior nursing staff.

Ward pharmacy services should be fully utilised. Any special needs of the ward will become apparent to the ward pharmacist but there is no substitute for active co-operation with the pharmacist. A climate of passive acceptance of a service is not conducive to achieving the highest standard of care for patients.

The senior manager

The continuing need to reduce the number of drug errors which take place should be the concern of those involved in policy making, management, and teaching as well as those in clinical practice.

Nurse managers spend a good deal of their time allocating staff to meet service commitments. Along with the many other demands which they try to meet, perhaps greater consideration should be given to the number of staff needed at the main medicine round times or when pre- and post-operative medications are to be given.

The extent to which two nurses should be involved in the administration of medicines continues to exercise the minds of nurse managers and nurses in clinical practice. In April 1985 it was reported that the UKCC was of the view that

'with the exception of Controlled Drugs and possibly a limited number of other locally defined exceptions, practitioners whose names are on the first level parts of the register and midwives, should be seen as competent to administer medicines on their own and responsible for their actions in so doing'. At the time of writing consultations are proceeding on this important aspect of nursing practice. Community nurses have, of course, always administered medicines single-handed.

Currently however, it is common for hospital policies to require that two nurses should be involved in the administration of medicines, one of whom should be a trained nurse. The possible advantages and disadvantages of this

Table 10.1 The advantages and disadvantages of the involvement of two nurses in medicine administration in hospital

Advantages	Disadvantages
Presence of second nurse provides an additional check which should improve patient safety by reducing drug errors.	Blurring of responsibility leading to confusion and perhaps error.
Presence of second nurse helpful if calculations of drug dosage are required.	Nurse learner may be reluctant to 'challenge' a trained nurse and assume that the trained nurse is always right.
Patient feels reassured that a second person is involved in checking the medicine.	May provide false sense of safety in medicine administration.
Provides important learning situation for procedures of medicine administration.	Medicine round may take longer because of double checking.
	Dilution of professional responsibility.
Impact of interruptions can be minimised since the medicine round can probably be continued by one nurse.	In some situations, e.g. night duty, staffing levels make it impracticable for two nurses to be routinely involved in medicine administration.
Some patients understandably wish to ask questions about their medicines during medicine rounds. This may be difficult for one nurse to cope with although even if two nurses are present some complex questions may have to be noted for answering later.	
Improved security of medicines during medicine rounds.	
Any emergency arising during the medicine round can be dealt with more promptly.	

approach are summarised in Table 10.1. It should be noted that there is little evidence in the literature to confirm or otherwise the views expressed, which is not surprising, since a valid comparative study would be very difficult to undertake with so many variables to influence the outcome.

Clearly the advantages and disadvantages outlined in Table 10.1 do not carry equal weight, but will serve as a frame of reference when local policies are being formulated. As with all other aspects of nursing care the procedure to be adopted will always be chosen with the best interests of the patient in mind.

The need for two nurses to be involved in the administration of medicines to children is dealt with in Chapter II.

Medicine management

Some thought should also be given in some wards and departments to the timing of medicine rounds and the number of rounds which are required. Even when a standardised system of prescribing and administration is in use, there should be room for flexibility to meet the needs of individual situations, e.g. rounds to relate with mealtimes or to coincide with the maximum number of staff available. Such flexibility must always reflect the need for effective drug therapy.

Equipment and fixtures used in the management of medicines such as medicine trolleys and storage facilities should be chosen with care so that the particular needs of the ward are satisfied. Nurse managers should always be prepared to take time to consult with practising clinical colleagues as to their requirements. Guidance from the pharmacist and supplies officer should also be sought. Policy makers must ensure that the tools of the trade, including prescribing and recording documents, are of similar design and relevant to the drug therapy used in all wards. Mechanisms are needed to ensure that there is an effective means of updating prescription charts and associated documents in such a way that the needs of a particular professional group are not overlooked. This will often require tact and diplomacy since the differing needs of doctors, nurses, and medical records officers may conflict.

As in many areas of nursing practice there is great need for operational research into many aspects of medicine management. Nurse managers have a duty to encourage their staff in this direction. Finally, the nurse managers must ensure that disciplinary procedures applicable in the event of errors in medicine administration are relevant and not seen as threatening by nurses.

Some teaching and service staff would like to see more widespread formal assessment of nurse learners in their conduct of a medicine round, as currently happens in England. While practical assessments may be somewhat artificial, a system which demands, at least at one stage, that staff learn the correct procedure, is to be encouraged. A further benefit would be that trained nursing staff and medical staff would also require to adopt high standards of practice. Whether a sufficient number of examiners could be made available for such an undertaking is debatable.

Continuing education on the subject is of course essential for all trained nursing staff along with updating of nurses returning to work after some years absence. Attendance at regular in-service lectures and seminars on medicine administration should now be compulsory.

In-service training
Considerable thought should be given to the format and content of in-service training designed to improve the overall standard of medicine management and thus to reduce errors. Rather than focus on narrow mechanistic task-orientated aspects, a much wider frame of reference is advocated. The reason for this is that the causes of errors in the administration of medicines are often complex involving the interaction of a number of factors. A study day format that has been found helpful by the authors consists of a preliminary session in which groups of nurses are asked to identify the overall aims and objectives in drug therapy coupled with a discussion of the role of the nurse in drug therapy. Groups can be asked to identify the practical problems faced by the nurse in achieving the aims and objectives and discharging the role to the full. The ideas generated by the groups are collated for discussion in plenary sessions. This material can then be used to draw up action plans designed to reduce or eliminate errors at ward level. An example of such a plan follows.

Action plan for eliminating/reducing errors in the administration of medicines

Short-term measures
Encourage by all practical means adherence to drug policy.

Pay particular attention to patient identification. Integrate verbal report on current ward drug therapy with nursing report.
Provide suitable drug information source at ward level e.g. BNF
Wherever possible increase involvement of patients in their own drug therapy.
Eliminate borrowing of medicines between wards.
Reduce interruptions during the administration of medicines.
Ensure equipment available for medicine administration is suitable in all respects.
Improve procedures for checking medicines prior to administration.

Long-term measures
Encourage the development of ward prescribing policies, reduction of ward medicine inventory. Make careful choice of new equipment e.g. medicine trolley. Establish regular in-service education for nurses on all aspects of drug therapy.
Develop ward pharmacy services.
Improve nurse staffing levels.
Establish educational programmes for medical students on procedural aspects of ward medicine management including prescribing.
Promote research into all aspects of medicine use.
Examine and if necessary improve disciplinary procedure for dealing with errors in the administration of medicines.

The final session can then be devoted to a discussion of actual drug errors both from the literature and local experience, care being taken to avoid disclosing any potentially embarrassing details. Course members can also be given an update on aspects of the hospital policy regarding prescribing and administration of medicines.

In conclusion, the question of error avoidance has to be approached in a very positive way without causing undue anxiety. The practical guidance which follows is in two parts; first, general advice which is widely applicable and second, advice which is more specific.

General advice to ensure correct administration of medicines

Patient
- *ensure correct identification of the patient*
- *take extra care at extremes of age*

With individual exceptions, the risks to infants and the very old are greater — partly because of the effects of the drugs but also because they may be unable to speak for themselves.

Prescription
- *use correct documentation* and report any inadequacies in the documentation design/layout.
- *follow the policy* and do not accept inadequate unclear instructions.
- *ask/check/ask again if not satisfied.* While wishing to trust colleagues, do not passively take the word of a senior member of staff as necessarily correct.
- *have all calculations checked*
- *report at once any suspicions* you may have that all is not in order, be it regarding the prescription, the product or the patient.

Medicine
- *ensure correct storage of medicines*, e.g. do not mix different ampoules in the same container.
- *report any apparent abnormalities*, e.g. changes in size, shape, colour of a product.
- *use the correct dosage form*, e.g. request a supply of 5 mg tablets rather than try to break a 20 mg tablet.
- *use the correct equipment*, e.g. measures, syringes.
- *be aware of drug interactions*, e.g. drug/drug; drug/food
- *avoid drug incompatibility*, e.g. when adding drugs to intravenous fluids.

Staff
- *avoid the use of abbreviations and chemical symbols*, e.g. when ordering stock.
- *be observant.* Here is the distinction between seeing and observing. The ability to take in the global view of, say, a chart or the contents of the medicine trolley as well as the details of one prescription or one product has to be acquired.
- *read the literature and keep up to date*; ask for more information if it is not provided.
- *make full use of pharmacy services* especially ward/clinical pharmacy service and drug information services.
- *encourage the development of a questioning, enquiring attitude*

Specific advice to ensure correct administration of medicines

Patient
- be especially careful when patients are mobile and where large groups of patients are sitting about at random, e.g. in day rooms.

Prescription
- be alert to sudden changes in dosage.
- if it appears that a dose has to be made up of several tablets/ampoules, check carefully that all is in order.
- pay particular attention to doses expressed in micrograms.
- take particular care with similar looking drug names.
- when two nurses are involved in the administration of medicines, read out the details of the prescription and the label so that each is aware of the other's interpretation of them. Also when administering a medicine for which a calculation has to be made, make the calculation independently before making comparison.

Medicine
- where there is no intravenous reconstitution service available and this task has to be undertaken by nursing staff, ensure correct volume of correct diluent is used. (This advice applies equally to oral dosage forms.) If in *any* doubt, ask advice from the pharmacy department.
- do not alter any labels on containers of pharmaceutical products.
- do not remove drugs from containers unless for administration.

- any drug removed from its container and not used, should be disposed of safely (see p. 152).

Staff
- when a telephoned order for medicines is unavoidable write the message down and repeat it to the caller.
- ensure adequate flow of information, e.g. to bacteriology department. Diagnostic tests may be influenced by patients' current or previous drug therapy.
- report/discuss/seek views of colleagues especially if patient safety is involved, e.g. unexplained side-effects of a drug.
- when two nurses are involved in administering medicines the more experienced nurse should check the decisions, calculations and actions of the less experienced nurse.
- whenever possible reduce the ward medicine inventory by encouraging the adoption of a ward formulary or prescribing policy.

Apart from actions taken by individuals or within a particular profession, it is essential to ensure that an active multidisciplinary Drug and Therapeutics Committee keeps under review all aspects of medicine management and issues guidance when necessary.

Conclusion

However accurate and detailed the prescribing, however efficient the pharmaceutical service, however effective the nursing management, there can be no substitute for the greatest care and attention to detail when a medicine is actually administered. Understandably the nurse who undertakes the final act feels in a very vulnerable position. This is because the administration of a medicine is so 'visible' and so final. The medicine has actually been taken by the patient or injected into the patient's tissues. At this stage any second thoughts are not capable of being translated into action (other than reporting the error or suspected error). Unlike written prescriptions, doses actually given cannot be changed. This situation should be recognised by all those who prescribe and dispense medicines and by

those who draw up policy and procedure documents. Errors in the administration of medicines are rightly regarded very seriously by nurse managers. However, it may well be that the application of rigid disciplinary procedures may not always be in the best interests of patients, since a tendency to conceal errors may develop.

Every effort must be made to ensure that the nurse who is required to administer medicines has all the skills, knowledge and support necessary to perform this vital duty safely and efficiently. Equally the nurse must adhere to the established procedures at all times. Deviations from this will, sooner or later, result in hazard, or worse, for the patient.

Unfortunately errors in the administration of medicines can never be completely eliminated. However, the development jointly by all the health professionals concerned, of safe, practicable guidelines for medicine management and adherence to these, will help to ensure that patients receive the standard of care to which they are entitled.

PATIENT COMPLIANCE

An essential component for the successful outcome of any treatment plan, drug or otherwise, is the patient's compliance with the prescriber's advice and directions. Patient compliance can be defined as 'the extent to which the patient's behaviour coincides with medical or health advice'. The term 'patient compliance' is often considered to be unsatisfactory, since it has overtones of coercion or compulsion. Alternative, less threatening terms that have been proposed include 'therapeutic alliance' and 'treatment adherence' (Blackwell, 1976). For the purposes of this discussion the term 'patient compliance' will be used because it is capable of exact definition, and given appropriate circumstances it can be measured. At no time will the term be used here with any threat, real or implied.

Nurses both in community and hospital practice are well placed to help patients comply with the medical advice and instructions they are given regarding drug treatment. Often, the nurse is the only health professional who has continuing contact with the patient over long periods. As a result, the nurse is able to gain an understanding of the patient's difficulties, to offer advice and to monitor compliance against this background.

Extent and significance of non-compliance
A very rough idea of the extent of non-compliance can be obtained when surveys are undertaken on the vast quantities of drugs collected during 'DUMP' (Disposal of unwanted medicines and pills) campaigns. Many studies have been published which have demonstrated in detail the extent of non-compliance with directions regarding drug treatment. In long-term therapy, compliance is often very poor, averaging about 50% (Evans & Spelman, 1983). With short-term therapy the position may generally be better. Studies by Donabedian & Rosenfeld (1964) and Mushlin (1972) showed that up to 75% of patients complied with their directions. Few studies relate the extent of non-compliance to the failure to achieve the desired therapeutic outcome. Nevertheless non-compliance should always be considered as a possible reason for treatment failure.

Measurement of non-compliance
Many difficulties are presented when measuring, or assessing patient compliance. The methods available vary from the basic tablet count to the use of fairly sophisticated monitoring devices (Norell, 1979), and the measurement of the drug (or metabolite) in body fluids. The methods available are listed under two headings, firstly methods that are normally available to the nurse and secondly those methods which require considerable technical back up, and are only applicable in structured investigations into patient compliance.

Methods of compliance assessment available to the nurse
1. Does the patient have the prescription dispensed?
2. General impressions of the patient's understanding of the drug regimen.
3. Tablet counts at suitable intervals.

4. Physiological markers, e.g. pulse rate in digoxin therapy.
6. Visible presence of drug or metabolites in urine or faeces e.g. rifampicin produces a reddish discolouration of the urine.

Other methods of compliance determination
1. Measurement of drug or metabolite in urine.
2. Measurement of pharmacologically inert chemical markers added to the medicine, in body fluids.
3. Medication monitors that record the withdrawal and time of withdrawal of a dose from the container.
4. Hair sampling. Some drugs can be detected by chemical analysis in the hair.

Significance of non-compliance
Does it matter that some patients fail to take their medicines as prescribed? There can be no simple answer to this question. Failure to comply may delay a patient's restoration to full health, (failure to complete a course of antibiotic therapy), or may be life-threatening (inappropriate use of a corticosteroid by an asthmatic patient). The active extent of non-compliance must also be taken into account since it may well be that for a particular regime an 80% compliance level by the patient may be adequate to achieve the desired therapeutic outcome. No general rules can be established. The whole situation must be assessed, since in many cases the patient's condition will vary and thus his need for medication will change also. Intelligent non-compliance has been described by Weintraub (1976) as occurring when patients either reduce the dose or stop taking a medicine altogether. The reasons for this behaviour may, when examined, be quite rational, such as the adjustment of a drug dose in response to the occurrence of side-effects.

Factors in non-compliance
Many factors have been identified as contributing to patient non-compliance. Haynes and Sackett (1979) cite more than 200 factors that have been studied, ranging from doctor/patient relationships to the colour and taste of the

prescribed medicine. The factors involved can be classified into three main groups; personal factors, social factors and factors related directly to the prescribed medicines. Rarely if ever, will non-compliance be due to a single identifiable factor. Often it will be attributable to a number of interacting factors.

Personal factors
Personal factors will include the patient's own beliefs as to the value or otherwise of the therapy. Ethnic aspects may be involved when the patient's beliefs in traditional remedies may conflict with mainstream Western medicine. Relationships with the health personnel involved, especially the patient's 'faith' in the prescriber will often influence the outcome. Loss of recent memory, physical disabilities and other factors often associated with the ageing process may contribute to patient non-compliance. Some psychiatric illnesses, such as schizophrenia, may also bring particular problems. Pressures of a busy life are not conducive to compliance, especially when several daily dosage intervals are involved. When the patient's understanding of the regimen is poor and the knowledge of his condition limited, poor compliance will often result.

Social factors
Social factors that may contribute to non-compliance include isolation arising from a breakdown in the family structure, deprivation and poverty. The patient who has to contend with a difficult journey to the surgery or pharmacy or who cannot afford prescription charges will probably need help and guidance, not only with the use of medicines but with the Social Security system also. Older people often have to contend with multiple deprivation, and are more vulnerable when things do go wrong with their medicine taking.

Factors directly related to medicines
Nurses should always be alert for difficulties a patient may experience in taking or using prescribed medicines. In many instances these will be practical problems, such as difficulty in using eye drops, or squeezing ointment from a tube. Problems with medicines will vary according to the presentation used e.g. large tablets and capsules may be difficult to swallow, very small tablets may be difficult for a patient with stiff fingers to pick up. Liquid medicines may have an unpleasant taste, colour or 'feel' in the mouth. Many liquid medicines that are used by older patients are formulated for children. Highly coloured, sweet, sickly flavours are generally not very acceptable to older patients, even if children find them acceptable, which often they do not. Measuring liquid medicines will be difficult for many patients, as will shaking a 500 ml glass bottle of liquid medicine which may weigh almost 1 kg. Topical preparations may be difficult to use (e.g. stiff ointments), and products that stain the patient's linen or bath may prove unacceptable. Inappropriate packaging of dispensed medicines may result in non-compliance. Child-resistant closures are difficult for many people, although the use of these has reduced accidental poisoning of children significantly. Labelling systems have been improved with the introduction of machine-printed labels for all dispensed medicines, but the small print on some labels may be impossible for some patients to read. Medicines prescribed for prophylaxis may not always be taken as prescribed because the patient does not feel the benefit directly. Unpleasant side-effects, such as headache, nausea etc. may, undoubtedly, be a cause of non-compliance.

The practical problems discussed above, although often contributing to non-compliance according to the strict definitions given, may also jeopardise the safe management of medicines by the patient e.g. child-resistant closures, once removed, may be left off, with consequent loss of security. Many patients find more unfamiliar presentations, such as suppositories and pressurised aerosols, very difficult to use properly.

The patient's response
In the face of the catalogue of difficulties described above, it is hardly surprising that many highly motivated patients, their carers, health and social workers involved develop their own 'aids to compliance'. Many different

approaches have been reported (Williams, 1979). The most common is probably the setting out of individual doses, in advance, in household containers such as egg cups, ice trays, egg boxes and the like. Sellotape has been used to stick tablets and capsules to suitable fixtures in the kitchen or living room to act as a reminder that the dose is due. Labels on the containers of dispensed medicines are often amended by the addition of lay terms such as 'water tablets', 'sleeping tablets', 'heart tablets' etc. as an aid to identification. Instructions on labels may be modified, additional labels being added often using large print or symbols to reinforce the dosage instructions. The start of a favourite TV programme may be used by a patient as a signal that a dose is due. A variety of charts, calendars etc. have also been used to assist the memory.

It would appear that many of these ingenious aids are of assistance to some patients and we should obviously not discourage this self-help approach. Equally, there can be no doubt that in some situations the 'homemade' devices will be a further source of problems which may not always be recognised by the patient. By transferring tablets from the original well-closed container, product security and stability will often be lost. If glyceryl trinitrate tablets are not stored in a well-sealed glass jar the volatile active ingredient will be lost. Some tablets absorb moisture from the atmosphere and may become unusable.

Nurses, pharmacists and doctors can learn from the patient's coping strategies, since these may emphasise inadequacies in the service provided, and give very clear pointers to the patient's difficulties.

Strategies to improve patient compliance

Before embarking on a course of action designed to improve patient compliance two main questions must be borne in mind. Firstly, does the patient really need drug therapy or is some other form of therapy more appropriate? Secondly, will improved compliance assist in the achievement of the therapeutic objective(s)? For instance, it may well be that improved compliance will result in an unacceptable level of side-effects. It is also vital to determine the real causes of non-compliance and to ensure that any strategies decided upon are within the patient's capabilities, otherwise further problems will be created for the patient.

The available strategies can be considered under three main headings.

- Labelling and packaging (presentation) of dispensed medicines (e.g. use of large print on labels).
- Provision of suitable aids to compliance (e.g. compartmentalised tablet dispenser).
- Educational, counselling approach (e.g. provision of information leaflets to patients).

In some situations a combination of strategies may be required, the patient being given a suitable aid and counselled as to the importance of the therapy. Whilst there is no sure way to identify the potential defaulter, it is essential to make every effort to identify the high-risk patient.

Presentation of dispensed medicines

Plastic, lightweight bottles with a cleft for ease of handling by an arthritic patient may be useful (Fig. 10.8.). Containers used for tablets should generally be at least the 32 ml size for ease of handling. Plastic containers are gener-

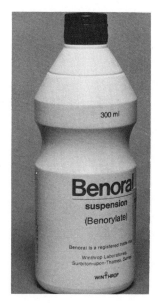

Fig. 10.8 Plastic bottle for arthritics

ally preferred by patients. Screw caps that can easily be removed have obvious advantages (Le Gallez et al, 1984) for some patients (Fig. 10.9) although there is great need to ensure that containers fitted with such closures are stored out of the reach of children.

A wide variety of labelling systems are available, all of which are designed to provide the information required for the patient in a clear unambiguous way. Ideally the label of a dispensed medicine should bear the following information.

- Full instructions about the drug and its required frequency
- Approved name of product and strength
- Name and address of dispensing pharmacist
- Date of dispensing
- Quantity dispensed
- Expiry date of product
- Lay term (e.g. water tablets)
- Warning — keep out of reach of children
- Any special storage instructions
- Any special precautions in use
- For external use only and/or other appropriate warnings

Examples of the way in which additional information, that cannot be included on a label, can be conveyed are illustrated (Fig. 10.10). Blind or partially sighted patients can be helped by using labels with specially large print and/or

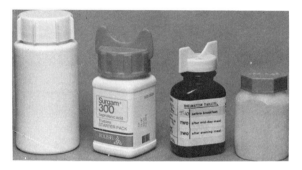

Fig. 10.9 Screw cap bottles

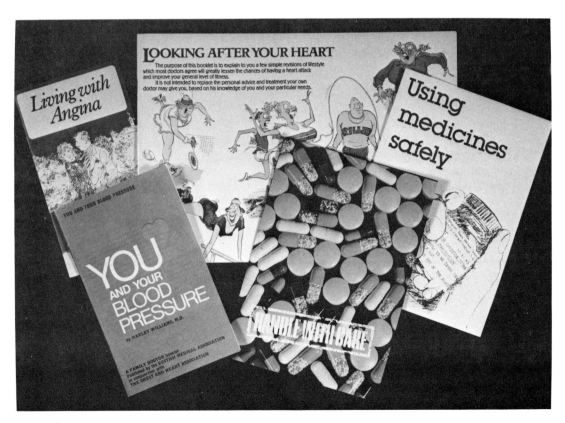

Fig. 10.10 Information leaflets

Braille (Fig. 10.11.). The needs of patients whose command of English is minimal will require attention. Labels written in their mother tongue will be required. The needs of the illiterate must be recognised and dealt with in a sympathetic way. Pictorial labels have been developed and these may prove useful in some situations. Nurses should discuss the needs of their patients with the pharmacist who will often be able to help once the problem has been defined.

Aids to compliance

A number of different aids have been developed (Williams, 1984) for both solid and liquid dosage forms.

Aids in the management of solid dosage forms

The well known 'Dosett'® tray (Fig. 10.12) has certain special features, notably the Braille markings and a detailed labelling facility on the reverse. Other compartmentalised trays of the 'Wiegand'® type (Fig. 10.13) are useful since each compartment can be labelled with the contents and any special instructions. The 'Pill Minder® (Fig. 10.14) has some degree of 'child resistance' unlike the other trays described above. Other products available include the 'Medidos'® system which has the advantage of being highly portable since each daily tray can be carried separately (Fig. 10.15).

Combination products (e.g. diuretic with potassium) may prove useful, since the number of tablets to be taken daily is reduced. Compliance packs (calender packs) are also made available for some products (e.g. oral contraceptives).

Aids in the management of liquid dosage forms

Measuring liquid medicines with the standard medicine spoon may prove difficult for many patients. Several alternative measuring devices are available, (Fig. 10.16). Blind patients may find a special measuring device helpful (Fig. 10.17).

Other aids in the management of medicines

A long-handled ointment applicator (see Fig. 8.4) has been developed for patients with physical disabilities. Occupational therapists have an important role to play in advising on the use of the various aids available.

Whilst the provision of an aid to compliance will help many patients, equally the mere provision of an aid without other supportive action is unlikely to achieve anything.

Educational and counselling approaches

Patient information

A study undertaken by the Office of Health Economics in 1980 showed that 50% of patients wanted more information about their prescribed medicines. Of this group, information on side-effects, both short- and long-term, composition of medicines and actions was wanted. Along with their professional colleagues nurses can play a key role in ensuring that patients have sufficient knowledge to enable them to manage their prescribed medicines safely and effectively and thus achieve therapeutic benefit. Herxheimer (1976) has outlined the knowledge

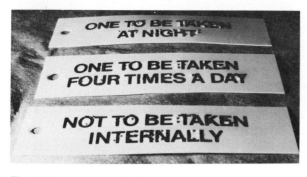

Fig. 10.11 Large print Braille labels

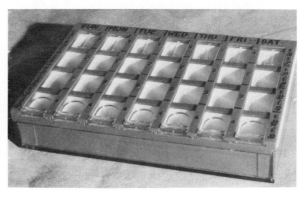

Fig. 10.12 Dosett® tray

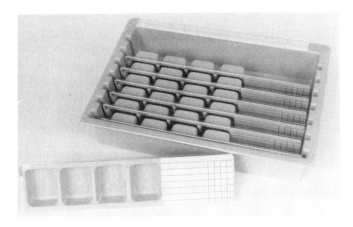

Fig. 10.13 Wiegand® tray

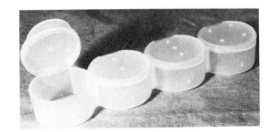

Fig. 10.14 Pill minder®

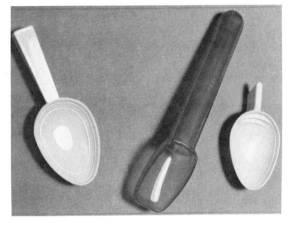

Fig. 10.16 Alternative measuring devices

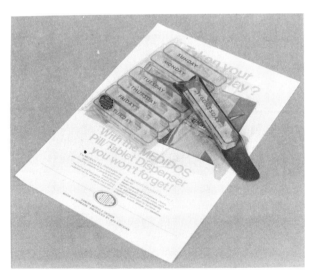

Fig. 10.15 Medidos® system

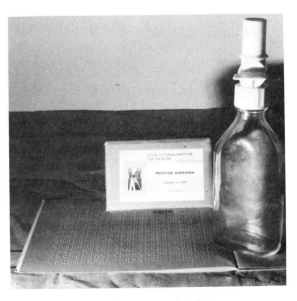

Fig. 10.17 Medicine dispenser for the blind

needed by patients, or by those responsible for their day-to-day care, in terms of the following questions to the prescriber.

- What for and how?
- How important?
- Any side-effects?
- How long for?

In turn these basic questions can be broken down further.

What for and how?
- What kind of tablets are they and in what way do you expect them to help?
- How should I take them? How many and how often?
- Will I be able to tell whether they are working?
- How do I keep them?

How important?
- How important is it for me to take these tablets?
- What is likely to happen if I do not take them?

Any side-effects?
- Do the tablets have any other effects that I should look out for?
- Do they ever cause any trouble?
- Is it alright to drive when I am taking them?
- Are they alright with other medicines I may need?
- Will alcohol interfere with them?
- What should be done if someone takes too many?

How long for?
- How long will I need to continue with these tablets?
- What should be done with any left over?
- When will I need to see you again?
- What will you want to know at that time?

In some situations, such as terminal care, it will not be appropriate to give the patient all the information listed above, but the list of questions does give much useful guidance to nurses, pharmacists and prescribers.

Pre-discharge training in self-administration of medicines

Many patients are discharged home with a complex drug regime to cope with. Whilst in hospital the patient has been given medicines at regular intervals by nurses, often regrettably with little real involvement of the patient, other than swallowing the dose. At a suitable time prior to discharge it may be helpful to involve the patient much more fully by setting up a self-administration programme with the aims of securing compliance following discharge home.

The conventional medicine administration systems used in many hospitals are, of course, highly structured and involve the patient in a passive role only. Possible methods of achieving more participation by the in-patient in medicine taking and management are briefly described below together with a discussion of the advantages and disadvantages of the various approaches. In each situation it is obviously essential to select the patients carefully and ensure that hospital policies are clearly laid down and understood. Legal and procedural difficulties can conflict with the needs of patients, but with full consultation and co-operation between disciplines these can be minimised.

Self administration systems

Individual patient dispensing system using a medicine trolley or individual patients' medicine cupboards

Medicines are dispensed (for a suitable period prior to discharge) for each patient on an individual basis. A system of labelling is used which reflects the patients' needs (e.g. use of lay terms, 'water tablets' etc.) and also normal professional requirements. The medicines are kept at ward level in an individual compartment within the ward medicine trolley. On the normal ward medicine rounds the patient is encouraged to ask for his medicines using terminology that the patient understands. The patient should be asked to remove the dose from the container, which gives the opportunity to assess if the patient can read and understand the label, open the container and measure the dose. The recording of the administration of the dose is undertaken by the nurse conducting the medicine round. (A suitable record is made on the recording sheet that medicines are to be self administered).

A similar system can be employed using an individual patient's medicine cupboard sited suitably in the ward. The ambulant patient is given the key to his cupboard at the appropriate time, or is encouraged to ask for it, and the self-administration is supervised to a limited extent, depending on the patient's needs. Using these systems a step-by-step approach can be adopted, with levels of supervision being reduced over a period of time as appropriate. With these systems there is little, if any, conflict with normally accepted hospital practices. Counselling on the more general aspects of the use of prescribed medicines prior to discharge can be undertaken in conjunction with this approach.

Setting out of individual dose in advance of administration

Individual doses are set out in advance of self-administration in four-compartment plastic trays (Wiegand® trays) which are suitably labelled. Patients are encouraged to ask for their medication at the appropriate time of day. This system is not ideal, since there is no opportunity to evaluate the patient's ability to manage medicines dispensed in the traditional manner. The setting out of doses in advance of administration is, to many authorities, unacceptable. By setting out only single doses the objections to this approach are reduced.

Inpatients having custody of their own prescribed medicines

Although this system has been used in some centres the risks and possible legal complications make it unsuitable for use in most hospital settings. However in certain situations (e.g. where patients have single rooms), there are few valid objections to the use of this approach. Adequate supervision is of course required.

The use of compliance aids

When a patient has particular difficulties using traditionally dispensed medicines it may be worthwhile considering the use of a Dosett, Medidos, or Wiegand 7 day tray. If such aids

are used it will be necessary to ensure security of the compliance aid in the ward. These containers would normally be filled in Pharmacy. The additional work load created by this approach is a factor that would limit the application of this system.

Both from an examination of published literature and general consideration of the problem, there would appear to be no entirely satisfactory procedure that can be used to enable self-administration of medicines to be carried out by in-patients. Further investigation of this matter is desirable, but in the meantime the methods described above can be advocated.

Patient information leaflets

A wide range of patient information leaflets is available (Sloan, 1984) which may be used to supplement and reinforce the counselling of patients. These range from general information on a particular condition and associated drug therapy to information packages designed to meet the needs of an individual patient (Palmer, 1979). A study by George et al, (1983) found that patients who received a leaflet were more likely to be completely satisfied with the treatment and with the information they had been given. It is vitally important that the information given to patients by different health workers is complementary and does not give rise to confusion.

Education packages

Nurses working in the community can play a wider educational role by presenting talks to organised groups in the community on aspects of the safe use of medicines. The topics covered by the talks would naturally be selected in line with the interests and needs of the group. In some situations however, a structured presentation in the form of a tape-slide or video package may be appropriate. As an example of this approach, a tape-slide package has been developed for groups interested in the care of older people. (Graves Organisation, 1984). An outline of the content is as follows:

- demographic aspects
- extent of use of medicines by older people

- physiology of the ageing process
- factors that cause older people to have difficulty managing their medicines.
- practical help in medicine management available to older people.

The presentation can be supported by a demonstration of aids to compliance. Leaflets giving general guidance on the safe use of medicines are made available to reinforce the message. It is of course difficult to measure the value of this approach, but at the very least it does provide the presenter with a valuable opportunity to gain an insight into the problems relating to medicines that many people may have, either as patients or carers.

Summary

Patient non-compliance has been widely described in the literature during the past 20 years. Few of the studies reported have attempted to correlate non-compliance with therapeutic outcome, but in many situations, patient non-compliance and inadequate management of medicines are serious problems. Patient non-compliance is not confined to patients in the community. It may occur in hospital in-patients also.

Nurses have an important and expanding role in identifying patient non-compliance, and in contributing to the achievement of patient compliance. Strategies to improve patient compliance are available and should be used selectively with the overall aim of improving therapeutic outcome.

REFERENCES

Blackwell B 1976 Treatment adherence. British Journal of Psychiatry 129: 513–531
Donabedian A, Rosenfeld L S 1984 Follow-up study of chronically ill patients discharged from hospital. Journal of Chronic Disorders 14: 847–862
Evans L, Spelman M 1983 The problem of non-compliance with drug therapy. Drugs 25: 63–76
Falck K, et al 1979 Mutagenicity in urine of nurses handling cytostatic drugs. Lancet 1: 1250–1

George C F, Nicholas J A, Waters W E 1983 Prescription information leaflets; a pilot study in general practices. British Medical Journal 287: 1193–1196
Graves Organisation 1984 A tape slide presentation. Older people and their medicines.
Haynes R B 1979 In: Haynes R B, Taylor D W, Sackett D L (eds.) Compliance in health care. John Hopkins University Press, Baltimore p 1–7
Herxheimer A 1976 Sharing the responsibility for treatment. Lancet 2:1294
Le Gallez P, Bird H A, Wright V et al 1984 Comparison of 12 different containers for dispensing anti-inflammatory drugs. British Medical Journal 288: 699–701
Ley P 1981 Professional non-compliance. A neglected problem. British Journal of Clinical Psychology 20: 151–154
MacPherson W, Andrew M, Brown M, Laing J 1983 Survey of drug administration by learners. Unpublished
Norell S E 1979 Improving medication compliance a randomised clinical trial. British Medical Journal 2: 1031–1033
Mushlin A I 1972 A study of physicians' ability to predict patient compliance. Master's thesis. John Hopkins University, Baltimore
Palmer B 1979 Patient education and drug therapy. Pharmaceutical Journal (1.12.79): 562–566
Sloan P J M 1984 Survey of patient information booklets. British Medical Journal 288: 915–919
Sontaniemi E A et al 1983 Liver damage in nurses handling cytostatic agents. Acta Medica Scandinavica 214: 181–9.
Weintraub M 1976 Intelligent and capricious non-compliance. In: Lasagna (ed.) Compliance p. 39 Futura, Mt. Kisco N.Y.
Williams A 1979 The role of the pharmacist in improving compliance in the elderly patient. Proceedings of the Guild 6: 1–22
Williams A 1984 Medicine Management. Nursing Mirror 159 Community Forum ii.

FURTHER READING

Aronson J K 1983 Adverse drug interactions. Prescribers' Journal. Vol. 23. (June) 3: 66–76
Clark-Mahoney J P 1984 Self-medication program improves compliance. Nursing 84. December p. 41.
Gatford J D 1982 Nursing calculations. Churchill Livingstone, Melbourne
Pirie S, Sullivan P 1984 Mathematics in the ward. Stanley Thornes, Cheltenham.
Scholes M E, Wilson J L, Macrae S 1982 Handbook of nursing procedures. Blackwell, Oxford.
The Royal Marsden Hospital 1984 Manual of clinical nursing policies and procedures. Harper and Row, London

11 OTHER ASPECTS OF DRUG THERAPY

DRUGS IN PREGNANCY

The thalidomide tragedy in the 1960s focussed attention on the great problems which can arise when drugs are used during pregnancy. Thalidomide, an effective sedative-hypnotic, caused horrific physical and internal organ defects in many babies whose mothers had been taking this drug in early pregnancy. Although some pharmaceutical companies were at this time testing new drugs for teratogenicity (causing congenital malformation), such tests were not standard procedures since the need for them had not been fully appreciated. The thalidomide tragedy caused widespread concern about possible fetal damage from other drugs taken by pregnant women. As a result, it was realised that the standards for predicting and preventing fetal damage were inadequate and required to be revised. By using laboratory animals it was shown that the teratogenic potential of thalidomide could have been discovered but it was also shown that there is great variation in the ways different species react to drugs.

During the first 2 weeks of human gestation the fertilised ovum already is sensitive to drugs and after this, drugs may produce congenital malformations in the fetus. The time of greatest risk is between the 3rd and the 11th week of pregnancy when differentiation of organs occurs. The development of the embryo is very rapid with continuous changes resulting from cell division, cell migration and cell differentiation. Each organ and each system undergoes a critical stage of differentiation at a precise period of prenatal development, e.g. the heart from day 20 to day 40 and limbs from day 24 to day 46. It is during this time that specific gross malformations can be produced by particular drugs.

During the second and third trimesters of pregnancy, complete closure of the palate occurs in the fetus at 8 weeks, differentiation of the external genitalia between the 4th and 5th month and further differentiation of the nervous system from the fourth month until after birth. Drugs administered during these trimesters may interfere with the normal development of the genitalia and nervous system.

As a general principle, drugs should not be administered to a woman during pregnancy unless the potential benefit to the mother outweighs the risk to the fetus. However, serious illness can occur during pregnancy and complications of pregnancy often need to be treated with drugs so that administration cannot always be avoided. The mother may suffer from a chronic condition which requires continuous medication. For example, patients with hypothyroidism require regular doses of thyroxine. Although the placenta is relatively impermeable to thyroxine (MacGillivray, 1975) adequate replacement in hypothyroid patients is extremely important for it has been shown that children of women who have inadequate replacement therapy, scored lower in tests of mental and fine motor development when compared to the offspring of women with adequate replacement therapy (Man et al, 1971)

The transfer of drugs across the placenta is accomplished in a similar manner to the distribution of drugs in body organs and tissues. Most drugs cross the placenta by simple diffusion from an area of high concentration to an area of low concentration. Biochemical and physiological changes occur in women during pregnancy and therefore, drug distribution, metabolism and excretion may be altered. Metabolism of drugs in the maternal liver is reduced during pregnancy and an increase in plasma volume in conjunction with a reduction in albumin content may increase the amount of free drug in the plasma. Since the fetus is in equilibrium with the maternal circulation, drugs and metabolites which readily cross the placenta and enter the fetal circulation, will also be in equilibrium and will then pass back into the mother's circulation when cleared by the fetus.

Care must be taken when drugs are administered shortly before term or during labour, since these may not have been cleared from the fetus before birth. A drug can no longer pass from the fetal to the maternal circulation after the umbilical cord has been clamped, and this may cause adverse effects on the neonate after delivery due to problems of metabolism and excretion. If treatment is required, drugs preferred are those which have been extensively used in pregnancy and appear to be safe. The smallest effective dose should be used. New or untried drugs should be avoided when an alternative with a known 'safe' history is available.

Since the thalidomide tragedy, drugs have been tested in animal studies for teratogenic effects and data collected when adverse effects occurred. Information on the possible or confirmed teratogenic effect of many drugs is now available from drug information centres and drug companies.

Some drugs are used which are known to be teratogenic e.g. isotretinoin, used for systemic treatment of severe acne, causes serious central nervous system malformations in the fetus. It is *essential* to ensure that the patient is not pregnant at the time of starting treatment and effective contraception must be carried out both during treatment and for at least four weeks after stopping treatment to allow drug clearance from the body to take place. Similarly, where etretinate is prescribed for treatment of severe psoriasis, effective contraception must be continued for one year after stopping treatment due to this drug's long half-life. Patients are advised not to donate blood during this period since the drug could be transferred to someone who is pregnant. Alkylating drugs and methotrexate also carry a high risk of teratogenicity.

Antimicrobial drugs are frequently used in pregnancy for the treatment of maternal infection. The penicillins are probably the safest antibiotics for use in pregnancy. Tetracyclines are irreversibly incorporated into fetal teeth resulting in discolouration and a tendency to develop dental caries. Although the benefits of anti-epileptics to the mother may outweigh the risk to the fetus, there is an increased incidence of congenital malformation in infants born to mothers receiving anti-epileptic drugs (Hill & Tennyson, 1982). There is no evidence that general anaesthetics are harmful to the fetus provided that maternal hypotension and respiratory depression are avoided.

Although a great deal of work is now being done on the adverse effects of drugs administered during pregnancy, the effects of many drugs on the fetus have yet to be determined. Much of the work has been done on animals which may react differently to humans. In addition, studies conducted in humans are usually retrospective and it is difficult to attribute adverse effects on the fetus to a particular drug.

Drug treatment should be avoided whenever possible during pregnancy especially during the first trimester and prior to delivery. Care should also be taken in administering drugs to women of childbearing age, as major harmful effects of drugs on the fetus will be produced very early in pregnancy, possibly before the woman realises she is pregnant.

DRUG THERAPY IN THE YOUNG

All children, and particularly neonates, differ from adults in their response to drugs. The immaturity of organs involved in drug metabolism and excretion may alter not only the pharmacokinetics but also the toxicity of many drugs. Great variability exists in absorption, protein binding, distribution, metabolism and excretion according to age and weight and important differences have been observed in premature neonates, full-term babies and older children. These differences become more complex where congenital anomalies or disease states exist.

Absorption of drugs

Gastrointestinal tract
The absorption of drugs from the gastrointestinal tract is influenced by the pH of the stomach contents and also by gastric emptying

time. The pH of the stomach at birth is 6–8 but falls to a pH of 1–3 in the first 24 hours. (In premature neonates this fall does not occur because the acid-secreting mechanism has not fully developed). The pH then returns to between 6 and 8 for 10–15 days since no more acid is secreted during this period. This relatively neutral pH of the stomach contents may result in higher blood levels of drugs such as penicillin due to reduced chemical decomposition resulting in increased availability for absorption. The adult value of gastric pH (approximately 3) is gradually reached between 2 and 3 years of age.

Gastric emptying time may be as long as 6–8 hours in neonates, reaching adult values at 6–8 months. This prolonged emptying time may have an important influence on the absorption rate of orally-administered drugs.

Intramuscular injection
The absorption rate of drugs following intramuscular injection is influenced by the changes in muscle blood flow which occur in the first days of life and by vasoconstriction resulting from temperature change or circulatory insufficiency.

Skin
Percutaneous absorption is greatly increased in neonates and young infants who have thin, well-hydrated skin. This increased permeability has led to toxic effects associated with the use of hexachlorophane soaps and powders (Tyrala, 1977) and salicylic acid ointments. The dangers of absorption of corticosteroids from topical preparations are also widely recognised.

Protein binding of drugs
Neonates have reduced plasma protein binding of various drugs. This is because of a reduced plasma protein concentration and neonatal albumin having a lower binding capacity for drugs than that of adults. These factors may vary in their effects and may lead to drug toxicity. On the other hand, the dose of digoxin required in infants is high compared to adults. An average daily maintenance dose for adults is 3–5 μg/kg body weight whereas in infants it is 10–25 μg/kg. This higher dose is required

because the digoxin has a lower binding affinity for digoxin receptors in the myocardium of neonates (Kearin, 1980). In addition to reduced plasma protein binding, another factor affecting drug distribution is the total body water in neonates which is 70%, compared to the adult value of 55%.

Hepatic metabolism of drugs

Drug metabolism by the liver may occur in a number of ways e.g. by acetylation, by conjugation. In the newborn the necessary enzyme systems are developed to varying extents. Conjugation involving glucuronidation is deficient in some newborn infants. (Stern et al, 1970) A number of drugs including chloramphenicol are metabolised in this way. Where chloramphenicol is administered in 'normal' doses based on weight, serious toxicity can occur which may result in death ('grey baby' syndrome). This deficiency in metabolism disappears in the first or second weeks of life.

Excretion of drugs

At birth, all aspects of renal function are diminished but become comparable to that in adults between six months and a year. (Morselli, 1976) Full-term babies have a reduced glomerular filtration rate compared to adults. Compounds which are not extensively metabolised and depend on renal function for excretion are eliminated more slowly in neonates. The maintenance dose must be adjusted depending on the child's kidney function, increasing as the kidney function develops. On the other hand, drugs such as diuretics which depend on the glomerular filtration to produce a therapeutic effect will require a higher dose at birth when the creatinine clearance is approximately 20 ml/min, but at age one month, when the clearance rate is 60 ml/min, the dose would be reduced accordingly.

Calculating doses

Many new drugs become available after having been tested predominantly in adults so there is little or no information about paediatric dosing. Various methods are used to calculate the dose based on body surface area and body weight.

Body surface area
Drug doses for children can be calculated from adult doses according to the formula.

$$\frac{\text{Surface area of child (in metres}^2) \times 100}{1.76 \text{ m}^2}$$
$$= \% \text{ adult dose}$$

where 1.76m^2 is the surface area of an average adult male weighing 70 kg. Percentage tables are available from the literature. The dose of paracetamol for adults is 500–1000 mg. What is the dose for an 18 month old infant weighing 11 kg? According to tables in the literature, the surface area of an infant weighing 11 kg is 0.53 m^2. Utilising the formula this equates to 30% of the adult dose.

i.e. $\dfrac{30}{100} \times 500 \text{ mg} = 150 \text{ mg}$

and $\dfrac{30}{100} \times 1000 \text{ mg} = 300 \text{ mg}$

∴ the dose range is 150–300 mg

Dosage calculation based on body surface area is generally regarded as the most satisfactory method because factors such as metabolic rate and glomerular filtration rate are more closely related to body surface area than to body weight or age. Paediatric doses calculated from adult doses on a surface area basis are higher than those calculated on a weight basis because of a large surface area per unit weight in infants and young children. Care must therefore be taken when the drug is known to have a low therapeutic index (e.g. amino glycosides) or is poorly tolerated (e.g. narcotics, atropine).

Body weight
Drug doses for children can be calculated from adult doses according to the formula:

$$\text{child's dose (in mg/kg)} = \frac{\text{adult dose in mg}}{70 \text{ kg}}$$

where 70 kg is the weight of an average adult male. The dose of paracetamol can therefore be calculated.

$\dfrac{500}{70}$ is approximately equal to 7 mg/kg

$\dfrac{1000}{70}$ is approximately equal to 14 mg/kg

The range is therefore 7–14 mg/kg of body weight.

A child weighing 11 kg would require 77–154 mg.

These doses are approximately half those estimated by surface area methods. The correct interpretation is that the smaller mg/kg dose is meant for older infants and children while the larger mg/kg dose is for smaller infants since small infants have a relatively larger surface area in relation to their weight. Doses based on body weight tend to produce lower and therefore safer doses in infancy, particularly where poorly tolerated drugs are involved. However, where a drug is known to have a high therapeutic index (e.g. penicillins, cephalosporins) it is better to use the surface area method since these give approximately twice the dose calculated by body weight. It is important not to underdose infants with antibiotics.

Modification of dose. An obese child should be given only three-quarters of the dose estimated for his weight since body fat plays virtually no part in metabolism. As in adult therapy, these dosages must be modified where renal or hepatic disease is present.

The administration of medicines to children

Although the same principles and procedures apply as when administering a medicine to an adult, certain special factors must be recognised in paediatric practice and appropriate action taken. The precise nature of the problem and action taken will depend on whether the patient is in hospital or at home. (see list below) Nurses in hospital practice will recognise the importance of ensuring that the parent (or guardian), and where appropriate the child, has all the necessary information to enable the prescribed medicines to be used safely and effectively when discharged home.

Factors	*Action*
Required dose may be contained in small volumes.	Use suitable measure, e.g. oral syringe or if parenteral therapy use tuberculin syringe. Special paediatric strength ampoules should be made available, especially digoxin.
Required dose may not be available from existing ward 'stock'	Calculation may be required, or better, obtain specially dispensed formulation from the pharmacy.
Suitable presentation may not be routinely available.	Obtain the required presentation from the pharmacy, dispensed for the special needs of the patient if necessary, e.g. sugar-free preparations may be required for diabetic children.
Patient may reject medicine due to unpalatability.	Consult pharmacist to obtain, (if possible), an alternative product/presentation. Anderson (1977) describes the use of medicated lollipops containing local anaesthetics.
A dose or part of a dose may be rejected.	Involve third party to ensure dose is actually consumed.
Consequences of drug error may be very serious.	Involve a second nurse or doctor in checking, especially if a calculation is involved. This is even more important in therapy for neonates.
Parental involvement	Ensure parent or guardian has all the necessary information on the use of the medicines, especially where complex regimens are prescribed. This will be especially important where conditions such as asthma are treated with corticosteroids. Well presented written information may be

	helpful to support counselling.
School time medicines	If practicable the doctor will prescribe a twice daily dosage. Ensure that if medicines have to be taken at school the arrangements are safe and clearly understood by all involved.
Liquid medicines	Since liquid medicines are often prescribed for children, ensure that measuring technique is accurate and that the measure(s) available are suitable. Liquid medicines (especially suspensions) must be well shaken before use. The addition of a 'lay' term on the label, describing the purpose of the medicine will often be helpful to parents. Bottles of liquid medicines should be wiped clean after use.
Syrups	Refrigerated storage is generally required for antibiotic syrups. Regular use of syrups may be a contributory factor in dental caries. Guidance may need to be given on dental hygiene. Some sugar-free preparations are available. Expiry dates must be observed.
Safety	The use of child-resistant closures is an obvious requirement, as is the safe storage of all medicines in the home. Unused medicines must be safely disposed of. Flushing away or return to the pharmacy are normally advocated.
Complex regimes, long term therapy.	Suitable warnings should be given if prescribed drugs are likely to interfere with normal healthy activities, e.g. cycling. It is worthwhile to involve a clinical pharmacist as part of a multidisciplinary team so that problems relating to formulation, presentation and compliance (amongst others) can be identified and action taken.
Need for compliance	Consideration should be given to the need for a compliance aid. Charts indicating dosage intervals may be useful. Compliance packs may be of value for short periods away from home. Where these are not available from the manufacturer the pharmacist may be able to provide these.
Method of administration	The addition of medicine to an infant feed is not recommended since rejection of part of the feed will result in underdosing.
Lack of patient co-operation	Efforts need to be made to secure the patient's co-operation, which may, in part, be achieved by diversional tactics. Positioning the patient suitably, and helping the patient to maintain

that position are also important. On completion of the procedure the patient is made safe and comfortable, reassurance being given if necessary.

DRUGS IN BREAST MILK

Breast milk is the only food the infant requires for the first 4–6 months of life. There are many benefits to be gained from breast feeding. The composition of human milk is tailored to organ development and growth and some protection against infection is obtained. Compared with cow's milk there is less likelihood of food allergy and it is more digestible. The advantages for the nursing mother, in addition to maternal bonding, are a lower cost than substitute products and convenience. This latter point is appreciated by the father who is not awakened from his slumbers in order to prepare the next feed for his demanding offspring. In 1975 only 24% of mothers were breast feeding 6 weeks after the baby's birth but by 1980 this figure had risen to 42% (Department of Health survey, 1982).

When drugs are administered to nursing mothers there may be a number of adverse effects. The contact of the baby's sucking serves to keep prolactin levels high (Nichols & Nichols, 1979) and may delay subsequent pregnancy. Prolactin secretion can be altered by drugs. It is decreased by levadopa and bromocriptine and increased by phenothiazines, methyl dopa and theopylline (Kulski et al, 1978; Vorherr, 1974a, b). The production of milk can be affected by diuretics. Bendrofluazide has been shown to stop lactation (Healy, 1961). Spironolactone however can be used safely.

Although most drugs are excreted to some extent in breast milk, the significance of their effects depends on the amount excreted in the milk. The newborn metabolise and excrete drugs very inefficiently. Pre-term infants are at greater risk than others but the risk decreases as renal and hepatic functions mature. Since infants have poorly developed renal and hepatic functions, they may be particularly sensitive to the accumulation of drugs. Where possible, drugs should be avoided during breast feeding and mothers should be warned of the possible dangers of self-medication.

Because of their potential toxicity, a number of drugs are absolutely contraindicated while the mother is breast feeding. These include antithyroid drugs, radioactive isotopes, lithium, chloramphenicol, ergot alkaloids, iodides and most anticancer drugs (Abramowicz, 1979; Hervada et al, 1978) If some form of drug treatment is essential, then alternatives to these must be used or breast feeding must be stopped. A number of other drugs are to be avoided or used with caution, e.g. atropine may cause intoxication in sensitive infants, phenindione may cause haemorrhage and calciferol in high doses may cause hypercalcaemia in the infant.

If drugs are excreted in milk in relatively low concentrations (e.g. penicillins), the advantages of breast feeding probably outweigh the marginal risks involved. Many drugs known to be excreted in breast milk do not appear to produce adverse effects in the infant (e.g. cephalosporins).

Generally, the mother should breast feed prior to taking medication. When a nursing mother takes a drug which is potentially hazardous to the infant, breast feeding may be temporarily discontinued where a single dose or short course is involved. Attention should be paid to the half-life of the drug. In this situation breast milk should be expressed regularly to maintain lactation, and then discarded.

When drugs are prescribed for a nursing mother, a number of principles are adhered to by the doctor and the nurse should be aware of them.

1. Never prescribe a drug unless it is essential.
2. Use the safest drug where alternatives are available.
3. Use the lowest effective dose for the shortest possible time.
4. If there is no alternative to drug therapy and the principles above are adhered to,

adverse effects on the baby should not occur. The mother may need reassurance and general guidance so that she is alert for any recognisable effects on the baby.

REFERENCES/FURTHER READING*

Abramowicz M 1979 Update, drugs in breast milk. Medical Letter 21: 21–24

Anderson S 1977 Special formulations used in children's hospitals in the United Kingdom. Proceedings of the Guild of Hospital Pharmacists 3: 68–82

DHSS Survey 1982 Breast feeding, HMSO, London

*Glasper A, Oliver R W 1984 A simple guide to infant drug calculations. Nursing Add-on Journal of Clinical Nursing. 2(22): 649–650

Healy M 1961 Suppressing lactation with oral diuretics. Lancet 1: 1353–1354

Hervada A R, Feit E, Sagraves R 1978 Drugs in breast milk. Perinatal Care 2: 19–25

Hill R M, Tennyson L M 1982 Significant anomalies in the antiepileptic drug (AED) syndrome. In: Janz, Dam, Richens et al (eds) Epilepsy, pregnancy and the child. Raven Press, New York, p 309

Kearin M 1980 Digoxin receptors in neonates. An explanation of less sensitivity to digoxin than in adults. Clinical Pharmacology and Therapeutics 28:346

Kulski J K, Hartmann P E, Martin J D, Smith M 1978 Effects of bromocriptine mesylate on the composition of mammary secretion in non-breast feeding women. Obstetrics and Gynaecology 52: 38–42

MacGillivray M H 1975 Thyroid disfunction in the neonatal period. Clinical Perinatology 2 15

Man E B, Holden R H, Jones W S 1971 Thyroid function in human pregnancy. VII. Development and retardation of 4-year-old progeny of euthyroid and hypothyroid women. American Journal of Obstetrics andd Gynaecology 109:12

Morselli P L 1976 Clinical pharmacokinetics in neonates. Clinical Pharmacokinetics 1:81

Nichols B L, Nichols V N 1979 The biologic basis of lactation. Comprehensive Therapy 4: 63–70

*Sallis J F 1985 Improving adherence to paediatric therapeutic regimens. Paediatric Nursing March/April: 118–120, & 148

Stern L, Khanna N N, Levy G, Yaffe S 1970 Effects of phenobarbital on hyperbilirubinaemia and glucuronide formation in newborns. American Journal of Diseases of Children 120:20

Tyrala F F 1977 Clinical pharmacology of hexachlorophane in newborn infants. Journal of Paediatrics 91:481

Vorherr H 1974a The breast morphology, physiology and lactation Academic Press, New York

Vorherr H, 1974b Drug excretion in breast milk. Postgraduate Medicine, 56: 97–104

DRUG THERAPY IN OLDER PEOPLE

The fact that we live in an ageing society will be well recognised by most practising nurses. In the community, nurses spend almost half their time caring for patients over 85 years of age. Patients over the age of 65 years occupy 56% of all non-psychiatric beds in our hospitals. Departments of geriatric medicine of course account for the majority of these patients, but as examples, up to 50% of general medical beds and up to 80% of general practitioner beds are occupied by patients over pensionable age. The proportion of older people in the community has risen during this century from around 7% in 1901 to around 16% in 1971. It must also be remembered that the population of older people is itself ageing. A 34% increase in the number of people over the age of 85 years is projected for the next 25 years. Clearly this represents a major challenge for the caring professions. Although we must avoid negative stereotypes, the fact is that with advancing years illness becomes more prevalent and, with this, the need for drug treatment increases. Older people are not a homogeneous group, and their needs differ. There will, of course, be common threads but the older patient should be given consideration as an individual with hopes and expectations just like patients in other age groups. Most older people (95%) live in private households, the remainder being cared for in institutions, 3.5% being in hospital care and 1.5% in residential care. Later in this chapter detailed aspects of the management of medicines in the community hospitals, day hospitals and residential care settings will be discussed.

Physiology of the ageing process

It is important to distinguish between the ageing process and disease states, although there is a close relationship between the two. The physiology of the ageing process that impinges most directly on drug therapy involves loss of body water, a gain in total body fat, reduced ability to metabolise drugs, and, most important of all, diminished renal function. These and other factors are discussed below, in the context of geriatric clinical pharmacology.

Other changes associated with the ageing process that may have a direct bearing on the management of medicines by the older person (and other aspects of daily living), include loss of short-term memory, poor vision, hearing loss, reduced physical dexterity and strength of grip. Factors that may predispose to drug adverse effects include impairment of body temperature control, impairment of blood pressure maintenance on change of position and an older person's reduced ability to respond to physiological changes that may be caused by administration of a drug.

Geriatric clinical pharmacology

The factors affecting the absorption, distribution, metabolism and excretion of drugs have been described in Chapter 7. Physiological changes that accompany the ageing process will, in some instances, have a profound effect on the way in which drugs are handled in the body.

Absorption of drug

Although this aspect has not been extensively studied, the available data suggest that the ageing process is not accompanied by major changes in the rate at which drugs are absorbed.

Distribution of drug

With the loss of lean body mass and body water that accompanies the ageing process there is also a gain in total body fat. It can therefore be expected that for a given dose, higher blood levels will result in an elderly person than a younger person. Ageing is accompanied by a lower plasma albumin level and as a result there is less plasma protein to bind with the drug. More free drug is therefore available for diffusion to sites of action in the body. This, like other aspects discussed here, is a very complex matter but in general the impact of the ageing process on drug distribution will tend to increase the levels of drug in the tissues, although this may not always be accompanied by an increase in pharmacological effect.

Metabolism of drug

Drug metabolism is one of the major routes of elimination of drug from the body. Hepatic metabolism of some drugs would appear to be altered as a consequence of the ageing process which results in a reduction of liver bloodflow, and reduction in liver mass. General rules cannot be formulated, but for some drugs it would appear that decreased hepatic metabolism does result in a longer half-life of the drug.

Renal excretion of drug

Diminished renal function is associated with the ageing process, and the extent of the loss of function can be measured by the creatinine clearance test. Also, as with other aspects of ageing, there will be considerable variation in loss of function from individual to individual. Whereas the effect on drug action of reduced hepatic metabolism is very difficult to predict, the effect of reduced renal excretion is more readily determined. Drugs whose renal excretion are age-related include digoxin, and tetracycline. From this discussion it follows that doses of drugs that are excreted in the urine should be adjusted where there is renal impairment. Patients over 75 years will generally be more at risk than those younger.

Physiological response

There is some evidence that suggests that older people are more sensitive to certain drugs such as benzodiazepines and potent analgesics than younger people.

Extent of prescribing for older people

The presence of multiple disease states in older people is well known. Wilson et al (1962) found that out of 200 admissions to a geriatric unit 78% of patients had at least four major diseases, and 13% had eight or more. This together with the effects of the ageing process itself often results in multiple drug therapy being prescribed. Das (1977) studied the number of medicines being taken by a group of 114 older patients and found that 43% of the group were taking five or more different medicines. Scott et al (1982) examined the prescriptions for 353 hospital in-patients of ages ranging from 60 to 99 years. The mean number of drugs prescribed was 3 (range 0–11). Sedatives and analgesics were the drugs most commonly prescribed and 18.5% received potassium supplements. Gosney (1984) found that elderly patients admitted to general medical and geriatric wards of a teaching hospital were receiving, on average 2.14 drugs on admission, 5.48 during inpatient stay and 3.47 on discharge.

The 1985/6 Data Sheet Compendium includes specific advice on prescribing for the older patient, covering doses, dosage intervals and likely reactions.

Some problems of drug therapy in the elderly

The central theme here is that older people are more vulnerable to the adverse effects of drugs than younger people. It is vitally important to ensure the older person is given all the necessary help and support so that any necessary drug therapy can be safely and effectively managed. The presence of multiple disease states often results in multiple drug therapy. Problems of non-compliance in groups of older patients have been reported. Williamson (1978) found that drug-related problems contributed to the need for hospitalisation in almost 10% of admissions of older people to geriatric units. The isolation, deprivation, and poverty that some older people have to endure mean that compliance with drug therapy may well not have a high priority in the mind of the older person. In Chapter 10 the reasons for patient non-compliance and approaches to improving patient compliance are discussed. Many of the strategies designed to improve compliance have relevance to the older patient.

Table 11.1 indicates possible side-effects when some drugs commonly prescribed for older people are administered.

Drug interactions (see also pp. 90–92)

Since older people often suffer from multiple disease states, multiple prescribing is common. This obviously increases the risk of drug interactions occurring. An examination of prescriptions for 353 elderly hospital inpatients (age range 60–99 years) revealed 30 potentially harmful drug interactions in 23 patients (Scott

Table 11.1 Some drugs commonly prescribed for older people and possible side-effects

Drug group	Example	Some possible side-effects
Analgesics	Ibuprofen	Dyspepsia, gastrointestinal intolerance and bleeding. Skin rashes.
Anticholinergic drugs	Emepronium bromide	Dryness of the mouth, ulceration of gums and mouth when tablet held in mouth for long periods.
Antidepressants	Dothiepin	Anticholinergic effects especially in early stages of treatment. Postural hypotension
Antihypertensives	Atenolol	Coldness of extremities, muscular fatigue, bradycardia.
	Methyldopa	Sedation, bradycardia, nausea, vomiting and rash.
Cardiac glycosides	Digoxin	Anorexia, nausea, vomiting, muscle weakness, visual disturbances, arrhythmias.
Diuretics	Frusemide	Rashes, tinnitus and deafness in impaired renal function, nausea, malaise, gastric upset. Potassium depletion. Latent diabetes may become manifest
Hypnotics	Chlormethiazole	Sneezing, nasal congestion and irritation. Conjunctival irritation. Gastrointestinal disturbances.
Potassium supplements	Potassium chloride (slow release tablets)	Gastrointestinal disturbances. In the presence of obstruction, ulceration or perforation may arise.
Phenothiazines	Chlorpromazine	Extra pyramidal — tremor. Jaundice. Photosensitivity (high dosage), occular changes (long-term therapy)

et al, 1982). Contraindicated or adversely inter-acting drugs were identified in 200 of 6160 prescriptions by Gosney (1984). This evidence suggests that there is a need for increased vigilance on the part of those involved in the prescribing, dispensing and administration of medicines for older people.

Management of medicines by older people in the community

By the very nature of her work the nurse is in an excellent position to help to ensure that older people are obtaining maximum benefit and minimum adverse effects from their drug treatment. There are certain times during the provision of care, such as prior to discharge from hospital or at the commencement of a new course of treatment when the nurse should be especially alert to the needs of the older person. However, as with all patients, the circumstances and condition of the patient may change, therefore continual monitoring of the situation will be also called for.

As has already been stated, an older person may experience problems using prescribed medicines, or may be experiencing untoward side-effects. As with other aspects of human behaviour, medicine use can be a complex matter, especially in the community where medicine taking is often part of daily living for many older people.

A checklist is offered which the nurse may find helpful in assessing the patient's problem, which, once identified, may be capable of resolution. In many instances the nurse will be able to provide assistance to the patient from her own skills and resources but will, on occasions, require the help and support of doctor, pharmacist or social worker. Last, but by no means least, the patient's relatives, friends and neighbours may be in a position to help. The overall objective of any action taken is to ensure that the older person derives full benefit from the prescribed medicines. While the check list is put forward in the context of assessing the needs of the older person many of the aspects listed will be of relevance to patients in other age groups.

Checklist: Medicines in the community

The patient

Age and sex	The 'older' old (over 75 years) are more vulnerable to drug adverse effects than the younger old. Women appear to be more vulnerable than men.
Mental status	Does the patient understand about the use of the prescribed medicines? Is the short-term memory failing?
Attitudes	What is the general attitude of the patient to the prescribed medicines? Does the patient 'believe in the medicines'? Are the patient's attitudes to the medicines influenced by relatives/friends/neighbours?
Knowledge	Is the patient's knowledge of the medicines adequate in order to achieve compliance? Are the health professionals involved giving guidance that is consistent and relevant?
Physical	*Vision* Can the patient read the labels and follow the instructions? Are spectacles required/worn? *Hearing* Can the patient hear any instructions regarding the use of the medicines given by the doctor, pharmacist or nurse? *Mobility* Does the patient find it convenient to obtain the medicines? Does the patient's lack of mobility contribute to non-compliance with say, diuretic therapy? *Manual dexterity* Can the patient open the container and use the dosage form? e.g. the handling of very small tablets or use of an inhaler may present problems.
General circumstances	*Family support* Is family support available to assist in medicine taking? Would it be reliable if available? *Access to service* Is the pharmacy readily accessible? Does collection of the prescription present a problem? *Use of 'over the counter'/lay medicines* Has the patient discontinued prescribed therapy in favour of a proprietary or lay treatment? Is there a possibility that the non-prescribed medicine may interact with the prescribed medicines?

Checklist: Medicines in the community (con't)

The patient

General circumstances	*Alcohol use*
	The use of alcohol concurrently with prescribed medicines may result in dangerous interactions.
	Nutritional aspects
	In some situations a poor nutritional status may be a contributing factor to drug adverse reactions. Is the absorption of the drug influenced by food? If so, does the patient take the medicine at the correct time in relation to food intake?
	Any history of drug/medicine allergy
	Careful questioning may indicate if there has been any previous history of allergy, hypersensitivity etc.

The medicines

Labelling	Does the label give the patient all the necessary information in a form the patient can read and understand? Would a modified label design be of assistance?
Container	Can the patient open and close the container? This applies not only to oral solid dosage forms but to other forms of therapy, e.g. eye drops.
Dosage form	*Solid oral*
	Can the patient swallow the tablet/capsule
	Liquid oral
	Are any problems being experienced in measuring the dose, shaking the bottle?
	Topical
	Can the patient apply the ointment/cream etc. in the correct amount?
	Other
	Particular attention may need to be given to the patient's ability to use less common dosage forms such as suppositories, inhalers etc.
	Storage
	Is the storage safe, convenient and appropriate, e.g. is refrigerated storage required?
	Disposal
	Is the patient able to safely dispose of unwanted medicines?
	Multiple therapy
	Particular care should be given to patients receiving multiple therapy, since drug interactions may occur.
	Side-effects
	The patient may be experiencing unacceptable side-

Checklist: Medicines in the community (con't)

The medicines

Dosage form	effects which may be a direct cause of non-compliance. In some situations it may be possible to eliminate or reduce these to an acceptable level, e.g. taking the medicine with food may eliminate gastrointestinal disturbances.
Type of therapy	Seldom if ever will 100% compliance be necessary or indeed attainable, but the purpose of the therapy should be borne in mind when assessing a patient's use of prescribed medicines, since this may influence the approach to be adopted should a problem be encountered. If the therapy is being given for the treatment of an active condition, the patient may need an explanation of the importance of the therapy especially if the benefits are slow to appear. Prophylactic treatment may require a special approach, since again the benefits may not be immediately obvious to the patient. The importance of taking replacement therapy as prescribed should be stressed and if appropriate an explanation given to the patient. Whilst most drugs are capable of creating problems for the older patient, particular attention should be paid to drugs acting on the CNS to which older people are more sensitive.
The patient's general practitioner	The nurse may in certain circumstances wish to reassure herself that the doctor is fully aware of what has been prescribed and the extent of the patient's compliance. These aspects are linked with methods used to control the issues of repeat prescriptions and drug audit of prescribing policies that may be undertaken.

Management of medicines in geriatric wards

Just as steps should be taken to ensure optimal drug therapy for older people in the community, it is equally important to take all the necessary steps to ensure that this is also achieved in hospitals. The following check list is offered as a guide to sisters and nursing officers in assessing drug management in their wards. It is emphasised that the approach may be equally worthwhile in other wards.

- Are ward drug storage arrangements satisfactory?
  Security, space available and location should be reviewed. Is refrigerated storage available?
- Are drug stocks checked regularly by the pharmacist?
  Regular checks by the ward pharmacist can do much to ensure stocks are not allowed to go beyond their expiry dates.
- Is the design of the drug trolley suitable?
  Inconvenience caused by say lack of space in the drug trolley can be a potential source of error.
- Does the design of the prescribing and recording sheets meet with the needs of the ward?
  Long-stay units may have particular requirements that are not reflected in the design of the documentation. Linked with this it may be worthwhile to examine if hospital drug policies and procedures are appropriate.
- Is the equipment used in medicine administration suitable?
  Measures, spoons etc. normally available may not be ideal for the purpose.
- What is the frequency of review of the prescribed therapy?
  Regular review of the patient's current prescriptions is essential to ensure that therapy is not continued when it is no longer required.
- Is there a ward prescribing policy?
  Ward prescribing policies have many advantages, notably in reducing the ward drug inventory. Doctors and nurses therefore become familiar with a limited range of products which is an aid to the safe management of medicines.
- Is there an effective policy on how to deal with medicines brought into hospital by patients on admission?
  The common practice of encouraging patients to bring their medicines into hospital on admission is helpful to pres-

cribers in determining the patient's current drug therapy. If these medicines are allowed to accumulate at ward level, or are returned to the patient without careful evaluation of the situation, problems may result.

- Are ward pharmacy services available and effective? Does the drug distribution system reflect the needs of the ward?
  Ward pharmacy services can be of particular value in geriatric wards, especially in assessment wards, where a wide range of drugs is in use. Whilst no one drug distribution system is ideal for all situations every effort should be made to ensure that the system used is the most suitable e.g. pre-discharge training of patients in the use of their medicines needs a high level of pharmaceutical support.
- Is a record of drug errors/incidents maintained at ward level?
  From time to time it may be useful to review the general level of 'performance', not in connection with disciplinary procedures but in order to monitor the situation and prevent recurrence of drug errors.

Management of medicines in day hospitals
The day hospital aims to provide facilities for assessment, diagnosis and rehabilitation of patients who do not require hospital admission, and also aims to maintain the level of rehabilitation achieved by patients discharged from in-patient care. Such departments have become an accepted component of health care for elderly people and also for psychiatric patients. In the geriatric field, the limited supply of beds in hospital and the need for an immediate service to patients following their discharge from hospital largely account for the development of day hospitals.

Day hospitals operate during daylight hours and cater for the needs of appropriately selected patients allowing them to remain in the community with their spouse, relatives or friends. Facilities are provided for medical examination, nursing treatments, physiotherapy, occupational therapy, speech therapy, diversional therapy, chiropody and hair-dressing. Attendance at a day hospital varies with the individual patient, ranging from several times a week to merely once a month.

Practical aspects

The management of medicines in a day hospital is many sided as elderly patients present a wide range of conditions which require to be assessed and treated.

On his first visit to the day hospital, the patient should be asked to bring all his medicines with him. It is customary for the patient to be given a full medical examination as part of being assessed. The medicines should be examined and the doctor questions the patient in detail about his medicine asking him what each is being taken for, the number to be taken, the frequency and so on. If there is any doubt about the patient's ability to cope with the medicines at home, appropriate action should be taken by the staff of the day hospital. This may involve contacting a relative of the patient, the general practitioner, the district nurse or the community pharmacist. If necessary, the liaison health visitor may be asked to visit the patient at home to try to assist with the problem. Since patients attending a day hospital are out-patients under the care of their general practitioner, the geriatrician, while allowed to withdraw medication immediately from a patient for a suspected adverse reaction, may only suggest the need for a medicine or a change in prescription to the general practitioner; he may not prescribe medicines for the patient. At this time, the patient should also be asked if he is able to gain access to the medicines or if he is experiencing any other difficulties with them.

On subsequent visits, the patient is only required to bring those medicines which have to be taken during the period of the visit. It is tempting for the patient to transfer to smaller containers only those medicines which he will require but this practice is to be discouraged. The contribution made by ambulance personnel and home helps in prompting patients to remember to pick up important items such as their medicines (and door key) before they

leave home should not be undervalued. Some of the patients attending the day hospital may be capable of remembering to take their medicines as well as undertaking the procedure involved. Others, who normally are supervised or assisted in taking their medicines by relatives or a neighbour, will need this support maintained by the day hospital staff. The nurse is in an ideal position to supervise patients taking their medicines giving guidance and encouragement as required. It is especially important that she uses her powers of observation during treatment and that she is alert to the possibility of unwanted side-effects which can have serious consequences in older people.

To provide for those occasions when patients forget to bring their medicines or require to have a symptom dealt with on the spot, a small stock of medicines should be stored in the department. Small amounts of medicines for the relief of unexpected discomfort in patients may be held, such as simple analgesics and antacids. Supplies of certain specific medicines which patients may forget to bring with them and which should not be omitted should also be kept. These may include such drugs as digoxin, metformin and glyceryl trinitrate.

Apart from medicines, other nursing procedures involving pharmaceutical products may have to be carried out. These may include urine testing, catheter irrigation, stoma care and surgical dressings. Resuscitative measures may have to be instigated if a patient collapses and so the nurse must ensure that relevant and updated emergency medicines are available. The importance of keeping accurate records of the medicines which patients attending the day hospital are taking and good lines of communication between all the personnel involved cannot be overemphasised. The principles and practice of medicine management apply to the day hospital as much as in other situations. The notable feature of the day hospital in this context, however, is that the patients form a mobile and ever-changing group making patient identification and staff stability of the utmost importance.

Management of medicines in residential care settings

Many community health care staff, even if not actually working in a residential home, will on occasions come into contact with medicine administration systems used outwith hospitals. Significant numbers of residents in homes for the elderly will require regular medication. For some residents of some homes it will be possible to make suitable arrangements for self-administration of medicines. For many residents, however, it is necessary for the officer-in-charge to arrange for medicines to be stored centrally and administered to residents by staff of the home. The type of system used will depend on a number of factors such as the number of residents, the number and range of medicines in use and the physical layout of the home.

Two basic systems of medicine administration are used. The first is analogous to the individual patient dispensing system described on page 23. The individual resident's medicines are stored in separate containers within a medicine trolley. The medicines are administered to the residents directly from the container in which the medicine was dispensed. This system has much to commend it but in many homes it is not possible to use a medicine trolley because of lack of space in the home and absence of lifts. Staff in some homes consider this approach too 'institutional'. The second method, which is widely used, is based on a modular system described by Downie and colleagues (1984).

Solid dose forms, tablets and capsules, are set out in advance in labelled four compartment plastic trays. Liquid medicines are premeasured into labelled plastic cups, fitted with secure lids. These are then held in a larger tray along with the trays containing the solid dose forms. This larger tray is used to carry the medicines during administration to residents. (Fig. 11.1).

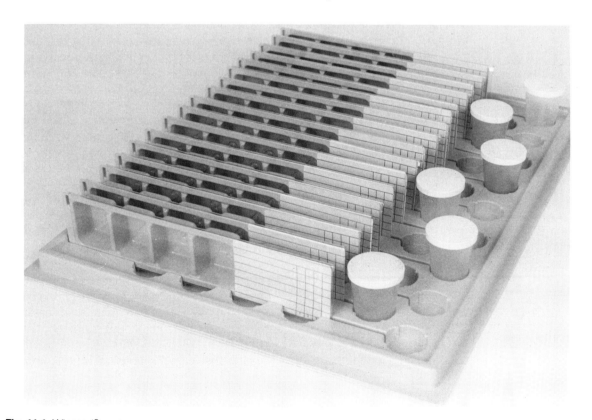

Fig. 11.1 Wiegand® system

The setting out of doses in advance whether by this or similar systems has understandably been criticised, since it is accepted practice to administer medicines directly from the container in which the medicine was supplied. In many residential homes the setting out of doses in this way is often the only practicable way to manage the distribution of medicines. Any medicine distribution/administration system used in a residential home should be supported by well designed documentation so that records are kept of all medicines supplied and administered. The documents used for hospital inpatients can be adapted to meet this need.

Alternative methods of medicine distribution and administration that have been advocated include the controlled dosage systems in which medicines are supplied in courses of treatment packed in blister packs (Rivers, 1985).

REFERENCES

Das B C 1977 Drug taking is a hazardous business for the old. Modern Geriatrics 1: 22–23
Downie G, Urquhart W W, Williams A 1984 Drug Administration — Safer than plastic cups. Health and Social Services Journal XCIV: 376
Gosney M, Tallis R 1984 Prescription of contraindicated and interacting drugs in elderly patients admitted to hospital. Lancet 2: 564–567
Rivers P 1985 An evaluation of a controlled dosage system as a method of supplying medicines to residential homes for the elderly. British Journal of Pharmaceutical Practice 7:252
Scott A, Stansfield J, Williams B O 1982 Prescribing habits and potential adverse drug interactions in a geriatric medical service. Health Bulletin 40(1): 5–9
Williamson J 1978 Prescribing problems in the elderly. Practitioner 220: 749–755
Wilson L A, Lawson I R, Braws W 1962 Multiple disorders in the elderly. Lancet 2:841

DRUG THERAPY IN TERMINAL ILLNESS

Research and practice, especially during the past 15 years or so, have resulted in high standards of terminal care being set by the hospice movement. With only 5% of deaths occurring in specialist terminal care centres, the need to attain equally high standards in the wider situation becomes obvious.

Care of the dying is now looked on as a specialised subject although the principles involved could be more widely adopted to meet the needs of patients in general hospitals and at home than is the case at present. In this field, probably more than in any other, there is the need to consider the patient in his entirety — physically, emotionally and spiritually — within the context of society generally and his family in particular. Attention to the many needs of the patient and of his family calls for a team approach. Energies previously directed towards cure are replaced by efforts to ensure the total comfort of the patient. This, in some instances, may necessitate such palliative measures as a small surgical procedure, a short course of radiation or doses of a cytotoxic drug. In all cases, however, the control of distressing symptoms is of the utmost concern.

Before embarking on any course of action to relieve symptoms it is essential to identify the problems which, in the patient's estimation, are the most pressing. Precise details of the problems should be established by the doctor with the help of nursing staff through questioning, observing and examining the patient. Analyses of admissions to hospices show that pain is the primary presenting symptom. Other troublesome symptoms experienced by dying patients include dry mouth, anorexia, nausea and vomiting, dyspnoea, cough, dysphagia, constipation, insomnia, anxiety and depression. The judicious use of medicines plays an important part in the control of these symptoms.

Pain control
The reasons for inadequate pain control are twofold; an inadequate concept of the nature of pain and ill-founded fears and fantasies concerning the 'addictive' nature of narcotic analgesics. In terminal illness whether pain is mild, severe or overwhelming, the need to evaluate the pain in detail is of paramount importance. A history of the pain should be taken from the patient whenever possible. Because different types of pain require different management, the exact location and distribution of the pain need to be identified.

In malignant conditions, infiltration by tumour into bone, nerve or viscera will produce differing painful effects. Bone pain may present as either a dull ache all over the bone or there may be a localised area of intense pain. It results from the production of prostaglandin by secondary cancer deposits. In vertebral collapse or post-radiation fibrosis, nerve pain occurs and is localised to definite dermatomes usually unilaterally. Visceral pain such as occurs in tumours of the liver, pancreas, kidney and lung are often caused by distension of the organ or stretching of its capsule. Likewise, the phantom pains which may follow amputation of a limb or the burning pain of the hands and feet following a course of vinca drugs are quite specific.

Nurses and doctors need to recognise the difference between acute pain and chronic pain. Acute pain is usually described vividly by the patient and has a clear-cut onset and predictable termination. By contrast, chronic pain which patients find hard to describe has no predictable ending and leaves the patient totally demoralised. It may be of help to the doctor at the time and for making comparisons at a later date to record details of the pain using a body chart. The patient should be asked to describe the character of the pain and any factors which alter its intensity. Each type of pain requires the appropriate analgesic and it is possible for one patient to need separate drugs for colic, raised intracranial pressure and bone secondaries.

As well as assessing the pain, the patient's demeanour should be considered. Anxiety, depression, mental isolation and fear can all exacerbate the misery of pain by lowering the pain threshold. Lack of sleep may compound the problem. Relief of these symptoms will reduce the amount of analgesics required.

Management of pain relief

When planning measures to relieve pain, several principles should be borne in mind. All analgesics narcotics or non-narcotics should be given on a regular basis, usually four hourly, to prevent pain from breaking through. It is important that nurses realise that each drug has a specific period of activity which should be reflected in the dosage intervals indicated by the prescriber. By titrating the level of analgesia against the patient's pain, gradually increasing the dose as required, freedom from pain can be reached. The formulation also should be suitable; it is desirable to give analgesics by mouth for as long as possible since injections are more hazardous, inconvenient and unpleasant for the patient. Solid dose forms may be given to swallow or for absorption sublingually. Some patients may prefer liquid preparations; dysphagic patients will require them of necessity. Use of the rectal route for analgesic drugs should not be forgotton. As a last resort drugs may have to be injected. Various battery operated pumps (Fig. 11.2) for the administration are now available. In hospital, a pump may be used attached to an intravenous cannula or to a subcutaneous needle, the latter being changed on alternate days. District nurses can maintain patients at home with a subcutaneous line in use and help to reduce the amount of medical supervision required. This type of pump is held in a holster slung over the patient's shoulder (Fig. 11.3) and although mildly restricting obviates the need for repeated injections and provides a steady level of circulating drug.

Extra analgesic cover may be required during a painful nursing procedure despite being timed to coincide with peak effect of regular analgesia. Nurses should be prepared to ask for an additional 'once only' dose to be prescribed for administration, for example, half an hour before a dressing is to be done. A self-

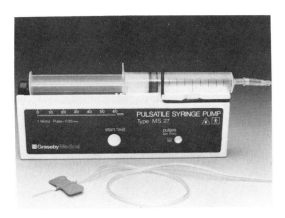

Fig. 11.2 Pulsatile syringe pump MS27

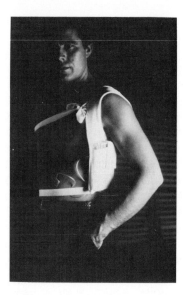

Fig. 11.3 Pump designed to be held in holster over patient's shoulder

administered mixture of nitrous oxide and oxygen containing 50% of each helps some patients in this situation.

Adjuvant therapy may also be prescribed. This takes the form of additional drugs whose purpose is to potentiate the effect of, in this case, an analgesic. Examples include chlorpromazine which has the additional benefit of being antiemetic, antipruritic and helpful in the control of hiccoughs and methotrimeprazine which is an analgesic in its own right as well as having antipsychotic properties. The need arises again therefore for nurses to be watchful for drug interactions.

Patients receiving regular narcotics require regular laxatives as constipation is inevitable. Should the first choice of analgesic fail to work, an alternative from another pharmacological group of analgesics should be prescribed in preference to adding another of the same group.

Some clinicians are reluctant to use narcotic analgesics such as diamorphine because they assume that tolerance will develop and result in the medication becoming ineffective, that the patient will become addicted to the drug or that respiratory depression is inevitable. On the contrary, studies have shown that the longer the duration of narcotic administration,

the slower the rate of rise in dose and the longer after starting this type of drug the patient survived, the greater the likelihood of an eventual reduction in dose. Indeed, the earlier low-dose opiates are started the better. Doctors and nurses should work in close harmony with their local hospice or regional pain centre, making best use of the experience and expertise for which they are now well known.

Even when a drug regime is established and appears to be working well, the nurse caring for the patient with as history of chronic pain must continue to observe and report changes in the patient's condition. It is the responsibility of medical staff to review drug regimes regularly but the continuing observations made by the nurse can assist in ensuring that alterations to the drugs or their doses are made whenever the need arises.

Proper management involving anticipation of pain, careful identification of pain, and application of basic pharmacology makes pain control possible in about 95% or more of dying patients. Nurses play a major role in this challenging aspect of patient care. The goal has only been reached when the misery of pain is replaced by comfort and contentment, alertness of mind, and dignity.

Symptom control
Many other symptoms can be troublesome to the person who is dying. Studies have shown that up to 50% of these symptoms are not mentioned by patients. A major role of health carers is the building up of a relationship with the dying person such that he feels he can ask about any problem which is troubling him, no matter how trivial. It is important to spend even a few minutes each day with the patient identifying anything that is distressing him. Daily meetings to review the patient's problems with staff immediately involved can be beneficial in establishing the true source of his distress and in working out strategies for overcoming them.

Simple remedies should be attempted first. Foremost, as with all patients, attention to the basic needs of living is essential. The patient cannot possibly be contented if he is not sleeping well. Sleep is prevented if the patient is in an uncomfortable position. Repositioning is only part of the answer unless the skin and the mouth feel right as well as the bladder and bowel. The meeting of each need is essential for the total satisfaction of all other needs.

Drugs play an important part in terminal illness in second place to, although still in conjunction with, nursing care. Anti-emetic drugs are very valuable and often required but will do little to quell nausea and improve the appetite as long as the smell of necrosing tissue permeates the air. Antidepressants are not intended to take the place of providing an opportunity for the patient to express sadness and disappointment. Used properly however, their place is important. Prescribing the medicine, selecting a suitable formulation, administering the medicine in an effective and acceptable manner to the patient, and keeping accurate records are skills in themselves. As always the drug(s) should be carefully chosen and looked at in context with the patient as a whole and any other therapy he may be receiving. Anticipating side-effects and being watchful for drug interactions are essential if the patient is to be spared further distress. The purpose that groups of drugs serve in terminal illness and some clinical implications are listed in Table 11.2.

Table 11.2 Groups of drugs used in terminal illness

Therapeutic group and examples	Indications for use	Clinical implications
Analgesics (non-opiates)		
buprenorphine	moderate to severe pain	Can be given by IM or slow IV injection, a sublingual tablet is also available; since buprenorphine is metabolised in the liver the action of the drug may be prolonged in patients with liver impairment.
mefenamic acid	mild to moderate pain	Also has an anti-inflammatory action; contraindicated in inflammatory

Table 11.2 Groups of drugs used in terminal illness (con't)

Therapeutic group and examples	Indications for use	Clinical implications
		bowel disease, peptic ulceration and hepatic impairment.
Non-steroidal anti-inflammatory drugs		
flurbiprofen indomethacin	pain due to bone metastases	Gastric irritation
Anticholinergics hyoscine	secretions causing death rattle	Given by SC injection
Antidepressants and anxiolytics	depression anxiety	See p. 210 for examples and discussion of these groups
Anti-emetics chlorpromazine	nausea, vomiting	Useful when given rectally to relieve hiccough
cinnarizine		May cause drowsiness and so alcohol should be avoided
cyclizine haloperidol		May cause drowsiness and dry mouth
metoclopramide		Extrapyramidal reactions have been reported
nabilone	useful in the treatment of nausea and vomiting caused by cytotoxic drugs	Contraindicated in patients with severe liver dysfunction; may impair mental/physical abilities; may interact with CNS depressants, alcohol and narcotic agents
prochlorperazine		May cause transient drowsiness and extrapyramidal effects
Antifungals amphotericin nystatin	candidiasis especially in patients who are debilitated on oral corticosteroids on systemic antibiotics	Oral hygiene should precede the treatment (see p. 134). It is essential to sustain contact with the lesions for as long as possible e.g. for oral candidiasis,

Table 11.2 Groups of drugs used in terminal illness (con't)

Therapeutic group and examples	Indications for use	Clinical implications
		following removal of dentures, a lozenge or pastille should be sucked. Patients should be encouraged to hold a suspension for as long as possible to coat the mouth before swallowing as candidal infections also commonly affect the oesophagus. Fluids and food should be withheld for 20–30 minutes. Fungal infections may occur in other sites
Corticosteroids betamethasone	as prednisolone	On a weight-for-weight basis is up to 10 times more active than prednisolone. Available as a soluble tablet and so may be useful when the swallowing of tablets presents a problem. Less likely to cause gastric irritation than the slightly soluble corticosteroids. Side-effects and contraindications are in general similar to those of other glucocorticoids.
dexamethasone	raised intracranial pressure caused by cerebral tumour mediastinal mass causing dysphagia	Side-effects include peptic ulceration, negative nitrogen balance due to catabolism and decreased carbohydrate tolerance.
prednisolone	anorexia	Enteric coated preparations should be used to reduce the risk of peptic ulceration.

Table 11.2 Groups of drugs used in terminal illness (con't)

Therapeutic group and examples	Indications for use	Clinical implications
	bronchospasm reduced sense of well-being pruritus in obstructive jaundice	As with all systemic corticosteroid treatment observe for signs of thrush.
topical corticosteroids	pruritus	See p. 101
Deodorising agents. antibiotics	sepsis arising from fungating growths	administered systemically
eusol	fungating growths	Lesions may be swabbed with $\frac{1}{2}$ strength eusol or a hydrogen peroxide solution.
hydrogen peroxide solution 3% or 6%		A few drops of deodorising solution may be applied to outer dressings avoiding contact with the lesion or alternatively a charcoal impregnated dressing may be used.
metronidazole	e.g. infected bronchogenic tumour, gastric carcinoma discharging sinuses stomas halitosis	Administered orally. Metronidazole suppositories may be inserted into large cavities. Hydrogen peroxide solution may be used to swab or rinse the mouth
Hypnotics temazepam	insomnia	Drugs with a long half-life should be avoided. 'Hangover' can be very distressing for patients (and relatives) Does not obviate the need for adequate pain relief.
Laxatives *Bulk forming* bran *Combined products* faecal softener stimulant	constipation	An adequate fluid intake is essential.

Table 11.2 Groups of drugs used in terminal illness (con't)

Therapeutic group and examples	Indications for use	Clinical implications
co-danthramer mixture		May cause pink discolouration of the urine.
Osmotic lactulose		Occasional nausea and vomiting
Stimulant sennoside B		May cause abdominal cramp and pink colouration of the urine.
Opiates morphine diamorphine	distress of dyspnoea anxiety and panic e.g. following episode of haemoptysis	To minimise side-effects simple oral solutions of morphine are preferable to multi-ingredient elixirs. Diamorphine hydrochloride has greater solubility than morphine sulphate allowing effective doses to be injected in smaller volumes (important in emaciated patients) Frequently cause nausea and vomiting and so a concurrent anti-emetic may be necessary. Beneficial side-effects of euphoria
Antipruritics antihistamines	itching	The drowsiness associated with antihistamine therapy will influence choice of drug. Topical antihistamine therapy should be avoided due to sensitisation reactions.
cholestyramine	pruritus due to obstructive jaundice	The dryness of the granules may create problems of swallowing

DRUG THERAPY IN PSYCHIATRIC PRACTICE

The introduction over the last 30 years of a wide range of psychotropic drugs has had, along with other changes, a profound effect on the provision of psychiatric care. Drugs in regular use in the mid-1950s included relatively unsophisticated sedatives such as the bromides and the barbiturates. These drugs would find only a limited, if any, place in present day practice. They have been replaced by a range of hypnotics, sedatives and anxiolytic drugs which are generally much safer in use and have fewer side-effects. The introduction of effective antipsychotic drugs and antidepressants also represents a major step forward. Prior to the introduction of drugs such as chlorpromazine and imipramine the treatment of the psychoses and depressive illness presented almost intractable problems.

Patterns of care have also changed markedly during the past 30 years. The availability of behaviour-modifying drugs has made it possible to maintain many patients in the community using out-patient clinics, day hospitals and community care in place of hospitalisation. In sharp contrast to the mainly custodial care of the past, when there was little or no active treatment, rehabilitation or discharge back to the community, the emphasis now is on all these aspects. The keynote today is flexibility of care in response to the needs of the individual patient. Where the required resources are available, some long-stay patients have been transferred to suitable accomodation in the community be it hostel, sheltered housing or private dwelling.

Whilst the number of patients of pre-retirement age who require hospitalisation is decreasing, an increasing number of older people who can no longer be cared for in the community, now require long-term hospital care. The increasing average age of the population of long-stay hospitals does in itself create many challenges for nurses and their clinical colleagues. Aspects of the drug treatment of older people are discussed in more detail earlier in this Chapter.

It is against the background briefly outlined above that the management and use of medicines in psychiatric practice will be discussed.

Classification of drugs used in psychiatry
Under each heading some examples are given together with brief notes on the general properties and some side-effects of the drug or group.

Hypnotics, sedative and anxiolytic drugs

Benzodiazepines Some benzodiazepines are used primarily as hypnotics (nitrazepam); others are used both as sedatives and anxiolytics (diazepam). In general, a small dose is used as an anxiolytic whilst a higher dosage has a hypnotic effect. Concern has been expressed on the widespread use of benzodiazepines in anxiety states because of the possibility of dependence developing. Hangover and drowsiness can be a problem with some of the longer-acting benzodiazepines such as nitrazepam.

Barbiturates The routine use of barbiturates is not advocated, owing to the many side-effects and the possibility of tolerance and dependency being created. The dangers arising from overdosage are also very considerable. (Phenobarbitone still has a place in the management of some form of epilepsy).

Antipsychotic drugs

Chlorpromazine and other phenothiazines are used in the treatment of schizophrenia. Patients with the acute form of the condition often respond well, normal behaviour being restored. Side-effects are, however, a cause for concern, especially extrapyramidal symptoms. A Parkinsonism-like syndrome may develop in time leading to the need for the concurrent administration of orphenadrine or benzhexol. Depot injections (see also p. 89) are widely used in the treatment of schizophrenia and related conditions. The choice of drug used will depend on the nature of the behavioural disturbances exhibited by the patient e.g. if aggression is present or the patient is with- drawn. Fluphenazine is available as a depot injection. Side-effects may include extrapyramidal symptoms and a Parkinsonism-like syndrome. Injections are repeated at suitable intervals generally ranging from a week to four weeks. The advantages of this form of treatment are considerable. Patient compliance is assured, and good control of symptoms of schizophrenia and related conditions is achieved.

Clopenthixol and flupenthixol (non-phenothiazines) are available as depot injections.

Antidepressant drugs

Amitriptyline. In addition to antidepressant activity, this drug has some sedative action and is useful when depression is associated with anxiety and agitation. Anticholinergic (atropine-like) side-effects are a particular cause for concern especially in older patients. The antidepressant action may take up to 30 days to develop.

Imipramine is a valuable drug for the treatment of several forms of depression. It has less sedative action than amitriptyline. Anticholinergic side effects in the early stages of treatment include dry mouth, eye disturbances, constipation and hesitancy of micturition. Postural hypotension, tremor and skin rashes may also be a problem.

Mianserin has similar clinical indications to amitriptyline. Side-effects are fewer and milder and there is less risk of drug interactions than with amitriptyline. Blood dyscrasias have been reported following treatment with this drug.

Monoamine-oxidase inhibitors (MAOI)

These drugs are used in the treatment of depressive illness. Side-effects include dizziness and hypotension. Severe hypertensive reactions can occur to certain foods, notably cheese, and some drugs. Patients taking these drugs should be advised as to the foods and drinks they must avoid. Verbal advice is normally supplemented with written information. If patients have previously been taking another antidepressant such as amitriptyline it is generally considered that a period of 14 days should elapse before commencing treatment with a MAOI. There are, however, differences of clinical opinion on this point.

Lithium

Although used for many years in psychiatric practice, lithium carbonate still remains an important drug. The main use of this drug is in the treatment of mania and hypomania. Certain forms of depression are also treated by lithium therapy. It is important to adjust the dose so that serum lithium levels are maintained within the therapeutic range.

General considerations

Patients receiving treatment for a psychiatric illness may, of course, also require treatment for a co-existing physical condition. This may lead to problems for prescriber, nurse and pharmacist in ensuring that the drug treatment for the psychiatric patient is both safe and effective. Some general points of guidance are given below.

- Particular care is required when prescribing for the older patient because of possible adverse effects resulting from poor renal excretion.
- Since many psycho-active drugs have significant side-effects the impact of unavoidable side-effects should be minimised.
- Drug interactions are of particular concern with many psycho-active drugs.
- Drug/food interaction although relatively rare, must be guarded against.
- The counselling of patients (and relatives) on the safe and effective use of their medicines is essential. This is especially important when the benefits of drug treatment may take many days to be felt by the patient.
- Patients may need to be warned that the therapy may cause drowsiness leading to impaired ability to drive or operate machinery.
- Steps may need to be taken to limit the quantities of medicines given to a patient at any one time.
- Drug policies and procedures should reflect the special needs of the psychiatric patient.
- Problems arising from patient non-compliance should be guarded against as far as practicable.
- Aids to patient compliance should be provided where appropriate
- Some patients (and their relatives) may be very concerned about the possibility of 'addiction' developing, and therefore will need reassurance and guidance on this aspect.
- The use of alcoholic beverages by patients must be limited, or in some cases discontinued.

Management of medicines at ward level

The same overall legal and procedural arrangements apply for the storage and administration of medicines as with general wards. However, in view of the flexibility of care previously mentioned it is necessary to establish procedures which enable therapeutic objectives to be achieved. For instance, it is often necessary, as part of a rehabilitation programme, to arrange for patients to be responsible, at least in part, for the management of their own medicines (see p. 186).

Patients are encouraged wherever possible to go on social outings either in a group or with relatives. Opportunities for such outings often arise at short notice. The provision of medicines for patients to take whilst on social outings may cause problems. The lack of advance notice, often precludes dispensing of the necessary medicines by the hospital pharmacy. For group outings a considerable number of individual doses of different medicines may be required which would be time-consuming to dispense. Even if the medicines are dispensed in the conventional manner this may not be appropriate, since informality must obviously be maintained on the outing. The presence of a collection of tablet bottles is hardly conducive to achieving an atmosphere of enjoyable relaxation especially in a public place. Nevertheless, safe medicine administration must be achieved at all times. The approach adopted will vary depending on circumstances. Wherever possible, depending on the kinetics of the drug, and length of outing, doses of some drugs could be given just prior to the commencement of the outing.

Where this is not possible supplies of the necessary medicines should be taken on the outing in pre-packed form, preferably strip or blister packed for ease of handling. Attention to the security of such medicines is of course essential.

For the individual patient going on a short outing (less than 24 hours) the necessary medicines (solid doses only) can be supplied as above or placed in a compartmentalised daily tray (see p. 184). In all cases a suitable record of medicines provided in this way, (or for use by a group), should be kept at ward level. The pharmacist's help and advice should always be sought on these and related problems.

Prescribing for patients who go home for weekends

At an appropriate stage in the rehabilitation process patients are encouraged to spend weekends at home. Where patients are receiving regular drug therapy it is important to make suitable arrangements so that essential therapy can be continued whilst the patient is away from hospital. In these circumstances the necessary medicines are dispensed by the hospital pharmacy. Many patients are able to go home for the weekend on a regular basis. In such circumstances a special prescribing system that is safe and easy to operate is required.

One such system, developed in Aberdeen, is based on a triplicate prescription form system. The first form (see Fig. 11.4) is the original prescription, the second form, (white, carbon copy), is identical apart from the fact that 'pharmacist's signature' replaces 'doctor's signature'. The third form is a second carbon copy (pink) identical to the first form. On the first occasion a prescription is raised for a patient going home for the weekend it is written on the top form, the doctor's signature appearing in the top part of the prescription. This form, together with the white copy are sent to pharmacy for dispensing. The white copy is retained on file in the pharmacy and the original returned to the ward with the patient's medicines. On second and subsequent occasions when the patient requires the medicines, the original prescription is sent to the pharmacy. On each occasion the prescription is to be dispensed, the form is signed by the doctor, and the period of supply indicated. Provided there are no changes in the patient's medicines one form can be used for 3 months. The second copy (pink) remains on the ward for reference. By using this, or a similar system, much time-consuming, repetitive, prescription writing is eliminated. At the same time the patient's weekend medicines can be regularly reviewed. Regular, repeat prescribing for patients going home for weekends can also be managed using microcomputer technology.

Management of medicines in psychiatric day hospitals

The procedures for the management of medicines in psychiatric day hospitals are essentially the same as those followed in other day hospitals (see p. 201). Since attendance at a day hospital is an important part of the rehabilitation process, most patients will be in control of their own medicines, just as if they were at home. Although it will be necessary to maintain adequate security of medicines brought into the day hospital, this will normally involve nothing more than commonsense precautions, such as not leaving handbags, jackets etc., containing medicines, unattended. The patient usually obtains all his medicines from his own general practitioner, other than any special medicines such as depot antipsychotic therapy, which will often be provided and administered in the day hospital. However, in certain situations, where a patient is considered, for whatever reason, to be 'at risk', the necessary medicines will be supplied from the pharmacy in such a way that the patient can be issued with one, two or more days supply at a time, depending on his condition. Strip-packed medicines presented in small, labelled cardboard wallets are ideal for this purpose.

The emphasis in the day hospital is on preserving, as far as possible, the patient's normal way of life, at the same time providing the level of support needed in the most appropriate way. The opportunity to contribute, through group discussions, to the support of others is also created.

WARD .... HOSPITAL ....

PATIENTS NAME ....

	Approx. Time	Date			Approx. Time	Date
FROM	.... a.m.	....	UNTIL		.... a.m.	....
	...........................p.m.				...........................p.m.	

MEDICINE (Block letters)	Type of Preparation	Dose	Times of Administration						Quantity Dispensed
			8	12	2	6	10	Other Times	

DOCTOR'S SIGNATURE ....

Date from	Date to	Doctor's Signature
(including times if different from above)		

Fig. 11.4 Prescriptions for patients who go home at weekends

Role of the community psychiatric nurse in medicine administration and management

The role of the community psychiatric nurse has two main elements, firstly after care, secondly prevention with crisis intervention if necessary. Specialisation is emerging, especially in relation to the care of the older patient. In addition to a case load which is well defined in advance by the consultant psychiatrist, patients may be referred to the community psychiatric nurse (CPN) by a general practitioner, social worker or nurse. Self-referrals may also have to be responded to from time to time. Working within a multidisciplinary team and acting as a co-ordinator is also a vital part of the CPN's role.

The CPN may undertake some general

nursing care in a given situation, but in the main, this type of care will be provided by the community nurse. In relation to the overall aim of achieving the safe and effective use of medicines the CPN will act as adviser and counsellor to the patient, (and, if necessary, to the patient's relatives), on all aspects of his medicines. Where required the CPN will also undertake duties more directly related to medicine administration. These duties will include the monitoring of the patient's response to the therapy with particular reference to dosage levels and the occurrence of side-effects. The prescriber, who is often the patient's own general practitioner, is kept informed and recommendations made as to any changes the CPN considers would be advisable. Where the patient is considered to be at risk, the CPN may undertake responsibility for ensuring that the patient receives his medicines in regular, but controlled amounts. This may be achieved by the use of strip-packed tablets, as described previously; or by using the Dosett® (see p. 184).

Increasingly, depot antipsychotic therapy is administered in the local health centre, clinic or general practitioner's surgery, but on some occasions, in cases of default or other difficulties the CPN would give these injections.

In the Grampian area, guidelines for community psychiatric nurses on the carriage, storage and administration of medicines are normally issued to the CPN as follows:

Community Psychiatric Nurses policy for the carriage, storage and administration of medicines

Administration
1. This is a policy statement issued by Grampian Health Board for the guidance of those nurses working in community settings who are required to carry and administer medication.
2. Medicines will be administered by the community psychiatric nurse (CPN) in response to a prescription made in accordance with current Grampian Health Board policy by the appropriate medical officer.
3. In situations where the CPN is involved in establishing a patient on new medication, the CPN will maintain observation, or return with 3–5 days, for a short period following administration to ensure adverse reactions are identified in the early stages of treatment.

4. The withdrawal of drug therapy will be treated with the same care as initial administration and the patient will remain under supervision for a period agreed with the doctor.
5. In situations where patients require assistance with the daily management of oral medicines, the CPN may be required to provide direct help, e.g. by the use of the Dosett box. The Nursing Officer should be asked to authorise this.

Carriage
6. Only single doses of the prescribed medication for a specifically named patient, together with the prescription sheet and drug administration record are to be carried by the CPN. A small reserve of the total projected day's requirements may be carried to allow for spillage or loss in use.
7. The CPN may collect and transfer medicines obtained by prescription from a community pharmacist to the patient's home.
8. Medicines taken into the community should be carried in the container issued for that purpose and should, where practicable, remain in the CPN's possession at all times. When left in a car they should be locked in the boot.

Storage
9. The nurse manager will identify a secure location from which the CPN may draw medicines required and return unused stock daily.
10. It is recommended that CPNs consult with the pharmacist on technical matters such as storage, stability etc, of all medicines. Storage requirements for individual products must be complied with.

Care and disposal of equipment and medicines
11. A safe system of disposal for used needles and syringes will be provided by the nurse manager for each CPN.
12. Return of unwanted medicines should be carried out in accordance with the guidance issued by the area pharmaceutical service.
13. In the event of needle pricks or contamination of a wound with blood, the CPN will comply with the requirements of current Grampian Health Board policy.
14. In the event of actual or suspected loss or theft the CPN will immediately inform the Nursing Officer or senior nurse on duty outside normal working hours.

Record keeping
15. The Grampian Health Board main prescription sheet, Form S150, will be used for the prescription of drugs for community patients. A record of drugs administered will be maintained using Form S151.

Review
16. It is considered good practice for the CPN, together with the patient's doctor to undertake regular and periodic review of prescribed medicines and ensure that the outcome is recorded.

ROLE OF THE COMMUNITY NURSE IN DRUG THERAPY

With the increasing trend towards care in the community, the role of the community nurse in relation to drug therapy has expanded over the last few years. Other factors have contributed to this expanded role not least of which is the ageing population (see also p. 196). The vital role of the community nurse in relation to drug therapy can be considered under a number of headings.

Storage and safe keeping of medicines in the home

The patient's general practitioner normally prescribes the necessary medicines although in certain special situations a consultant may retain this responsibility. It is important to remember that the medicines are the patient's property and should always be regarded as such by the community nurse. Patients should be advised on the safe storage of medicines especially the need to keep all medicines out of the reach of children. Any special storage requirements such as refrigeration should also be borne in mind. On occasions the nurse may need to advise the patient, or patient's relatives, to destroy any accumulations of unwanted medicines. If a Controlled Drug is involved the nurse should not take possession of these since the nurse is not authorised to receive Controlled Drugs in this way. The nurse should not take possession of other unwanted drugs. In both situations the nurse should give the necessary guidance to the patient or patient's relatives and a record of the destruction should be made. The record should be witnessed and signed by the nurse and a member of the patient's family or carer. On some occasions it may be possible for the patient to sign.

Administration of medicines

Essentially the community nurse has the same responsibilities as the hospital nurse. There is of course a difference of emphasis but the principles are the same. The detailed guidelines given on pages 150–152 apply equally to the community nurse but of course a second nurse will not be present to carry out the checking procedure. Full records of medicines administered, normally only parenteral forms, are maintained and signed by the community nurse.

The responsibility for taking oral medicines rests with the patient but in some situations older people may need guidance and help from the community nurse especially when the patient's short-term memory is failing. Despite strenuous and ingenious efforts by the nurse, severely confused patients may be beyond immediate help. Hospital admission may be required in the patient's best interests.

Monitoring drug therapy

The community nurse gets to know her patients especially well and as a result is in a good position to assist in the monitoring of all drug therapy. As part of planning nursing care a note is made in the patient's records of possible side-effects that may arise from the prescribed drug therapy. When planning a visit, this specific information is taken into account by the nurse. This provides a basis on which judgements can be made relating to changes in the patient's condition which may or may not be due to the side-effects of drug therapy. The nurse will be especially concerned about this aspect of her role when a new course of drug therapy is commenced. The occurrence of side-effects should of course be reported to the prescriber so that, if necessary, changes in therapy can be made.

Provision of information to other health care workers

On occasions it may be necessary for the community nurse to provide information on a patient's drug therapy to colleagues in the community. For hospital colleagues this is often conveyed via the liaison health visitor. Information can now be transferred, using microcomputer technology, through the public telephone system (Health Net British Telecom) so that a printed message is available without the delay often associated with a letter.

Provision of information to patients

The patient may receive conflicting advice about his medicines from well-meaning neighbours, relatives and friends. This may cause confusion in the patient's mind which may lead to non-compliance. Community nurses are often able to give the patient suitable guidance with the help of the general practitioner and community pharmacist where necessary.

Compliance aspects

Since the general practitioner prescribes the vast majority of all medicines it follows that the scope for improving patient compliance in the community is almost unlimited. Many of the strategies for improving patient compliance discussed in Chapter 10 can be used by the community nurse.

Proprietary and 'lay' medicines

Many patients will purchase proprietary medicines which may in some instances conflict with prescribed medicines. For example aspirin-containing preparations potentiate the effect of oral anticoagulants and should obviously be avoided by patients receiving this therapy. Normally the general practitioner and community pharmacist will give the patient guidance but the patient may be unaware of the presence of aspirin in a proprietary product. The introduction of selected list prescribing under the NHS will no doubt result in more patients buying medicines from a pharmacy. If the community nurse is aware of the proprietary medicines a patient is taking, suitable advice can be given.

Patients may also have faith in a 'lay' remedy or some form of alternative medicine. This aspect is briefly discussed in Chapter 2.

Care of the patient following cytotoxic drug therapy

In order to respond to the special needs of the patient who has received cytotoxic drug therapy in hospital the community nurse will require detailed information of the nature of the therapy.

Administration of controlled drugs

The necessary drugs will be prescribed by the patient's general practitioner, supplied by the community pharmacist, and kept in the patient's home. The community nurse keeps a record in the home of doses administered together with the balance of ampoules (or other dosage form) remaining.

Security of medicines and equipment

Normally the community nurse does not carry with her any medicines other than those which may be required in the emergency treatment of anaphylaxis. Checks are made at regular intervals to ensure that these preparations have not passed the expiry date. Syringes and needles are not left in the patient's home and suitable arrangements must be made for safe disposal by the nurse.

Extended role of the nurse in the community

Although it is customary for vaccinations to be administered by health visitors in clinics, the administration of immunological agents by nurses is regarded as part of the Extended Role of the Nurse which requires authorisation from the medical practitioner involved. Other procedures that come into this category include tuberculin skin tests, intravenous and intra-arterial medication.

The triple duty nurse

The guidelines above apply equally to the triple duty nurse working in remote areas of the country.

Specialised therapy in the home

Apart from haemodialysis and peritoneal dialysis, a discussion of which is beyond the scope of this book, several sophisticated forms of therapy (see below) are now carried out in the patient's own home. The number of patients involved is not large but it would appear that this trend will develop in the years ahead. The extent to which the community nurse is involved in the therapy will depend on several factors. In a number of situations patients will be taught to carry out the technique for themselves but will need support and guidance from the nurse who will also carry out periodic checks on the patient's technique. Technical support services (e.g. equipment maintenance) will also be required by the patient.

Home intravenous antibiotic therapy
Patients suffering from cystic fibrosis or advanced bronchiectasis have been taught to self-administer intravenous antibiotics using an intravenous cannula inserted in the hospital where the treatment was initiated.

Home parenteral nutrition
This form of therapy (see also p. 142) is used for patients with severe intestinal failure. In most instances the therapy is required in the short term where the condition is reversible but in some patients therapy must be continued for life.

Home ambulatory IV cytotoxic therapy
Research is currently being undertaken on this aspect of home drug therapy. Community nurses may become involved in the maintenance of Hickman Catheters introduced to save frequent venepunctures for out-patients receiving cytotoxic therapy.

Continuous subcutaneous infusion of insulin
The administration of insulin by continuous subcutaneous infusion is made possible by the availability of portable external insulin pumps. There are theoretical advantages in using such a drug delivery system as compared to the traditional daily or twice daily injections. Further evaluation of the use of these pumps will no doubt be undertaken.

Continuous IV administration of drugs using a syringe driver
This technique is available for use in the patient's home for pain control in terminal care, and other specialised forms of therapy.

Intermittent IV administration of drugs using a syringe pump
A battery-operated syringe pump is also available for the injection of drugs in boluses at regular but infrequent intervals.

Home nebulisers for the treatment of asthma
Nebulisers are occasionally prescribed for asthmatic patients who have been found unresponsive to conventional treatment. Dangers associated with this form of treatment have been identified particularly when the nebuliser in use has not been prescribed.

The forms of home therapy briefly described above have a number of advantages, the greatest of which is the fact that many patients are able to resume a reasonably normal lifestyle with this form of treatment. In addition, home therapy is more economical than hospital-based therapy. Obviously, care in patient selection for any form of sophisticated home therapy is extremely important as is the need for training and continuing support. In certain situations the community nurse may need special instruction on the techniques involved, which can best be provided in the ward where the treatment is initiated. Community nurses are responding to this technological revolution working to ensure that their patients receive maximum therapeutic benefit.

Index